# The Biological Basis of Clinical Observations

Fully updated for its fourth edition, *The Biological Basis of Clinical Observations* provides readers with the understanding needed to perform clinical observations, make accurate judgements about the patient's condition and make good decisions concerning patient care.

This essential textbook supports safe and effective clinical practice by explaining the techniques involved in making clinical observations, alongside the biological knowledge which gives them meaning. For each topic, it explains the pathological basis for variations in observed results, focusing on relevant anatomy and physiology, genetics and pharmacology, and the basic principles of care. A greatly expanded chapter on pharmacology reflects the increased importance of this subject in the nursing curriculum. Topics discussed include:

- temperature
- cardiovascular observations
- respiratory observations
- urinary and bowel observations
- neurological observations
- nutrition
- fluid balance
- skin
- pharmacology
- pregnancy.

*The Biological Basis of Clinical Observations* is a unique text which integrates explanations of essential procedures with the biological knowledge that underpins practice. It is essential reading for all nursing and healthcare students preparing for clinical practice.

**William T. Blows** was formerly a nurse tutor and lecturer at City University of London, UK where he taught biology to nurses.

# The Biological Basis of Clinical Observations

Fourth Edition

**William T. Blows**

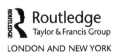
Routledge
Taylor & Francis Group

LONDON AND NEW YORK

Designed cover image: Getty Images

Fourth edition published 2024
by Routledge
4 Park Square, Milton Park, Abingdon, Oxon, OX14 4RN

and by Routledge
605 Third Avenue, New York, NY 10158

*Routledge is an imprint of the Taylor & Francis Group, an informa business*

First edition published by Routledge 2001 as *The Biological Basis of Nursing: Clinical Observations*
Third edition published by Routledge 2018

*British Library Cataloguing-in-Publication Data*
A catalogue record for this book is available from the British Library

ISBN: 978-1-032-48446-4 (hbk)
ISBN: 978-1-032-48440-2 (pbk)
ISBN: 978-1-003-38911-8 (ebk)

DOI: 10.4324/9781003389118

Typeset in Optima
by Apex CoVantage, LLC

# Contents

# Figures

# Plates

# Tables

# Preface to the fourth edition

*William T. Blows*

Medical science has been fighting for many years against three enemies: aging, disease and ignorance.

On the face of it, aging is inevitable, but science is making progress in creating healthier and disease-free elderly. There is no reason why aging must always result in ill-health. The goal is to have a healthy and happy life, even if you live beyond 90 years of age!

Fighting disease has always been the main thrust of medical research, and there have been successes in both treatment and prevention of disease. This will continue with increasing pace as a result of advances in many areas, notably genetics, pharmacology, diagnostics, vaccinations, epidemiology and, perhaps surprisingly, computing science, artificial intelligence and robotics. There are still many hurdles to overcome, especially in cancer medicine, neurological and genetic conditions and viral pandemics to mention just a few.

Ignorance is still a major problem. What we know about the health risks linked to smoking, illicit drugs and obesity should be enough to prevent these conditions from ever happening again. But there are still many smokers and illicit drug takers and the population generally, especially in the west, is gradually increasing in weight. There are also specific problems that arise, such as vaccine deniers and pandemic conspiracy theorists who set up barriers to promoting health. Over the years political actions, such as banning smoking in restaurants, have helped to make advances in health promotion. Maybe there is a case for putting health science on the school curriculum from an early age.

Biological studies are a major part of any healthcare training programme because the sciences are vital for working as an autonomous practitioner. The client's problems will be affecting a biological system, and the assessment and treatment will have a biological basis.

Medical sciences have never seen such a remarkable flood of new knowledge as we are seeing today, knowledge that is already changing the way we treat disease. If healthcare professionals are going to remain at the front of this revolution, they must be familiar with the sciences and technologies that underpin the changing face of the care they give.

Clinical decision-making is based on accurate observations. A thorough understanding of the underpinning sciences is essential to broaden the number of choices available and to facilitate making the correct choice.

This book takes clinical observations and explores the biology underpinning them. It gives the possible pathological basis for variations in the observed results. It looks at both fundamental and advanced observations, e.g. neurological observations. This book will also be of use to educators and trained professionals with students under their leadership. The fourth edition has been updated with new information on many topics, including signs of a patient's deteriorating condition (red-flag tables) and an expanded pharmacology chapter, with drug tables added to several chapters.

William T. Blows
May 2023

# Acknowledgment

The author wishes to thank Dr Ian Hill-Smith and Dr Gina Johnson for allowing me to use information from their excellent book *Little Book of Red Flags* which was published by the National Minor Illness Centre, Bedfordshire, in 2021.

# 1 Temperature

- Introduction
- Heat gain
- Heat movement and loss
- Heat regulation: gain versus loss
- Temperature scales and normal temperature variation
- Taking the body temperature in adults
- Temperature in children
- Abnormal high body temperatures
- Abnormal low body temperatures
- Thermal injury
- Key points
- Notes
- References

## Introduction

Stabilising the internal environment of the body, e.g. temperature, is a process called **homeostasis** (see page 10). At 37°C, the temperature is balanced to provide the optimum conditions for tissue metabolism. Cooler temperatures would slow down the rate of cellular chemistry and function. Many chemical reactions require enzymes to speed up the process to a level necessary for life. When these temperature-sensitive reactions are cooled, the slowing of metabolism becomes dangerous to health. Hotter temperatures cause metabolic systems to become inefficient and enzymes to become denatured. **Denaturing** is a heat-related change in protein structure which leads to failure of cellular activity.

This essential stabilisation of optimum temperatures happens despite changes in the environmental temperature, i.e. the **ambient temperature**. External factors such as shelter, clothes and fires allow humans to survive in low or high temperatures that

DOI: 10.4324/9781003389118-1

would otherwise be hostile to the body. Extremes of external temperature put great pressures on the body's thermoregulatory systems, and sometimes they fail to cope. A dangerous change in the internal temperature is the cause of many deaths in very hot or very cold conditions. The very young and the elderly are the most vulnerable to these changes.

Measurement of body temperature becomes important for two reasons. First, it gives insight into the metabolic and homeostatic activity of the body; second, it may also provide information about the possible cause of any abnormal state, contributing to an accurate diagnosis. Balancing body temperature requires mechanisms to ensure that the heat gained is equal to the heat lost.

## Heat gain

Heat production is part of the energy obtained from the use of the high-energy molecule **ATP (adenosine triphosphate**; Figure 1.1) in cellular metabolism. All cells use ATP, but some use more than others, e.g. liver and muscle cells, and therefore they liberate more heat. ATP itself is constructed from **ADP (adenosine diphosphate)**, plus additional **inorganic phosphate (Pi or PO$_4$)** to make triphosphate, using energy from dietary nutrients. Enzymes within the **mitochondrion**, i.e. the powerhouse of the cell, produce ATP from the metabolism of glucose and fat.

### Glucose

Glucose (Figure 1.2A) is the final product of dietary carbohydrate breakdown by the digestive tract. One gram of glucose yields about 4 kilocalories per gram (4 kcal/g, or 17 kJ/g) of energy, known as the **Atwater number** for carbohydrates. Glucose undergoes glycolysis in the cytoplasm of the cell. **Glycolysis** is the breakdown of glucose to the substance **pyruvate** (Figure 1.2B), which enters the mitochondrial matrix and joins the **tricarboxylic** (the **Krebs** or **citric acid**) **cycle**. Pyruvate first becomes **acetyl coenzyme A (acetyl-CoA)**, the entry point for substances joining the cycle. Throughout the cycle, a series of reactions occurs that results in a return to acetyl-CoA (Figure 1.3).

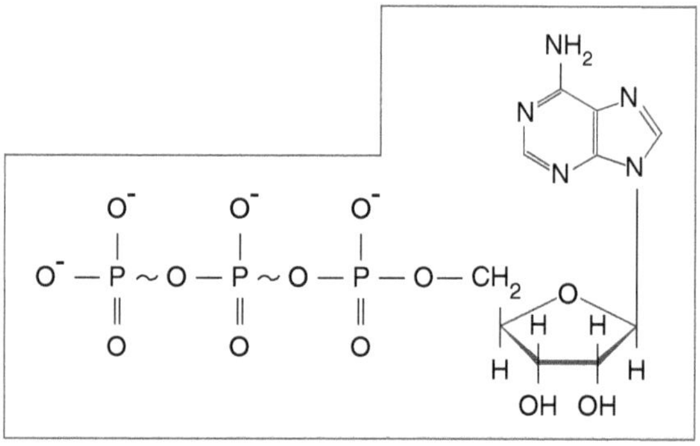

*Figure 1.1* The adenosine triphosphate (ATP) molecule is composed of an adenosine component (right side of box) with three phosphates (PO$_4$) attached (left side of box). Two of those attachments are high-energy bonds (shown as wavy lines ~).

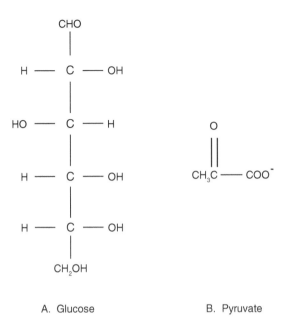

A. Glucose                    B. Pyruvate

*Figure 1.2* A. Glucose molecule ($C_6H_{12}O_6$). B. Pyruvate molecule ($C_3H_3O_3$). Glycolysis is the break-down of glucose (with 6 carbons) that results in 2 pyruvate molecules (3 carbons each). Do not get pyruvate muddled with pyruvic acid (not shown) which is pyruvate with an additional hydrogen ($C_3H_4O_3$).

The purpose of this cycle is twofold. First, it is a means of shedding excess carbon (C) by combining it with oxygen ($O_2$) to form the waste gas carbon dioxide ($CO_2$). Second, it produces hydrogen (H) atoms that are transported to a chain reaction series, the **electron transport system** (Figure 1.4). Two molecules move the hydrogen from the Krebs cycle to the electron transport system on the inner mitochondrial membrane, i.e. **nicotinamide adenine dinucleotide** (**NAD**) and **flavine adenine dinucleotide** (**FAD**). These bind to hydrogen to form **NADH** and **FADH₂**. At the first component of the electron transport chain, the hydrogen atoms split into **ions**, i.e. particles having a positive or negative charge, in this case a **proton** ($H^+$) and **electrons** ($e^-$) (Figure 1.4).

The protons are pumped out of the matrix to a position between the inner and outer mitochondrial membranes (Figure 1.5), and the electrons are passed down the electron transport system (Figure 1.4). Using enzymes bound to the inner-membrane folds (**cristae**) of the mitochondrion (Figure 1.5), this transport system releases electron energy in stages and immediately traps this energy by the conversion of ADP and inorganic phosphate ($P_i$) to ATP (Figure 1.6).

This generates some heat, but more heat will be liberated later when the ATP is used by the cell for other activities, i.e. the ATP is reduced again to ADP and $P_i$ (Figure 1.6). Heat is then available for contribution to body temperature. The hydrogen ions previously pumped out return to the matrix, and an enzyme, **ATPase**, converts ADP+$P_i$ to ATP, thus storing energy. Electrons and protons reunite to form uncharged hydrogen at the end of the process, i.e. $2H^+ + 2e^- \rightarrow 2H$. Further oxygen joins the hydrogen to create water, i.e. $2H + O \rightarrow H_2O$, which contributes to body hydration or is excreted (see Chapter 6).

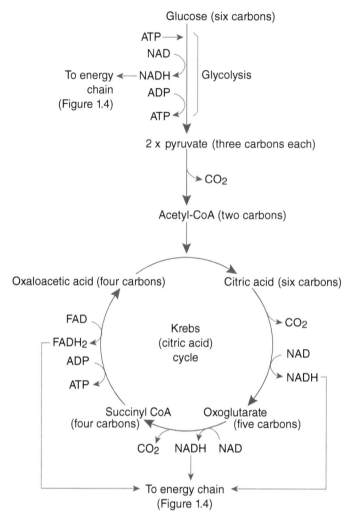

*Figure 1.3* The Krebs (citric acid or tricarboxylic acid) cycle. Two pyruvates are obtained from each glucose as a result of glycolysis. Some adenosine triphosphate (ATP) is needed to start the process. From pyruvate, acetyl coenzyme A (acetyl-CoA) feeds into the cycle by binding to oxaloacetic acid to form citric acid. The carbon count of each step is shown, and at various points carbon is lost by combining with oxygen to form $CO_2$. Nicotinamide adenine dinucleotide (NAD) and flavine adenine dinucleotide (FAD) combine with hydrogen at the points shown to transport this energy-rich hydrogen to the energy chain (Figure 1.4). Adenosine diphosphate (ADP) becomes energy-rich ATP during glycolysis and the cycle.

## Fats

Unlike glucose, fats provide energy differently. The Atwater number for fats is about 9 kcal per 1 g, more than twice that of glucose. Fats occur in the diet as **triglycerides**, i.e. three **fatty acids** attached to a single **glycerol** molecule. The whole molecule takes on the shape of the letter E (Figure 1.7).

Fatty acids can be split from the glycerol by the enzyme **lipase**. Free glycerol can be converted to glucose by the liver, a process called **gluconeogenesis**, i.e. genesis = creation,

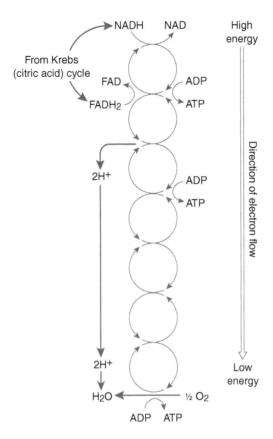

*Figure 1.4* Electron transport chain. A simplified diagram of the cyclic reactions that electrons pass down from the high-energy end to the low-energy end. Hydrogen ions (H⁺) and electrons arrive from the Krebs cycle transported by nicotinamide adenine dinucleotide (NAD) and flavine adenine dinucleotide (FAD). As the electrons flow down the chain reactions, they lose energy, which is used to convert adenosine diphosphate (ADP) to adenosine triphosphate (ATP). The hydrogen ions pass directly to the end of the chain reaction where they rejoin with their electrons and join with oxygen (half of $O_2$) to form metabolic water ($H_2O$). This takes place on the inner membrane cristae of the mitochondrion.

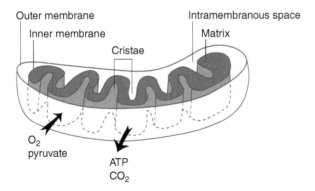

*Figure 1.5* The mitochondrion. Pyruvate enters the matrix from the outside where glycolysis takes place. The matrix is the site of the Krebs cycle. The energy transport chain occurs on the cristae of the inner membrane. Oxygen ($O_2$) enters and combines with carbon to form carbon dioxide ($CO_2$). Adenosine triphosphate (ATP) leaves and passes to all parts of the cell.

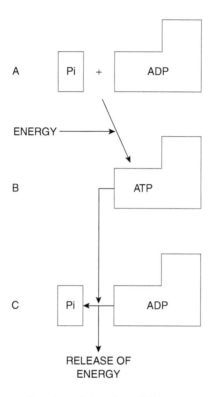

Figure 1.6 The conversion from adenosine diphosphate (ADP) and inorganic phosphate (Pi) to form an ATP molecule involves establishing a high-energy bond (i.e. it requires and stores energy). Release of that energy occurs when that bond is broken to create ADP and Pi once more.

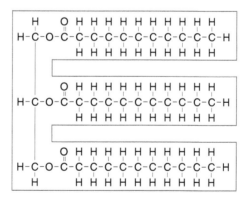

Figure 1.7 The E-shaped triglyceride molecule. A glycerol backbone holds together three long carbon (C) chain fatty acids saturated with hydrogen (H) and some oxygen (O).

neo = new; the creation of new glucose or creating glucose from a non-carbohydrate source. This new glucose can be used by the liver and the rest of the body in the same way as glucose from carbohydrates. Free fatty acids from the triglyceride molecule can be used by the liver for the Krebs cycle but not from pyruvate. Instead, they enter the Krebs cycle

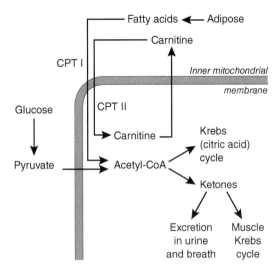

*Figure 1.8* The entry of fatty acids into the Krebs (citric acid) cycle is an alternative pathway to glucose as an energy source. Movement of fatty acids across the inner mitochondrial membrane is effected by binding with carnitine, which is recycled. Binding with carnitine requires one form of the enzyme carnitine palmitoyltransferase I (CPT I), and removal of carnitine requires the other form, CPT II. Some acetyl-CoA goes on to become ketones, which can be used for muscle energy or excreted.

by converting to **acetyl-CoA**. Fatty acids provide an alternative, more direct input into the cycle other than via pyruvate (Figure 1.8).

Large quantities of fatty acids arriving in the liver, as in **diabetes**, cannot all become acetyl-CoA, so they go through a different process leading to **ketone** formation, mostly **acetone**. Acetone is excreted in the urine or breath. Normally, muscles can take up ketones from the blood for use as energy, but in diabetes this use of ketones may be blocked (see *diabetes*, Chapter 8).

*Protein*

Proteins, a vital nitrogen source, can also be used for heat production if absolutely necessary. Normally, carbohydrates are the first source of energy, followed by fats if carbohydrates are not available (e.g. in **starvation**) or cannot be used by the body (e.g. in **diabetes**). If fats are not available either, e.g. because of depletion of stored adipose, protein will be used as a last resort. Whereas fats used for energy results in weight loss, protein used for energy causes **muscle wasting** (Chapter 7), and the patient is in a very serious state of ill health. Muscle wasting is seen in those who are dying from a terminal disease. This is a condition called **cachexia** (Chapter 7), which results in debility, weakness, emaciation and a mental state of hopelessness.

In order to use **amino acids** as an energy source from proteins, the liver must first remove the **nitrogenous** component, the **amino group**, a process called **deamination** (Figure 1.9). The rest is converted to glucose (**gluconeogenesis** again, this time glucose from protein).

The glucose can be used as blood sugar to provide energy for cells, giving protein the same Atwater number as carbohydrates (i.e. 4 kcal per 1 g). The nitrogen within the amino

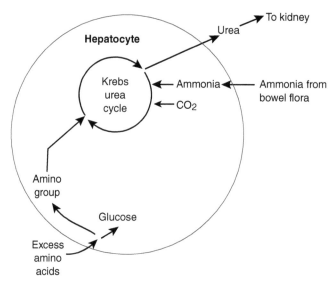

*Figure 1.9* The Krebs urea cycle in liver cells (hepatocytes). Excess amino acids are split to release ammonia ($NH_3$). The remaining component can then be converted to glucose. The cycle provides a means of eliminating the excess nitrogen in the form of urea, $CO(NH_2)_2$. Ammonia from bowel flora also joins the cycle with $CO_2$ to form urea for excretion.

group is in the form of **ammonia** (**$NH_3$**). Ammonia is toxic and should not be released into the blood in large quantities. Most of the ammonia is further converted in the liver to **urea**, i.e. **$CO(NH_2)_2$** via the **Krebs urea cycle**.[1] Urea is a safer compound to enter the blood, but it can still be toxic if blood levels are constantly raised, e.g. when the kidneys fail to excrete it.

*Metabolism*

**Metabolism** is the total of all the chemical reactions in the body that use energy and liberate heat. There is a minimum rate of metabolism below which cellular activity will fail, with a subsequent threat to life. The **basal metabolic rate** (**BMR**) refers to the minimum total internal energy expenditure when awake but at rest or the minimum metabolic rate at rest needed to sustain life. More heat energy is produced in areas of the body where cells undergo high metabolic rates, e.g. the liver and the brain, or undertake movement, e.g. the muscles during exercise. These areas demonstrate rapid release of energy, creating heat as an extra product. The body creates an average of about 420 kilojoules (100 kcal) of heat per hour. This would raise the body temperature by 2°C per hour if it were not lost at a rate equal to that at which it is produced (Blows 1998). Cells rich in mitochondria are produce high metabolic rates and more heat production. The trunk of the body has the greatest number of cells positioned away from the surface, where heat cannot escape directly into the environment, and it is therefore warmer (Figure 1.10). They would be much hotter still if heat were not moved away from the core by the blood. Blood leaving the brain, the liver and active muscles is significantly hotter than the blood entering these organs.

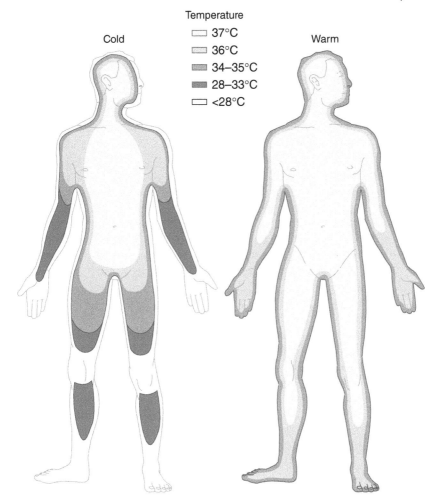

*Figure 1.10* Temperature profile in a cold and in a warm environment. Notice the restricted core temperature (37°C) in the cold environment, keeping vital organs warm while mini-mising heat loss from the extremities. Under these conditions, the temperature of the extremities can be as much as 10°C lower than the core.

## Heat movement and loss

About 1°C difference exists between the **core temperature** and the **peripheral tem-perature**, but this difference can increase in cold environments to the extent that the hands and feet can be as much as 10°C cooler than the trunk (Figure 1.10). As more heat is produced it is moved away from the core to the surface tissues by the blood. Moving heat in this manner is crucial to prevent very active tissues, such as the brain, muscle and liver, from overheating and virtually cooking themselves in situ. Tissues in direct contact with the external environment, mostly the skin of the extremities, will not produce enough heat in extreme cold conditions to survive, so they rely heavily on heat transported to them by the blood. Should the blood supply to the extremities fail, as in extreme cold conditions, the tissues can die, causing **gangrene** (an area of dead tissue). Loss of fingers and toes from gangrene in extreme cold conditions is not uncommon.

Heat loss from the body is mostly through the skin and to a lesser extent through mucous membrane, faeces, urine and exhaled air. Visible sweating is a very important means of heat loss. About 2 million sweat glands exist in a single individual, with greater concentrations in specific areas such as the axillae and palms. Extra body heat is used to convert the sweat from a liquid state at body temperature to a vapour also at body temperature. The heat used for this purpose does not raise the temperature of the sweat, and therefore it is called the **latent** (**hidden**) **heat** of evaporation. It is 'hidden' because it cannot be detected on a thermometer. A similar situation is seen when latent heat is required to convert boiling water at 100°C to steam, also at 100°C. Sweat vapour passes into the air taking heat with it. In high-temperature situations, such as a hot day or a high body temperature, e.g. infections or excessive exercise, sweating[2] becomes a vital means of cooling the skin, which can then accept more heat from the core. An environment of high humidity severely reduces the skin's ability to vaporise sweat, which then remains as a liquid on the skin, and as the skin temperature rises, so does the core temperature.

Other means of skin heat loss are conduction, convection and radiation. **Conduction** is the passage of heat from the skin into any cooler object touching the skin. The body warms the bed, the clothes, the seats and so on, by conduction. It is all heat lost from our cells. It is the smallest amount of heat lost during the day unless the body is suddenly immersed in cold water. Then, rapid conduction causes quick and severe **hypothermia** (low body temperature). **Convection** involves the warming of air next to the skin. Warm air rises and moves upwards and is replaced by colder air from below. This continuous process makes humans mobile convector heaters, warming any environment they inhabit. This warm air layer is rapidly removed by the wind, and if this it cold wind it causes the body to chill quickly, known as the **wind chill factor**. **Radiation** of heat is also continuous, where heat passes directly out from the skin into any object it hits, warming that object. Gas or electric fires heat a room, and the sun warms the Earth in the same way. Much of this heat is in the form of **infrared radiation**, and this is what infrared thermometers use to identify the presence of heat. It is also infrared that is picked up by thermal imaging cameras used in rescues and night vision.

### Heat regulation: gain versus loss

The body must switch from increased heat production when it is cold to increased heat loss when it is hot. This process is sensitive to small changes in both the internal and the external temperature**. Homeostasis** is the maintenance of a stable internal environment, the aim being to stabilise the normal temperature at 37°C (98.4°F, often called **normo-thermia**). The blood distributes heat evenly to all the tissues. It involves sensory feedback to the brain and an output to **effector organs**, i.e. organs that can effect a change (Figure 1.11).

Thermoregulation is a *negative* feedback mechanism in which the system reverses the direction of the original stimulus, i.e. if the temperature goes up, the mechanism drives it down, and vice versa. The area of the brain responsible for this is the **hypothalamus**, the body's thermostat. The **preoptic nucleus** of the hypothalamus is rich in both heat- and cold-sensitive neurons. These can monitor the temperature of the blood that passes through the nucleus and initiate any necessary action. The heat-sensitive neurones fire impulses faster as temperature rises, with a similar response from the cold-sensitive neurones to

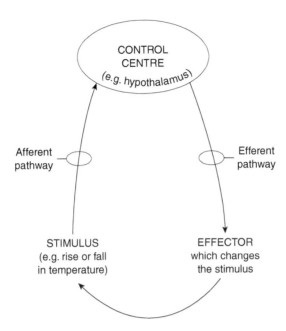

*Figure 1.11* The homeostatic mechanism begins with a stimulus affecting a receptor at the start of the afferent pathway. This pathway carries nerve impulses from the receptor to the control centre, which is usually part of the brain (and in the case of temperature, it is the hypothalamus). The control centre triggers action in response to the stimulus. Nerve impulses then pass from the centre, via the efferent pathway, to an effector organ (i.e. something that can change the stimulus). This then makes the appropriate changes to correct the stimulus. Most homeostatic mechanisms are negative pathways (i.e. they reverse the stimulus, e.g. if the temperature rises, the effector organ will take action to lower it, and vice versa).

cooler temperatures (Hall 2016). Peripheral and ambient temperatures are also monitored by both cold- and heat-sensitive receptors in the skin, and internal temperatures are monitored by sensors within the spinal cord, the abdominal organs and around the major veins. In all these areas, cold receptors dominate, indicating the need for the body to avoid low rather than high temperatures. They feed back to the hypothalamus which has complete second-by-second information on the total body temperature (Hall 2016). The hypothalamus maintains a **set point** of 37.1°C and initiates any changes necessary to stabilise the temperature at this set point. Any situation where the body temperature rises above the set point, i.e. **hyperthermia**, **pyrexia** or **hyperpyrexia** (see page 15), causes the hypothalamus to activate the **sympathetic nervous system** which stimulates sweating. Also it *reduces* sympathetic **vasoconstrictor tone** (Figure 3.3, page 45) causing vasodilatation of the skin vessels coupled with relaxation of the precapillary sphincters. Together, these allow more blood and more heat to reach the body surface, causing the skin to be hot and flushed. Skin blood flow can vary from 250 ml to as much as 2,500 ml per minute, depending on thermoregulatory needs (Watson 1998). Sympathetic stimulation also results in an associated increase in heart rate, ensuring faster delivery of blood to the skin and an increase in the respiratory rate to expel more heat in the breath. Behavioural changes means the individual removes clothes or bedding to get comfortable and takes a cold drink or a cooling shower.

In **hypothermia** the body temperature is below the set point, i.e. 35°C or lower. The hypothalamus initiates sympathetic activity that increases cellular metabolism to generate more heat, and it *increases* sympathetic **vasoconstrictor tone** (Figure 3.3, page 45). This will constrict the peripheral blood vessels in the skin to reduce the heat loss. Sweating is shut down as much as possible but some water loss through the skin is maintained. Respirations are also reduced to minimise the loss of warm air and water vapour in the breath.

It may seem contradictory that the sympathetic nervous system can be activated in both the extremes of body temperature – hot and cold – and yet have different effects. This is because the sympathetic nervous system uses the neurotransmitter **noradrenaline** at the termination synapse, and this binds to different receptors with often contradictory results. Hair erector (or **pilomotor**) muscles cause hairs to stand on end, a process that traps more air next to the skin for improved insulation. Its use is limited in humans due to the sparseness of hair compared with animals and because humans wear clothes. It does cause *goose pimples* that clearly indicate that the skin is chilled. The **motor nervous system** supplying the skeletal muscle is used to increase muscle tone[3] (Figure 14.7, page 294) that induces shivering to boost heat production, as all muscle activity does. The motor system also enhances conscious behavioural responses, such as turning on heating systems, exercising and dressing warmly.

## Temperature scales and normal temperature variation

The body temperature is measured in degrees **Celsius** (or **centigrade**, **°C**) as part of the **Standard International** (**SI**) **system**. Strictly speaking, the SI unit for temperature is the **Kelvin** (**K**), but this is rather impractical for clinical use since 0°K is *minus* 273°C (–273°C, called *Absolute Zero*) i.e. the coldest possible temperature, which would make normal body temperature 310°K (Figure 1.12).

Celsius uses 0°C as the freezing point of water and 100°C as the boiling point of water at one atmosphere of air pressure (generally accepted as sea level). This last point

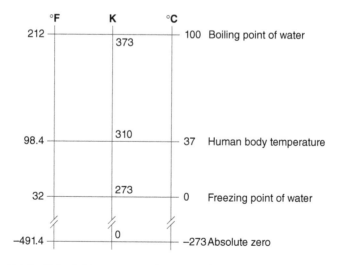

*Figure 1.12* The Kelvin (°K), Celsius (centigrade, °C) and Fahrenheit (°F) temperature scales. The correlations between absolute zero, the freezing point of water, the human body temperature and the boiling point of water are shown.

is important since boiling point is dependent on the air pressure. Water boils at reduced temperatures as air pressure drops, i.e. when ascending away from sea level. The Celsius scale has taken over from the **Fahrenheit** (**°F**) system, which had the freezing point at 32°F and the boiling point at 212°F. The body temperature at 37°C was previously measured at 98.4°F, a figure that may still be found in older texts. The conversion of Celsius to Fahrenheit uses the formula 1.8 (°C) + 32 = °F, i.e. taking the normal body temperature of 37°C as an example, 1.8 × 37 = 66.6; then 66.6 + 32 = 98.6°F (Figure 1.12).

Normally, small local changes in peripheral body temperature are to be expected with variations in the external air temperature or contact with hot or cold surfaces. Such circumstances arise in very hot or very cold weather or work environments involving molten metal or refrigeration. These variations can cause thermal injuries if over-exposure occurs. A normal **diurnal (24-hour) pattern** of fluctuations also occurs, with lowest temperatures in the morning and highest in the evening. The body is also hotter after a warm bath or shower, and the core temperature will be temporarily increased by a hot drink, making oral measurement at this time deceptive.

## Taking the body temperature in adults

Routes for taking the temperature include the mouth, axilla, groin, rectum and ear. The traditional means of taking the temperature, i.e. the oral route, measures the temperature of the blood in the carotid artery, blood that is coming directly from the core temperature (Watson 1998). The peripheral and core temperatures are different because the periphery has the role of losing heat into the environment and therefore it can fluctuate with changes in the ambient temperature. The core temperature must remain constant and is therefore the most accurate and stable temperature to measure. It is also the temperature at which the vital organs must exist to function normally. Which route is used depends on several factors, particularly in relation to specific client groups or certain situations when oral temperatures are inappropriate. The confused elderly, the mentally disturbed and very young children are those where the oral route is not appropriate.

**Disposable** thermometers are used mostly in paediatric units as they are more suitable for use with young children, especially in paediatric emergency care. A series of temperature-sensitive chemical colour change dots provides an easily read system (Figure 1.13). The dots change from orange/red to blue, and the temperature is read as the highest-valued dot to turn blue.

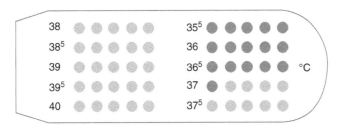

*Figure 1.13* Tempadot thermometer reading. The dots change from red to blue according to the temperature recorded. Each dot represents 0.1°C. The one illustrated here shows 37°C (i.e. normal body temperature).

There are also multi-use colour strips that are placed on the forehead. These are read while in contact with the skin because the colour changes reverse if it cools down. They are less accurate than most other thermometers and therefore can only be considered as a guide to the temperature in small children at home. They are also measuring the temperature of the skin (peripheral) rather than the core temperature, and because of this they are not used by the NHS (Gallagher 2023).

**Electronic** devices are available for use in the ear and forehead (non-contact) use. They display a **digital** result. Electronic **infrared** thermometers are primarily for use in the ear, measuring the infrared radiation from the eardrum, but some measure infrared emitted from the skin without touching the skin (forehead, non-contact). The temperature is instantly calculated by the thermometer based on the infrared level detected. The eardrum shares the same blood supply as the hypothalamus, which makes it very close to core temperature, equating well with pulmonary artery temperature (O'Toole 1998). It is also easily accessible with a short probe that fits into the external canal of the ear. The lens on the tip of the probe must face the tympanic membrane and a good seal should be obtained around the probe to ensure that only body heat is sampled. The presence of **cerumen** (earwax) may give a false reading that is lower than reality. The infrared probe is better used on adults and older children who not only have reasonably formed external ear canals but will cooperate better with the procedure. Accuracy is generally good. An assessment of various types of thermometers and their accuracy is given by Gallagher (2023).

### *Why mercury thermometers are a thing of the past*

**Mercury** thermometers had been in use for a long time, but mercury use in newly manufactured thermometers has been banned in the UK since 2009 (Gallagher 2023). This is due to the hazard of released mercury which is toxic, especially if inhaled as vapour. Mercury can remain in the environment for months after a mercury spillage. Skin and mucous membrane absorption of mercury is low, but the vapour is well absorbed through the lungs. Acute mercury poisoning (within 30 minutes of exposure) causes thirst, nausea, vomiting, abdominal pains, diarrhoea with blood and ultimately renal failure. Chronic mercury toxicity involves irritability, excessive salivation, loose teeth, gum disorders, slurred speech, tremors and unsteady gait (see Chapter 14). Broken glass was an additional risk. It is not surprising that the mercury-in-glass thermometer has become a museum piece.

### Temperature in children

Maintaining the child's temperature at normal levels during the perinatal period reduces infant mortality (Lyon 2006). Very young children loose heat quickly, especially by evaporation, but they are unable to replace the heat due to limited movement, i.e. heat from muscle activity. They also have an immature hypothalamus and therefore have difficulty in stabilising their core temperature through normal homeostatic responses. Illness or preterm immaturity makes this situation worse (Lyon 2008). Babies are born with a high proportion of **brown fat**, which generates additional heat through metabolism, particularly when stimulated by **melatonin**, a hormone produced from serotonin in the pineal gland of the brain. This is unlike the usual white fat, which only stores energy but lacks the metabolism to produce heat. However, the brown fat is inadequate to maintain the body's temperature on its own, and it gradually diminishes with age, at the same time as increasing muscle activity produces more heat as the child develops walking, climbing etc. Very young children may not have developed the ability to shiver, and they cannot therefore gain heat from this mechanism. These children are dependent on warm environments and clothing to prevent hypothermia.

### Abnormal high body temperatures

**Fevers** are high temperatures (i.e. above 38°C) (Blumenthal 1998). A **pyrexia** is recognised as a continuous body temperature above 37.5°C up to 39.9°C, and a hyperpyrexia is 40°C or above (Harker and Gibson 1995). Raised temperatures are both a symptom of a disorder and a natural body defence mechanism which reduces the severity and longevity of a disease.

Raised temperature may be caused by a wide range of disorders, e.g. toxins or drug reactions, viral and bacterial infections, reactions to vaccination, prolonged exposure to a hot environment, brain disorders affecting the hypothalamus, neoplasms, autoimmune diseases or the penguin effect[4] (Blows 1998). Infectious diseases are common, especially in children and can range from self-limiting viral infections, e.g. the common cold, to life-threatening disorders such as meningitis and sepsis. The body may fail to control the temperature when the hypothalamic set point is exceeded. In fever, the hypothalamic set point is driven up to a higher level (e.g. 39°C) in a regulated manner, unlike hyperthermia, in which there is an unregulated temperature rise (Henker *et al.* 1997). Because the control centre has been reset higher in fever, it perceives normal temperature of 37°C as being too low (Figure 1.14). Homeostatic mechanisms will then drive the temperature up to its new set level.

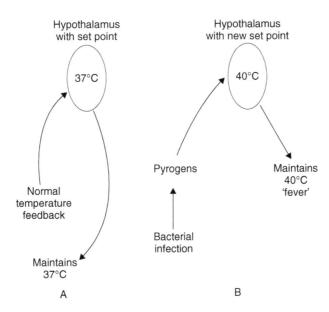

*Figure 1.14* The mechanism for fever. (A) The normal body temperature is maintained by the hypothalamus having a set point of 37°C and by feedback from the body indicating any changes to this temperature, which the hypothalamus will correct. (B) In fever, pyrogens released from bacteria reset the hypothalamic set point to a higher value (here, reset to 40°C, but it can be other high figures), and the hypothalamus attempts to maintain that higher temperature.

The set point rise is due to the action of **pyrogens,** chemical agents that can readjust the hypothalamus. Pyrogens include various toxins, including proteins or their degraded products, and some endotoxins from bacteria, e.g. the **lipopolysaccharide, LPS,** layer from outside the cell wall of gram-negative organisms. After death of the organism, the endotoxin is phagocytosed, and the phagocyte itself (usually a **macrophage**) releases **interleukin 1**. This passes to the brain where it stimulates the formation of a **prostaglandin**, and this acts to reset the set point of the hypothalamus to a higher level. This is a rapid process, the temperature rising within 8 to 10 minutes of the release of interleukin 1. The endotoxin LPS only needs to cause the production of a few nanograms of interleukin 1 to cause fever. The involvement of prostaglandins may explain how **antipyretics**[5] such as **aspirin** and **paracetamol** may help to reduce the body temperature (see Antipyretics, page 18).

As a defence mechanism, a raised body temperature improves the immune system response to infections and may even reduce viral replication and virus release from the cells.

It appears to do more damage to infected cells than to normal cells. The debate about 'should we provide treatment for fever or not?' continues (Wrotek *et al.* 2021).

**Hyperthermia** is a group of high body temperature disorders that includes **heatstroke** (Edwards 1998; Harker and Gibson 1995). This is a rapid rise in body temperature (to 40°C or more) caused by exposure to a hot environment, and the hypothalamic set point is soon exceeded. Sweating fails to control the temperature. Symptoms include hot, dry skin, full and bounding pulse, headaches, confusion, dizziness and failing consciousness. The **penguin effect** is a similar heatstroke caused by a reduced ability to sweat in the centre of a tightly packed crowd. Examples of this occur in crowds at a major event, such as a pop music concert or people packed together in a commuter train on a hot day. It is named after penguins that crowd together to conserve heat in Antarctica. Emotional excitement, dancing and possibly drugs are features at pop concerts that can cause excess heat production with reduced ability to sweat. On crowded commuter transport, standing passengers may collapse but remain pinned upright, risking a loss of life because there is no means to lay them flat. The penguin effect can cause many casualties at once, all suffering from the heat and also from fluid and electrolyte losses (see chapter 6) (Blows 1998). **Heat exhaustion** is associated with exposure to hot environments where the hypothalamus has been able to keep the temperature at relatively normal levels for most of the time by sweating. However, continued heat exposure and profuse sweating result in excessive fluid and electrolyte loss which eventually leads to collapse with headaches, weak and rapid pulse, confusion, nausea, cramps and pallor. One of the important differences between heatstroke and heat exhaustion is time, i.e. heatstroke happens quickly; heat exhaustion happens after several hours. **Malignant hyperthermia** is a complication associated with an inherited muscular disorder triggered by administration of inhalant anaesthetics and muscle-relaxing drugs. It occurs mostly in the young. The muscles maintain a state of contraction soon after induction of anaesthesia, and this muscle activity generates heat that can raise the body temperature by as much as 1°C every 5 minutes. About 20% of sufferers can die from the effects as it also induces acidosis, tachycardia and hypotension.

**Febrile convulsions** in children under 7 years of age indicate two things: (1) a pyrexia usually caused by an infection; and (2) a hypothalamus that is too immature to cope with the high temperature. The most common causes are chest and ear infections, but any infection can trigger a fit at this age and assessment should consider the possibility of sepsis.[6] The mechanism that responds to a high temperature by causing a fit is not well understood. The overall management is two-pronged: (1) treating and terminating the fit quickly, which involves reducing the temperature whilst maintaining a clear airway; and (2) investigating and treating the underlying infection. Preventative measures require early detection of pyrexia and cooling the child gently before a fit is triggered. Thermometers are not so important. It is usually sufficient for parents to feel the child's head and trunk to recognise they have a high temperature. It is important to remove excess clothing, cool down the environment if it is too hot, and get medical help. Tepid sponging is not recommended and temperature reduction resulting in hypothermia is a possible danger (Doyle and Schortgen 2016). In the clinical environment, accurate temperature measurement becomes important and is easily achieved. Reassuring the parents is important including allowing the parents be with the child for as long as possible. Long-term epilepsy from febrile convulsions occurs very rarely.

Treatment of heat disorders has involved cooling along with fluid and electrolyte replacement where necessary (see Chapter 6 for *fluid and electrolytes*). Reducing the high temperature is problematic since cooling too rapidly can induce shock – or more likely shivering – which would cause more heat production. The temperature should be reduced gradually, i.e. at a rate no faster than 1°C per hour, although this has been difficult to achieve and record. Tepid sponging is not recommended because sponging the skin to reduce fever, especially in children, is counterproductive, since it generates heat through shivering and is also uncomfortable for the child (Anon 1999; Blumenthal 1998). Given that fever is a regular response to infection or inflammation, some evidence indicates that rapid reduction of the temperature may not be beneficial and could cause unwanted difficulties (Edwards 1998; Harker and Gibson 1995). Generally, provided adults are sweating, they cope better with high temperatures than children. Sweating is a sign that the hypothalamus is still doing its job and drying sweat from the skin is counter-productive. Children below 7 years of age are the most likely to suffer convulsions, so try to prevent the temperature from going very high in this age group. Remove unnecessary clothing and provide a cool environment to promote natural heat loss. Cool drinks are of value because they reach the core temperature quickly and replace lost fluids. It is vital that the child is conscious and able to swallow. Be aware of the risk of shivering (e.g. **rigors**[7]) and try to prevent this. Shivering indicates the body has lost peripheral heat too quickly and is trying to generate more heat. The skin is getting colder than the core, and the hypothalamus is responding to the peripheral temperature rather than the core temperature, i.e. it is trying to warm up the skin. Electric fans help to cool a hot environment, but they should never be aimed directly at the patient. This would cool the skin and send cold sensations

*Table 1.1* Red flag warnings of deteriorating condition

♆ **Red Flag = Serious situation which needs urgent medical attention.**

| Flag warning | Details |
| --- | --- |
| ♆ **Red Flag** | **Temperature below 36°C (pending hypothermia) in anyone currently ill.** **Temperature of 38°C (pyrexia) or higher (e.g. hyperpyrexia) in babies younger than 3 months (possible risk of sepsis).** **Rigors: fever with visible shivering (possible risk of sepsis).** **Fits in children with fever, especially below 7 years of age.** |

(After Hill-Smith and Johnson 2021, with permission)

from the skin thermal receptors to the brain. The hypothalamus then tries to prevent heat loss from the body and tries to generate more heat, i.e. as seen in shivering. Cold air from a fan could cause peripheral vasoconstriction, which then prevents heat in the blood from reaching the skin. Although tepid sponging is not generally recommended, it may be useful when applied to hyperpyrexic patients who have lost the ability to sweat, i.e. the patient is hot and dry. Failure to sweat suggests that the hypothalamus has failed to respond, probably because the set point has been adjusted to a higher level than normal.

### Antipyretic drugs

Antipyretic drugs (e.g. paracetamol, ibuprofen and aspirin) are used to reduce elevated temperatures in those capable of taking oral medication. These drugs block the enzyme **cyclo-oxygenase** (**COX**) which produces prostaglandins from a cell wall fatty acid called **arachidonic acid** (See *non-steroidal anti-inflammatory (NSAI) analgesic drugs*, Chapter 12, page 257) (Figure 1.15). **Aspirin** is a useful antipyretic, but it should never be

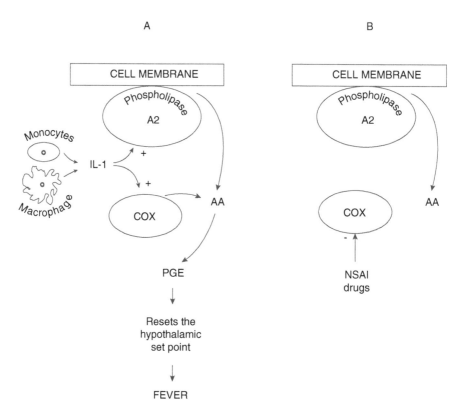

*Figure 1.15* The mechanism of antipyretic (anti-inflammatory) drugs. A. The enzyme phospholipase A2 releases arachidonic acid (AA), from cell membranes. Arachidonic acid is converted to various prostaglandins (PG) including prostaglandin E (PGE) by the enzyme cyclo-oxygenase (COX). Interleukin-1 (Il-1) from macrophages and monocytes promotes (+) the action of phospholipase A2 and COX. PGE causes inflammation and raises temperature by resetting the hypothalamic set point to a higher-level, causing fever. B. NSAI drugs block (–) the action of COX preventing the production of PGE.

given to children below the age of 12 years as this can induce **Reye's syndrome**, a severe neurological disorder. **Paracetamol** is a useful alternative to aspirin for children. If paracetamol appears to be ineffectual, **ibuprofen** may be a better option. Paracetamol and ibuprofen should not be given together simultaneously but used as alternatives to each other. Antipyretics alone are unlikely to prevent febrile convulsions, and other measures are required.

### Abnormal low body temperatures

Exposure to cold leads to a general loss of body heat, known as **hypothermia** or a local heat loss, called **frostbite**. Hypothermia can happen in anyone, but the largest numbers of cases occur in the very young and the very old. This is due to problems with the hypothalamus. In the very young the hypothalamus is still immature and cannot fully control their temperature balance (see page 10). The effects of cold increase gradually, and the early stages of hypothermia may not be recognised at first. Children feel cold to the touch and they may shiver, especially older children. They may also appear limp and quiet and may have cyanosed lips and extremities. They can collapse and possibly die from respiratory or cardiac failure. Children with wet skin and clothing are especially vulnerable since the water will evaporate quickly from the skin taking body heat with it. Because of poor insulation from very little body hair, combined with low heat production from reduced muscle activity, babies are very vulnerable to heat loss and are dependent on warm environments and insulation provided by clothing. **Incubators** have saved the lives of new born babies who cannot sustain normothermia by their own volition, e.g. such babies as **preterm** or **failure to thrive**. Incubation maintains the infant's environmental temperature usually a few degrees higher than average body temperature until the hypothalamus is mature enough to stabilise its own homeostatic control of heat loss. Since incubators must be opened occasionally to allow essential access, the room temperature must also be warm enough to prevent sudden chilling of the infant.

The elderly have age-related changes to the hypothalamus which gradually declines in function. The temperature control centre becomes less able to respond to body-temperature changes quickly. It cannot always provide heat regulation when environmental temperatures are above or below average for prolonged periods of time. Although hot environments can be harmful to the elderly who can die in a heatwave, it is the cold that causes most problems and deaths. Cold weather kills many elderly people annually, and special consideration must be given to older people during winter months, especially those who live alone in poorly heated homes. It is worse for those with limited mobility and those who are vulnerable to falling. An old person lying injured on a floor after a fall will lose heat quickly from their skin and may die from hypothermia before being found. Children will suffer from the effects of cold quickly, whereas elderly people deteriorate gradually as a result of prolonged cold exposure.

An important cause of potential hypothermia is surgery. During the **perioperative period**, patients are exposed to cool environments and may suffer a significant body temperature loss. Intensive care may also put some patients at risk of hypothermia, mainly because patients are inactive. They may be exposed for procedures and their total energy input for the day may be considerably less than what their body is used to. In these specialised clinical areas some units carry out **total temperature management** (**TTM**) as a means of preventing hypothermia. This involves continual monitoring of the patient's core temperature by electronic probes placed inside the body, in sites such as the pulmonary artery, oesophagus, rectum or urinary bladder. The temperature can be read at any time as a digital figure on a screen that shows other physiological readings. TTM also involves maintenance of normothermia in the patient during lengthy exposure or surgery using specialised electrically warmed blankets. Very strict control of the environmental temperature is maintained, often at an above average level, with rewarming of fluids or blood before or during intravenous infusion. Because body temperature, metabolism and healing are all linked, the healing process itself relies on maintaining a state of normothermia.

The dangers of hypothermia are caused by the low core temperature at which the vital organs must try to function. Any attempt to rewarm the person by applying heat to the periphery, i.e. warming up the skin, can be counterproductive and dangerous. The use of heat close to the skin, e.g. hot water bottles, heaters or electric blankets, will make the person look better and feel warmer to touch, but they only serve to dilate peripheral blood vessels, which then takes the vital blood and heat away from the core, cooling the core temperature further. This is not the same as using the specialised heated blankets identified in TTM, when the core temperature is normal, and the emphasis is on preventing hypothermia, not treating it. The main points about rewarming the established hypothermia are: (1) The person involved must be urgently removed to a warmer environment to prevent further heat loss. Trying to rewarm someone in a very cold environment is a struggle that the patient may lose. (2) Wet clothing must be removed and the skin dried. Water on the skin acts like sweating by removing further heat quickly. (3) The body should then be covered in dry clothing and the person preferably put to bed. (4) Warm drinks with sugar, given to the conscious person who is still able to swallow, would be beneficial. (5) Monitoring of the temperature by an electronic thermometer. The oral route may be dangerous in a patient who is in an altered state of consciousness. (6) Rewarming should be gradual, often quoted as 1°C rise per hour. Rapid rewarming, like rapid cooling, is harmful as it can induce shock. Once cooled, the core temperature is only raised by heat produced from tissue metabolism, and this will take time to be effective.

Thermal injury

Frostbite is a local thermal injury, and it is akin to burns because tissue is destroyed by an extreme temperature abnormality. The intense local cold causes vasoconstriction to the point of occlusion of blood flow, with resultant **anoxia** (lack of oxygen) of dependent tissues. All cellular metabolism stops when oxygen and nutrient delivery is shut down, wastes accumulate in the cells and enzymic reactions can no longer function. Apart from feeling cold, early signs of frostbite can include **paraesthesia** (tingling sensations) and numbness and pallor of the affected tissues, which may turn blue (**cyanosis**) and ultimately black. This is when the tissues are dead (**necrosis** or **gangrene**) and may slough off. An infection of the area involved can then follow, with life-threatening results. If the tissues involved survive and recover, they become red, blistered and painful. Emergency treatment involves prevention of the condition worsening by removal to a warmer environment as soon as possible and gentle rewarming by placing the affected parts against warmer areas of the body. Removal of any tight clothing or restrictive jewellery is essential to promote good blood flow and to avoid rubbing the injury, which can cause tissue trauma. Light dressings may help, and medical treatment is usually essential. Frostbite will mostly affect toes and fingers because these parts are at the distal extremes of the cardiovascular system, i.e. they are at the point of lowest tissue perfusion pressure, the **mean**

**arterial pressure** or **MAP** (see Chapter 3, page 48) and therefore will suffer more damaging vasoconstriction than those parts closer to the core. Distal extremities are thinner than central parts, i.e. compare the thickness of a toe with that of the thigh or the trunk. Cold can penetrate extremities faster, i.e. they have less body mass per unit of surface area than thicker parts of the body. Since it is the surface area that is exposed to the cold, it has less mass of tissue below it to chill than the same surface area of, for example, the thigh. This smaller mass of tissue is not capable of heat production to counteract the cold on the same scale as bulkier parts. The distal extremities are more dependent on heat delivered by the blood than any other parts of the body. This is why feet can get cold quickly and hot water bottles are used by some people to warm their feet in bed. It is also the reason why the temperature of extremities is a good indication of the status of the circulation in that limb. Warm hands, feet, fingers and toes indicate good circulation, whereas cold extremities indicate poor circulation. This is a useful observation on limbs encased in plaster casts where the toes or fingers are exposed or where an injury or vascular complication may disturb blood flow to that extremity. Using hand or foot temperature, along with the **capillary refill time** (see Chapter 3, page 48) to assess the circulation on the unaffected side will identify what the normal circulatory state is at that time. Since both limbs are normally equal, this will indicate what the circulatory state should be in the affected limb. Such a comparison made between the good limb and the affected limb may identify a serious problem on the injured side that requires urgent attention, e.g. possibly the plaster or bandages are too tight.

### Key points

- Body temperature is generally stabilised at 37°C, with a homeostatic negative feedback mechanism in place to maintain this.
- Homeostasis, such as temperature control, consists of a receptor, an afferent pathway, a control centre, an efferent pathway and an effector organ.
- The hypothalamus in the base of the brain is the central control of the temperature regulation, with input from temperature-sensitive sensory nerve endings in the skin and around vital organs.
- Normally, the body gains heat by cellular metabolism from energy-rich food and loses heat by evaporation of sweat, elimination, conduction, convection and radiation.
- Sweating is often a cardinal sign of overheating (pyrexia).
- Shivering is a cardinal sign of the body being too cold (hypothermia) or a sign of rigors.
- The core temperature is the most accurate to record since this is the temperature at which the vital organs must function.
- The peripheral temperature is usually lower than the core temperature since it responds more to the ambient temperature and humidity.
- Disposable, electronic and infrared thermometers have now replaced mercury thermometers in clinical use.
- Younger children are more vulnerable to temperature changes than adults and may suffer febrile convulsions.
- Electric fans are useful for cooling the environment but must not be directed at the patient.
- Tepid sponging may be uncomfortable for the patient and may be of little value, except in those circumstances of rapid body temperature rise where sweating has failed to control body temperature.

- Rewarming in hypothermia, like cooling in pyrexia, should be gradual, often quoted as 1°C rise per hour. Rapid rewarming, like rapid cooling, is harmful as it can induce shock.
- The temperature of extremities is a good indication of the status of the circulation in that limb. The warm hand or foot has a good circulation, whereas cold extremities indicate a poorer circulation.

## Notes

1  Be careful not to get the Krebs Cycle and the Krebs Urea Cycle muddled up. They are different cycles.
2  Not all sweating relates to temperature control. Sweating can occur for other reasons as well, notably in shock, where the patient may actually be cold. It is the result of overstimulation by the sympathetic nervous system.
3  Muscle tone is a state of tension in a muscle that prepares it for contraction. Muscles without tone are loose and floppy and don't contract well. Exercise increases tone and lack of exercise reduces tone (Figure 14.7, page 294).
4  Penguin effect is high temperature caused by being trapped in the middle of a crowd of moving people, e.g. at a pop music concert where everyone is dancing (i.e. generating heat; see page 16).
5  Antipyretics are drugs used to reduce high temperatures (see page 18).
6  The assessment and management of child disorders is a highly specialised skill, and full coverage is beyond the scope of this book. If there is any concern regarding a child with a high temperature that child should be referred to a doctor at the earliest opportunity (see also Table 1.1).
7  Rigor is a feeling of cold with visible shivering whilst the body temperature is actually above normal.

## References

Anonymous (1999) Fever analysis remains a burning issue. *Nursing Times, 95*(9): 47.

Blows W.T. (1998) Crowd physiology: The 'penguin effect'. *Accident and Emergency Nursing, 6*: 126–129.

Blumenthal I. (1998) What parents think of fever. *Family Practice, 15*(6): 513–518.

Doyle J.F. and Schortgen F. (2016) Should we treat pyrexia? And how do we do it? *Critical Care, 20*: 303. https://doi.org/10.1186/s13054-016-1467-2

Edwards S.L. (1998) High temperature. *Professional Nurse, 13*(8): 521–526.

Gallagher, P. (2023) Best digital thermometers 2023: Which? best buys and expert buying advice. *Which?* www.which.co.uk/reviews/digital-thermometers/article/how-to-buy-the-best-digital-thermometer-aiuBk7T48tjz?source_code=911CRJ&gclid=CjwKCAjw0N6hBhAUEiwAXab-TRweTk-k2iV_IFmSZiTETH3cRrAjH5mNb9XKVtvKwp1k5Vl6i7T8eXhoCkLgQAvD_BwE&gclsrc=aw.ds (updated: 6th April 2023) (Accessed 14th April 2023).

Hall J. (2016) *Guyton and Hall Textbook of Medical Physiology* (13th edition). W.B. Saunders, Elsevier, Philadelphia, PA.

Harker J. and Gibson P. (1995) Heat-stroke: A review of rapid cooling techniques. *Intensive and Critical Care Nursing, 11*: 198–202.

Henker R., Kramer D. and Rogers S. (1997) Fever. *AACN Clinical Issues, 8*(3): 351–367.

Hill-Smith I. and Johnson G. (2021) *Little Book of Red Flags*. National Minor Illness Centre, Bedfordshire.

Lyon A. (2006) Applied physiology: Temperature control in the newborn infant. *Paediatrics and Child Health, 16*(6): 386–392. http://doi.org/10.1016/j.cupe.2006.07.017

Lyon A. (2008) Temperature control in the neonate. *Paediatrics and Child Health, 18*(4): 155–160.

O'Toole S. (1998) Temperature measuring devices. *Professional Nurse, 13*(11): 779–786.

Watson R. (1998) Controlling body temperature in adults. *Nursing Standard, 12*(20): 49–55.

Wrotek S., LeGrand E.K., Dzialuk A. and Alcock J. (2021) Let fever do its job: The meaning of fever in the pandemic era. *Evolution, Medicine, and Public Health, 9*(1): 26–35. https://doi.org/10.1093/emph/eoaa044

# 2 Cardiovascular observations (I)

The pulse and electrocardiogram (ECG)

- Introduction
- Heart physiology
- Observations of the pulse and apex beat
- The pulse in children
- The electrocardiogram (ECG)
- Heart sounds
- The anti-arrhythmic cardiac drugs
- Key points
- Note
- References

## Introduction

The heart cycle creates two parameters that can be measured: (1) the number of times it beats per minute, the **pulse**; and (2) the pressure of blood leaving the heart, i.e. **blood pressure** (see Chapter 3). These are inseparably linked; the pulse is dependent on blood pressure since it is the pressure of blood exerted against the arterial wall in waves corresponding to heart contractions. The pulse varies with the blood pressure i.e. if the blood pressure falls the pulse rate rises to compensate, because low pressure will deliver inadequate blood to the tissues, and the heart will speed up the delivery.

## Heart physiology

The heart is a muscular pump that is divided vertically by an internal wall, the **septum**, into separate left and right sides (Figure 2.1). Each side has a smaller upper chamber, the **atrium** (plural **atria**) and a larger lower chamber, the **ventricles**. Valves exist between the atria and ventricles, the **atrioventricular** (**AV**) valves, which close to prevent backflow of blood during heart (ventricular) contraction. These are the **bicuspid** (bi = two, cuspid = cusps or flaps) valve on the left and the **tricuspid** (tri = three) valve on the right.

Blood is received into the right atrium from the **venae cavae**, the major veins returning blood from the body to the right side of the heart. On the left side, the atrium receives

DOI: 10.4324/9781003389118-2

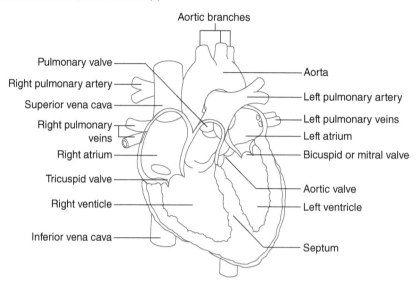

*Figure 2.1* Cross section through the heart (viewed anteriorly).

blood from the **pulmonary veins** returning blood from the lungs. From both the atria, blood passes through the AV valves and fills the ventricles. Contraction of these ventricles pushes blood through **semi-lunar valves**, which prevent backflow to the ventricles: the **aortic valve** on the left and **pulmonary valve** on the right. The **aorta** is the main artery taking blood from the left side of the heart for distribution around the body. The first branches of the aorta are the **coronary arteries**, which supply the heart wall itself with blood. Partial or complete blockage of these arteries deprives the myocardium of blood, leading to **angina** or **myocardial infarction**, both forms of heart attack. The **pulmonary artery** carries blood from the right side of the heart to the lungs for oxygenation. The result is a double circulation i.e. a **systemic** circulation from the left side of the heart to the entire body tissues and back to the right side of the heart, and a **pulmonary** circulation from the right side of the heart to the lungs and back to the left side of the heart (Figure 2.2).

The systemic circulation is much larger, involving all the systems of the body, and it is sustained at a high pressure of blood. The much smaller pulmonary system operates at lower pressures because blood has only to pass from the heart to the lungs and back, entirely within the chest.

The heart wall consists of a muscle layer, the **myocardium**, an inner smooth lining of **epithelium**, called the **endocardium** and an outer membrane, called the **pericardium**. The myocardium has specialised muscle cells that are linked by branches, and this allows them to contract simultaneously, acting as a single unit, known as a **functional syncytium**. Myocardial cells contract during stimulation by nerve impulses that pass through the heart from the **sinoatrial (SA) node**, the pacemaker of the heart (Figure 2.3). The SA node is capable of triggering regular cardiac contractions without outside control (called an *inherent power of rhythmic contraction*). Despite this, the SA node does have external regulation by the **autonomic nervous system (ANS)**, which maintains the heart rate at an average level (about 72 beats per minute). The **sympathetic** component of the ANS increases the heart rate, whereas the **parasympathetic** component (via the **vagus nerve**) decreases the heart rate. They work together to stabilise the heart rate, but

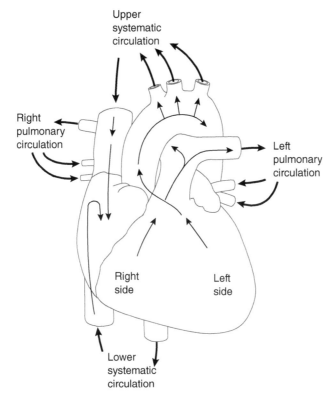

*Figure 2.2* Double circulation of the blood from the heart. The systemic circulation passes from the aorta to the upper and lower parts of the body. The pulmonary circulation passes from the pulmonary arteries to the left and right lungs.

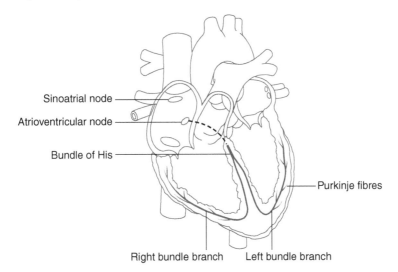

*Figure 2.3* The cardiac conduction system. Impulses arise from the sinoatrial node and pass across the atria to the atrioventricular node. From here, impulses pass down from the bundle of His (also called the atrioventricular bundle) and into the left bundle branch and right bundle branch. The Purkinje fibres are wide terminal branch cells that distribute the impulses to the myocardial cells.

at the same time the presence of both sympathetic and parasympathetic components allows the heart rate to be increased or decreased as the tissue's demand for blood changes. During physical activity, limb muscles in particular force an increase in heart rate to supply more blood, and the sympathetic component will be dominant. At rest, especially during sleep, the parasympathetic component dominates to slow down the heart rate.

The **cardiac cycle** is the sequence of events the heart goes through from one beat to the next. Contraction of the ventricles is **systole**, when blood is pushed out of both sides of the heart, followed by ventricular relaxation, or **diastole**, the ventricular refilling phase. These events are linked to the electrical conduction activity that starts at the SA node and passes through the myocardium. As it crosses the **atria**, they contract and push some blood downwards to top up the ventricles. The impulse arrives at the level of the AV valves, but it does not progress through the muscle any farther downwards beyond this point. At this level, the next node, the **atrioventricular** (**AV**) **node**, is activated. This node picks up the impulse and transmits it down the ventricular septum via conduction tissue called the **bundle of His**, which divides into the left and right **bundle branches**. From the lower end of the septum, the impulse passes via the **Purkinje fibres** at the end of the bundle branches to the ventricular muscle. The impulse passes upwards across the ventricles, causing them to contract (Figure 2.3).

So, the heart beats in two directions; the atria contract first, forcing blood downwards into the ventricles, then the ventricles contract upwards, forcing blood upwards towards the ventricular escape valves (aortic and pulmonary valves). This creates a repeated cycle: down-up . . . down-up . . . down-up . . . Each 'down' (atrial contraction) is followed by an 'up' (ventricular contraction).

Regulation of the heart is maintained by the **cardiac centre**, one of the *vital centres* in a part of the brain called the **medulla** within the **brainstem**. If any injury or disorder were to affect the cardiac centre, the heart would stop beating immediately.

The **cardiac output** (**CO**) is the **heart rate** (**HR**) multiplied by the **stroke volume** (**SV**) (CO = HR × SV), i.e. the volume of blood pumped out of each ventricle in one minute. The stroke volume is the amount of blood pushed out of each ventricle per contraction, which averages about 70 ml. The ventricles contract on average 72 times per minute (the heart rate, HR), so the cardiac output per ventricle is 70 ml multiplied by 72 beats per minute (i.e. 5,040 ml per minute). The cardiac output per ventricle is just over 5,000 ml (5 L) every minute. Considering the total blood volume in circulation is on average about 5,000 ml, it means that each ventricle pushes out the entire blood volume every minute and does this for 70+ years. This makes the heart one of the best pumps ever to have evolved, but it also makes it very difficult to build an artificial replacement heart.

### Observations of the pulse and apex beat

#### The pulse rate and strength

The **pulse** is caused by pressure exerted on the arterial wall causing expansion of the vessel for the brief moment that the wave of pressure passes. The pressure wave is caused by contraction of the ventricles on the left side of the heart forcing blood into the systemic arteries. The artery expands, stretching the muscular wall as the wave of blood from the heart passes by, then contracts back due to the muscular wall returning to its former state. The heart rate, about 72 beats per minute at rest, becomes the average adult pulse rate. *All* arteries demonstrate a pulse, but they are not all accessible for observation. For clinical purposes, the **radial** pulse is mostly used. This is found on the inner aspect of the wrist, on the thumb (= radial) side of a ridge (created by a tendon) that runs almost centrally down the distal end of the inner arm into the wrist. Pulses are normally taken by the observer's middle three fingers, not the thumb, to avoid the observer from feeling their own pulse, which is more prominent in the thumb. Taking the radial pulse is acceptable because it is non-invasive, not embarrassing for the patient (as some pulses may be) and for the most part it is accurate. It only loses accuracy when the blood pressure drops too low, when there are circulatory constrictions placed around the arm (e.g. during blood pressure cuff inflation) or if the arm is too obese to allow palpation of the pulse. Other pulse sites are possible, but they are associated with difficulties and are reserved for specific circumstances (Figure 2.4).

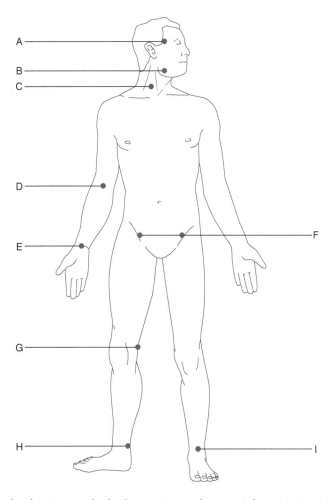

*Figure 2.4* Arterial pulse sites on the body. (A) Temporal. (B) Facial (on jaw). (C) Common carotid. (D) Brachial. (E) Radial (thumb side, the usual pulse for clinical practice). (F) Right and left femoral. (G) Popliteal (behind the knee). (H) Posterior tibial. (I) Dorsalis pedis (see Figure 2.5 for H and I).

The **brachial** pulse occurs along the inner aspect of the upper arm, beneath the brachial muscle, with the pulse being felt against the **humerus** (the upper arm bone) just above the elbow. The **temporal** pulse can be found on each side of the head just anterior to the upper margin of the ear. The **femoral** pulse is about midway across the groin and is used sometimes as a pulse check during cardiac arrest procedures, when embarrassment of the patient is not an issue. The **carotid** pulse lies in the soft tissues on each side of the larynx and is also used in cardiac arrest. Using this pulse on conscious patients, as may sometimes be necessary if the radial pulse is obscure, requires an explanation so that the patient will not be concerned. This pulse must be felt with only gentle pressure, since the carotid artery is part of the blood supply to the brain and must not be obstructed.

The **pedal** (= foot) pulses, mainly the **posterior tibial** and the **dorsalis pedis** (Figure 2.5), are important for assessing the blood supply to the leg and foot, and should be used in any limb vascular disease or during the management of all lower limb injuries and during surgery.

They are also essential after any application of potentially restrictive treatments, such as support bandages or splintage material, especially if limb swelling is still likely (see *capillary refill time*, Chapter 3, page 48). Pedal pulses and the radial pulse are considered to be peripheral pulses, i.e. they are on the extremities of the body. The femoral and carotid pulses are considered to be central pulses (i.e. nearer to – and in direct line with – the heart). In everyday clinical use, peripheral pulses are excellent, but they tend to diminish and even disappear when the cardiac output is low, e.g. in shock and cardiac arrest, and central pulses are then more useful.

The pulse rate is normally elevated during exercise and hard physical labour, and a fast rate is also part of the response to fear and excitement. **Tachycardia** is a fast pulse rate (e.g. 100 beats per minute or more), and **bradycardia** is a slow rate, usually below 50 beats per minute. During tachycardia, because more beats are packed into 60 seconds, each beat has to be shorter. This is achieved by shortening the filling phase of the heart (the **diastole**; see Chapter 3). The normal *maximum* heart rate is about 180 beats per minute, i.e. the maximum above which normal filling of the heart cannot take place. At this rate, the entire cardiac cycle lasts just 0.33 seconds. To achieve adequate ventricular filling during diastole requires a minimum diastolic phase of about 0.12

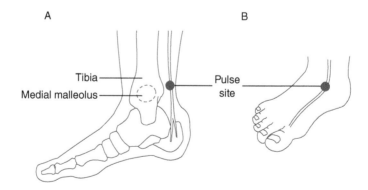

*Figure 2.5* Pedal (foot) pulses. (A) Post-tibial artery (immediately behind the medial malleolus on the tibia). (B) Dorsalis pedis (on the top of the foot midway between the lateral and medial malleolli).

*Table 2.1* The differences in the systolic and diastolic phases at heart rates of 67 and 180 beats per minute (bpm)

|  | Heart rate 67 bpm | Heart rate 180 bpm |
|---|---|---|
| Systole | 0.35 seconds | 0.2 seconds |
| Diastole | 0.58 seconds | 0.13 seconds |

seconds. The heart rate of 180 beats per second reduces the diastolic phase close to this minimum (Table 2.1). Heart rates in excess of 180 beats per minute would reduce this diastolic phase even further, bringing it below this minimum filling requirement. The cardiac output would then be reduced and the heart would be functioning below optimum efficiency (Table 2.1).

Tachycardia is a feature of systemic infections, especially associated with fever, and it is a compensatory mechanism for improving the tissue blood supply when a patient is in shock. It also occurs as a feature of fear and panic as well as excitement. Bradycardia can occur during **heart block** i.e. when the impulse from the SA node does not always reach the ventricles, and the ventricular contraction rate slows down.

The strength of the pulse is dependent on two factors: (1) the force applied to the blood by the left ventricle during contraction and (2) the stroke volume. The force of contraction can vary normally and in diseases such as **left heart failure** (**LVF**), where the myocardium is unable to achieve a full stroke volume (Gordon and Child 2000a, 2000b). Excess blood may be retained inside the heart at the end of each systolic phase. This can result in a reduced output to the arteries (known as the **forward problem**) and a backlog of blood unable to enter the ventricles because they are partly filled already and can only accept a limited blood volume from the veins (known as the **backward problem**). The stroke volume will decline in **hypovolaemic shock** (hypo = below normal, vol = volume, aemic = blood), where the blood volume in circulation is less than normal as a result of bleeding or burns. A weak, rapid pulse is characteristic of shock: weak due to a low stroke volume and rapid because the heart tries to compensate by pumping faster, which is part of the sympathetic response. **Thyrotoxicosis** (raised blood levels of the hormone **thyroxin** from the thyroid gland) and heart block can increase the force of contraction. **Palpitations** are heartbeats felt by the patient on the chest wall. They may be associated with arrhythmias but are often normal, being caused by extreme exercise or occasional extra beats (see page 33).

### Apex beat

The radial pulse rate taken at the wrist is a record of the number of times the left ventricle contracts per minute. Another way to measure this would be to listen through the chest wall, via a stethoscope, to the heart itself, counting the heart sounds per minute. It is important to listen to the ventricle (usually the left) at the outermost and lowest point of the heart (the apex of the heart); this is known as the **apex beat**. The radial pulse and the apex beat sounds should be equal in number, but sometimes the ventricular contraction is so weak (i.e. low cardiac output) that the force is insufficient to create a pulse at the wrist (see peripheral pulses, page 28). The difference between the radial and apex beats can be measured by two nurses working together. One takes the radial pulse in the usual way while the other listens to the apex beat. This is found by placing the diaphragm of a stethoscope over the space between the left fifth and sixth ribs close to the **midclavicular line**, an imaginary line drawn down the chest from a point midway along the left clavicle. Using the same watch and counting over the same 60 seconds, both the radial and the apex beats are recorded. Any deficit may show an apex beat higher than the radial beat, and subtracting the radial from the apex, the deficit can be calculated. As an example, an apex beat of 84 and a radial pulse of 74 indicates a difference of 10 beats (i.e. the ventricles have had 10 contractions during that minute that were not strong enough to create a radial pulse). Sometimes the radial count is recorded as higher than the apex beat, but this is not possible since the radial pulse depends on ventricular contractions. Such a result is clearly an error and the observation should be repeated.

### The pulse in children

The cardiovascular system in children must cope with its own growth while catering for increased demands on it as a result of growth in all other parts of the body. In children, the heart rate falls gradually from approximately 100–160 beats per minute at less than one month old to 60–90 beats per minute at more than 12 years of age (Table 2.2).

Breathing causes more pronounced changes in the heart rate in children than in adults, a difference of up to 30 beats per minute, slowing down during inspiration and accelerating during expiration.

It may be recommended in some paediatric units for the nurse to use the brachial or temporal pulse with the younger child, as this may be easier to find in a less than cooperative child and will therefore be more accurate. For the older child, when cooperation by the child is achieved, the radial pulse can be used. Using the carotid pulse in children is not justified since it carries specific risks regarding the blood supply to the brain and should not therefore normally be used in children of any age.

Rapid heart rates can be caused by heart failure, a complication of **congenital heart defects**. These are distortions of the heart anatomy that the child is born with. **Atrial** or **ventricular septal defects** (**ASDs** or **VSDs**), known as the *hole in the heart*, abnormally allow blood to pass from one side of the heart to the other. If blood passes from the right ventricle to the left ventricle through a VSD, deoxygenated blood (i.e. lacking oxygen) fails to go to the lungs for oxygenation from the right ventricle and is pumped by the left ventricle back to the body again. Efforts by the heart to improve the oxygen supply to the body result in an increase in the cardiac output, usually by a rise in the heart rate. Ultimately, if this is not corrected, the heart can enlarge and fail.

*Table 2.2* Heart rate in children of different ages when awake and asleep

| Age | Heart rate (awake) | Heart rate (sleeping) |
| --- | --- | --- |
| <1 month | 100–160 | 90–160 |
| 1 month–1 year | 100–150 | 90–160 |
| 1–2 years | 70–110 | 80–120 |
| 3–5 years | 65–110 | 65–100 |
| 6–11 years | 60–95 | 58–90 |
| 12–15 years | 60–90 | 50–90 |

### The electrocardiogram (ECG)

Willem Einthoven (1860–1927), a Dutch physiologist, was awarded the 1924 Nobel Prize in Physiology or Medicine for pioneering electrocardiography. In 1909, Augustus Waller demonstrated to the Royal Society in London the recording of an **electrocardiogram** (**ECG**) from a pet dog called Jimmie (Levick 2010). This procedure is an important, fast, accurate, non-invasive means of diagnosis of cardiac disease that can be carried out almost anywhere. The ECG records the electrical activity of the heart muscle as it occurs at skin level having passed through the extracellular tissue fluid between the heart and the body surface. Electrical activity (called **depolarisation**) at the SA and AV nodes is too small to create recordable changes at the skin surface, but the electrical activity within the larger myocardial muscle bulk can be recorded throughout repeated heart cycles. The tracing represents different views of the heart, similar to seeing different aspects of the same object when viewed from varying angles. The leads attached to the patient provide these different views of the heart (Figure 2.6).

The recording is a measure of the electrical difference between one electrode and another (i.e. bipolar = two electrodes are used) in leads **I**, **II**, **III** (Figures 2.6 and 2.7). This is between the fixed points of the right arm (**RA**), left arm (**LA**) and the left leg (**LL**). The fixed points (RA, LA and LL) form the **Einthoven triangle** (Figure 2.7). Lead I views the heart from RA to LA, lead II views the heart from RA to LL and lead III views the heart form LA to LL (Figure 2.6 and 2.7). The **aVR**, **aVL** and **aVF** are unipolar (one pole) leads measuring the electrical difference between a single fixed point (either RA, LA or LL) and the point at the centre of the triangle, as follows:

- aVR measures the difference between RA and the average of LA + LL
- aVL measures the difference between LA and the average of RA + LL
- aVF measures the difference between LL and the average of RA + LA.

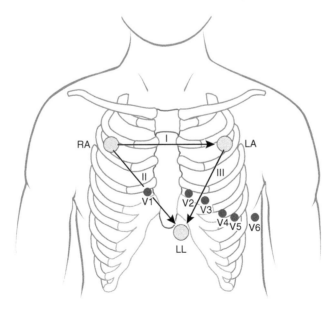

*Figure 2.6* ECG lead positions I, II, III (forming the Einthoven triangle) and sites for leads V1 to V6 across the chest.

In each case the centre of the triangle represents the average of the other two points (Hampton and Hampton 2019) (Figure 2.7).

The **V** leads (**V1** to **V6**) use a free-moving electrode placed at specific sites on the chest wall (Figure 2.6) that measure the electrical activity at each site (i.e. unipolar = one roving lead).

The main direction of electrical flow through the heart, called the **electrical axis**, runs down the heart from the SA node to the ventricles (Figure 2.8). This varies in position between the direction of leads I and aVF in different individuals. The chest leads are therefore snapshots of this axis seen differently from these various views.

The baseline of the tracing is **isoelectric** (i.e. zero voltage). Any deflection above this line indicates a view looking in the direction of the axis (i.e. positive, +), and a deflection below the baseline indicates a view that is more than 90° away from the axis (i.e.

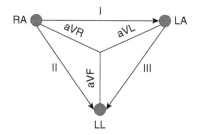

*Figure 2.7* The Einthoven triangle showing leads I, II and III, aVR, aVL and aVF.

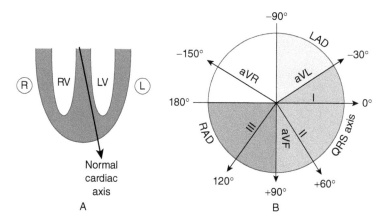

*Figure 2.8* The cardiac axis. A shows the general direction of the normal electrical impulses as they flow through the heart, called the cardiac axis. It lines up approximately with +60 degrees on the diagram in B. B shows the normal QRS axis as the widely shaded area between leads aVF and aVL. The normal axis falls somewhere in this area, but usually aligns closely with +60 degrees. B also shows the areas of left axis deviation (LAD) and right axis deviation (RAD). If the cardiac axis falls within either of these areas, it may sometimes be due to a cardiac pathology. If you line up diagram B with Figure 2.7 and then with Figure 2.6, the point in the centre is the same point on the chest. Leads I, II and III in Figure 2.7 and in B are pointing in the same directions, indicating that the leads are showing the direction in which each lead is viewing the heart.

negative, −). The normal pattern of activity is called **sinus rhythm**. Abnormalities of the tracing can be detected and identified as specific heart disorders (Figure 2.9). Atrial depolarisation (normally accompanied by atrial contraction) is recorded on the ECG as the **P wave**, followed by the **PQ interval**, an isoelectric event as the impulse passes down the bundle of His. The **QRS complex** is the depolarisation event of the ventricles (ventricular contraction, or systole), followed by ventricular repolarisation, identified as the **T wave** (ventricular relaxation). From the start of the P wave through to the start of the next P wave is a full **cardiac cycle**. It consists of a **systole** (the QRS complex or ventricular contraction) while all the rest of the cycle (including the P and T waves) are **diastole** (the filling phase of the heart).

**Arrhythmias** are deviations of the ECG pattern seen in various cardiac disorders and are used to aid the diagnosis (Haissaguerre *et al.* 2016). **Supraventricular tachycardia** (**SVT**) is the term used to describe an abnormally fast heart rate, typically over 100 beats per minute and often much faster, caused by an abnormality with the SA node or conduction across the atria (i.e. above the ventricles). It can occur in episodes for no apparent

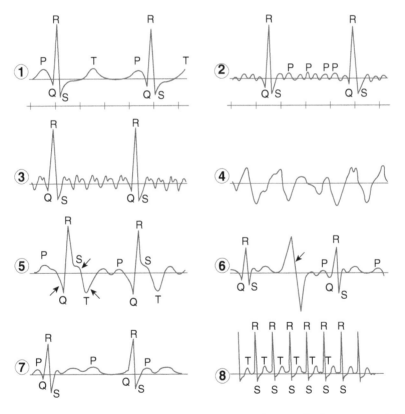

*Figure 2.9* Normal and abnormal ECG tracings. (1) Normal sinus rhythm. (2) Atrial fibrillation with multiple P waves between the QRS complexes. (3) Atrial flutter with the sawtooth appearance between the QRS complex. (4) Ventricular fibrillation, causes no cardiac output and requires urgent resuscitation. (5) Myocardial infarction with large Q waves, ST elevation and inverted T waves. (6) Ventricular extrasystole (ectopic beat, arrowed). (7) Heart block with P waves occurring at any point. (8) Supraventricular tachycardia with closer packed QRS complexes.

reason, followed by a return to a normal heart rate. The term includes **atrial fibrillation**, **atrial flutter** and **paroxysmal supraventricular tachycardia** (Figure 2.9). It also occurs in **Wolff-Parkinson-White syndrome**, a congenital problem with the heart's conduction system.

The major arrhythmias are (Figure 2.9):

- **Ventricular extra systoles** (also called **ectopic beats**) are extra systoles sometimes generated within the damaged ventricular myocardium after a myocardial infarction. These extra beats can occur anywhere with the ECG pattern and usually appear larger than the normal tracing.
- **Paroxysmal supraventricular tachycardia** (**PSVT**) is a period of heart rate often greater than 150 beats per minute and possibly as fast as 240 beats per minute. The ECG shows multiple narrow QRS complexes packed close together (see fast pulse rates, page 29) and the P wave is not seen.
- **Atrial fibrillation** occurs when instead of fully contracting, the atrial wall is only flickering in an irregular manner. This is caused by random chaotic firing of impulses from anywhere within the atrium. These flickering mini-contractions record as multiple small P waves on the ECG.
- **Atrial flutter** occurs when there is a fast atrial contraction rate, often faster than the ventricular contraction rate, so there may be, for example, three or four atrial contractions for every one ventricular contraction. It differs from atrial fibrillation by being normal regular full contractions, albeit at a faster than expected rate. It shows on the ECG as a characteristic regular 'sawtooth' pattern of contractions throughout the diastolic phase.
- **Ventricular fibrillation** is the one type of **cardiac arrest** where the ventricles are not contracting fully but are simply quivering. There is no substantial cardiac output, hence cardiac arrest. It requires defibrillation as part of resuscitation. On the ECG, a chaotic and irregular tracing is seen, with no distinct QRS complexes.
- **Heart block** occurs when there is a loss of synchronicity between the atrial contractions and ventricular contracts. This is because the impulse from the SA node is blocked from descending the bundle of His, and the ventricles are no longer responding to the SA node. The atria do respond to the SA node, but the ventricles contract in their own independent rhythm, which is generally too slow, causing a bradycardia. On the ECG, because the atria and ventricles are beating independently, the ventricles show a slow rate (with long diastole) and P waves that can occur anywhere on the tracing.
- **Myocardial infarction** (**MI**) is an area of dead tissue within the myocardium of the heart due to absence of coronary artery blood supply to that part of the heart. The term **infarction**, or **infarct**, is an area of dead tissue anywhere due to absence of blood supply. In the case of MI, this dead area cannot contract (and therefore cannot assist to pump blood) and it cannot conduct the electrical impulses. An MI area can be any size from tiny (which may not even be noticed) to large, life-threatening areas. Changes on the ECG due to MI are large Q waves, ST elevation (i.e. the section between S and T is raised above the isoelectric baseline) and inverted T waves (i.e. T waves dip below the isoelectric baseline).
- **Asystole** is the absence of a systole, which means no pumping phase of the heart, and therefore no cardiac output. This is another type of **cardiac arrest** and requires immediate resuscitation. On the ECG, this is seen as a dead flat isoelectric baseline, with no – or very little – evidence of cardiac activity.

*The ECG in childhood*

Children normally show variations in the ECG from that seen in adults. The Q wave amplitude may increase from birth up to a maximum between 3 and 5 years of age, reducing thereafter to a point close to the amplitude seen at birth. The QRS axis (Figure 2.8, page 32) in the neonate averages about 75 degrees, but over the first year this changes to around 65–70 degrees. There are also changes in the R and S waves. Chest leads placed on the right side show the R wave amplitudes reducing with age but increasing on the left side. The S wave shows a similar gradual change but the wave is inverted. Positive (upright) T wave deflections in leads V1 and V3R (i.e. a lead placed in the V3 position but on the right side of the chest) seen in the first few days of life will normally invert to negative values by day 7. Persistence of a positive T wave after 7 days of life should be viewed with suspicion of abnormality. In leads V2 and V3, the T waves usually begin inverted and slowly progress with age to an upright position. In leads V5 and V6, the T wave is upright at any age (Dickinson 2005).

Holter monitoring is an ECG recording device worn beneath the child's clothing over a 24-hour period. It records any arrhythmias that may occur and these can be matched to symptoms that may arise within the same time span (Shiels and Brugha 2020).

## Heart sounds

**Auscultation** (listening through a **stethoscope**) is used to identify abnormal heart sounds, and their identification is important. The closure (*not* opening) of the heart valves causes normal heart sounds as the valve cusps vibrate. Several heart sounds are recognised: the first (said to sound similar to 'lubb . . .') is the closure of the AV valves (tri- and bicuspid valves), and the second (said to sound similar to 'dubb . . .') is the closure of the semi-lunar valves (aortic and pulmonary). The complete cardiac cycle gives the sounds 'lubb . . dubb . . .' followed by a short gap, before being repeated. If the aortic valve closes just before the pulmonary valve, the second sound can be split into two sounds, as is common in healthy young people during inspiration. Breathing in causes increased filling of the right ventricle, and therefore a raised right ventricular stroke volume. This takes longer to eject during systole and the pulmonary valve closure is delayed. A third sound caused by the entry of blood into the relaxed ventricles at the start of diastole is also common in young people. A fourth sound is audible just before the first and is due to the atrial systole.

Valvular disorders create turbulence in the blood flow through the valve, and this disturbed flow causes extra sounds known as **murmurs**. **Stenosis** is a narrowing of the valve openings because the flaps will not part sufficiently to allow all the blood through. This occurs in diseases such as **endocarditis** (inflammation of the inner lining of the heart, the **endocardium**) because the valve flaps are made from extensions of the endocardium. Endocarditis causes growths to occur on the valve flaps, which impede their function. **Incompetence** occurs when a valve will not close properly and it allows backflow of blood (i.e. the valve is *leaky*). Since there are four valves and each is capable of either stenosis or incompetence, a total of eight disorders are possible, resulting in eight murmurs within the heart. But not all murmurs are due to disease. In young people, sometimes during pregnancy or in strenuous exercise, a **benign murmur** can occasionally be heard due to turbulence of the blood leaving the heart, and this is not a problem.

## The anti-arrhythmic cardiac drugs

Various cardiac drugs affect the pulse rate, blood pressure and conductivity of the heart. **Antiarrhythmic drugs** may be grouped into several classes according to function:

Class I: Sodium channel blocking drugs (Table 2.3; Figure 2.10)
Class II: Beta-receptor blocking drugs (Table 2.4)
Class III: Potassium channel blocking drugs (Table 2.5)
Class IV: Calcium-channel blockers (Table 2.6).

*Class I: Sodium channel blocking drugs (Table 2.3; Figure 2.10)*

Class I drugs are subdivided into IA, IB, IC and others. Amongst these is **Lignocaine (lidocaine) hydrochloride**, a class IB drug that suppresses the incidence and intensity of cardiac arrhythmias (Figure 2.10). This is important because both the incidence and intensity of arrhythmias can escalate into potentially fatal consequences, notably cardiac arrest. Lignocaine also lowers the sensitivity of the myocardium to electrical impulses within the

*Table 2.3* Class I: Sodium channel blocking and other anti-arrhythmic drugs

| Drug | Possible side effects | Use and other notes |
|---|---|---|
| **Class IA** | | |
| Disopyramide | Abdominal pain, reduced appetite, bowel disturbance, dizziness and nausea. | Ventricular/supraventricular arrhythmias. |
| **Class IB** | | |
| Lidocaine hydrochloride (Lignocaine hydrochloride) | Anxiety, confusion, drowsiness, euphoria, headache and hypotension (Chapter 3). | Ventricular arrhythmias, given by intravenous (IV) injection (child or adult) or infusion. Not licensed for use in children younger than 1 year. |
| Mexiletine | Angina pain, ataxia, dizziness, drowsiness, headache, bowel discomfort, constipation, hypotension (Chapter 3). | Serious ventricular arrhythmias. For use by specialist only in hospital. |
| **Class IC** | | |
| Flecainide acetate | Arrhythmias, dizziness, fever, oedema, visual disturbance, dyspnoea. | Supraventricular and ventricular arrhythmias. Used by direction of consultant. Not licensed for children under 12 years, |
| Propafenone hydrochloride | Anxiety, arrhythmias, nausea, vomiting, blurred vision, sleep disturbance, palpitations, bowel disturbance, chest pain. | Ventricular arrhythmias and supraventricular tachyarrhythmias. Used by specialists in hospitals. |
| **Others** | | |
| Adenosine | Abdominal and chest discomfort, dizziness, headache, hypotension (Chapter 3), dry mouth. | Paroxysmal supraventricular tachycardia. Given by intravenous (IV) injection. Some restrictions in use for children. |
| Vernakalant | Cough, dizziness, headache, nausea, vomiting, skin reaction. | Conversion of atrial fibrillation to sinus rhythm under specialist control. |

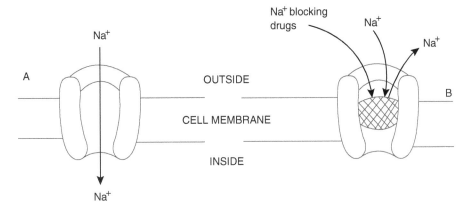

*Figure 2.10* Antiarrhythmic Class I sodium channel drugs. A. Sodium (Na⁺) enters the neuron during the first part (depolarisation) of an action potential (Chapter 11, Figure 11.10). B. Sodium channel blocking drugs prevent sodium entry down the channel. This reduces the action potentials, slowing the rate of conduction through the heart.

*Table 2.4* Class II: Beta-receptor blocking drugs

| Drugs | Possible side effects | Use and other notes |
|---|---|---|
| Esmolol hydrochloride | Anxiety, reduced appetite, drowsiness, poor concentration. | Short-term treatment of supraventricular arrhythmias, atrial fibrillation and flutter and tachycardia. |
| Sotalol hydrochloride | Anxiety, chest pain, fever, mood changes, muscle spasms and palpitations. | Ventricular tachycardia, prevention of paroxysmal atrial tachycardia or fibrillation. Not licensed for use in children under 12 years. |

conduction system, which makes it useful to slow the heart, and therefore important in treating ventricular tachycardia.

*Class II: Beta receptor blocking drugs (Table 2.4; Figure 2.11)*

**Beta-blocking drugs** block the **beta-adrenergic receptors**[1] that are normally acted upon by the sympathetic nervous system, reducing the sympathetic stimulation of the heart and therefore slowing the heart rate (Chapter 3, Figure 3.10). These drugs are used to treat **angina** (i.e. chest pain caused by restricted blood flow down the coronary arteries as a result of arterial disease). By slowing the heart rate, the myocardium needs less blood, and this puts less demand on the coronary artery supply, reducing the chest pain.

*Class III: Potassium channel blocking drugs (Table 2.5; Figure 2.11)*

Although Amiodarone is classed as a potassium channel blocker, it also contributes by blocking the other channels (sodium and calcium) and is therefore a valued anti-arrhythmic drug.

*Table 2.5* Class III: Potassium channel blockers

| Drug | Possible side effects | Use and other notes |
|---|---|---|
| Amiodarone hydrochloride | Liver problems, nausea, skin reactions, hyperthyroidism. | Arrhythmias where other drugs are unsuitable. Used under specialist control. Not licensed for children under 3 years. |
| Dronedarone | Slow pulse, bowel discomfort and diarrhoea, nausea and vomiting, skin reactions. | Maintain sinus rhythm after atrial fibrillation treatment. Used under specialist control. |

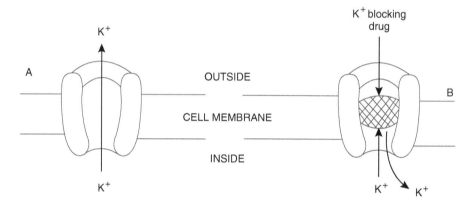

*Figure 2.11* Antiarrhythmic Class III potassium channel blocking drugs. A. Potassium (K+) channels allow outflow of potassium following the inward flow of sodium (Figure 2.10) during the second part (repolarisation) of an action potential (Chapter 11, Figure 11.10). B. Potassium blocking drugs stop the flow of potassium through the channel, prolonging action potentials and slowing the heart rate.

*Table 2.6* Class IV: Calcium channel blockers

| Drug | Possible side effects and interactions | Use and other notes |
|---|---|---|
| Verapamil hydrochloride | Hypotension (Chapter 3) and bradycardia with IV use. *Serious interaction with beta-blockers.* | Supraventricular arrhythmias by oral or slow intravenous (IV) infusion, angina and hypertension (Table 3.10). |

*Class IV: Calcium channel blocking drugs (Table 2.6)*

Verapamil is a **calcium-channel blocker**, preventing the entry of calcium into muscle cells and thus reducing heart contractility. It relaxes the muscle in blood vessel walls so they can expand and hold more blood, which means the heart has less blood volume to cope with at any given moment.

*Positive inotropic drugs (cardiac glycosides)*

**Digoxin** (Figure 2.12), increases the force of contraction and slows the heart rate and is therefore used in **heart failure**. It is also useful in the management of atrial flutter and atrial fibrillation. Care must be taken not to allow the pulse rate to drop persistently below 60 beats per minute. Bradycardia is a sign of **digoxin toxicity**, and nurses should check the patients pulse rate before administration of this drug. In addition, patients taking this drug, especially the elderly, should be observed for confusion, nausea and **coupled beats**, i.e. two pulse beats together followed by a pause before the cycle begins again.

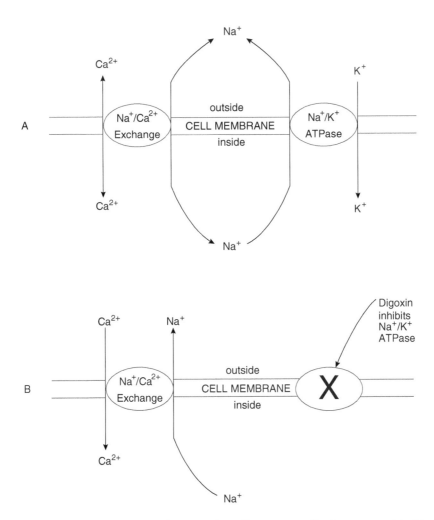

*Figure 2.12* Action of digoxin in cardiac muscle cells. A. Normally the enzyme Na⁺/K⁺ ATPase moves sodium ($Na^+$) out of the cell, and potassium ($K^+$) into the cell. Sodium is involved in the Na⁺/Ca²⁺ exchange. B. Digoxin blocks the Na⁺/K⁺ ATPase causing a rise in intracellular sodium, so the Na⁺/Ca²⁺ exchange pumps more calcium into the cell. This slows the heart rate, increases the force of contraction and increases ventricular filling.

*Table 2.7* Red flag warnings of deteriorating condition

**♆ Red Flag = serious situation which needs urgent medical attention.**

| Flag warning | Details |
|---|---|
| **♆ Red Flag** | **Anyone with central chest pain and sweating.**<br>**Anyone with palpitations, a rapid or slow pulse or an irregular pulse, especially if they have a family history of cardiac arrest or are taking cardiac drugs.** |

(After Hill-Smith and Johnson 2021, with permission)

*Anti-arrhythmic drugs in children*

Selected drugs are available for use in children, notably lidocaine hydrochloride, flecainide acetate, amiodarone hydrochloride, adenosine, sotalol hydrochloride and digoxin. They have restrictions in dosage and route of administration and various restrictions related to the child's age and must therefore be used only under specialist supervision.

**Key points**

*Cardiac physiology*

• The heart wall has a muscular myocardium, an inner endocardium and an outer pericardium.
• The sinoatrial (SA) node can trigger cardiac contractions with external regulation by the sympathetic nervous system (increases the heart rate) and the parasympathetic nervous system (the vagus nerve, decreases the heart rate).
• The cardiac cycle consists of systole (ventricular contraction) followed by diastole (ventricular relaxation).
• Electrical conduction starts at the SA node and passes through the atrial myocardium, which contracts. The AV node picks up the impulse and transmits it down the ventricular septum via the bundle of His, and then to the left and right bundle branches and on to the Purkinje fibres in the ventricular muscle, which then contracts.

*Pulse*

• For clinical purposes, the radial pulse is mostly used.
• The normal adult pulse rate is 65–72 beats per minute.
• Tachycardia is a fast pulse rate and bradycardia is a slow rate.
• The apex beat is found on the left outermost and lowest point of the heart: the space between the left fifth and sixth ribs close to the midclavicular line.
• A weak rapid pulse is characteristic of shock.
• The heart rate falls in children from 110–160 beats per minute below 1 year of age to 60–100 beats per minute over 12 years old.
• The brachial or temporal pulse should normally be used for younger children and the radial pulse should be used for older children; the carotid pulse should not be used in children.

*Electrocardiogram (ECG)*

- The ECG P wave occurs with depolarisation of the atria (atrial contraction), followed by the PQ interval as the impulse disappears down the bundle of His; the QRS complex is depolarisation of the ventricles (ventricular contraction, or systole) followed by ventricular repolarisation, the T wave (ventricular relaxation).
- Sinus rhythm is a normal ECG pattern; arrhythmias are abnormal deviations from the ECG pattern.

*Pathologies*

- A cause of cardiogenic shock is myocardial infarction (MI); an area of dead or dying myocardium (the infarct) results from occlusion of the coronary arteries.
- Valvular disorders create turbulence in the blood flow through the valve causing extra sounds (murmurs), e.g. stenosis, a narrowing of the valve opening or incompetence, when a valve will not close properly.

*Drugs*

- Bradycardia, confusion, nausea and coupled beats are signs of digoxin toxicity, and nurses should check that the patient's pulse is not below 60 beats per minute before administration of this drug.

## Note

1 Beta-adrenergic receptors normally bind to the neurotransmitter adrenaline, stimulating and increasing the sympathetic activity on the heart. Beta-blocking drugs reduce this cardiac stimulation.

## References

Dickinson D.F. (2005) The normal ECG in childhood and adolescence. *Heart*, *91*(12): 1626–1630.

Gordon K. and Child A. (2000a) Systems and diseases: The heart, part 9: Heart failure 1. *Nursing Times*, *96*(12): 53–56.

Gordon K. and Child A. (2000b) Systems and diseases: The heart, part 10: Heart failure 2. *Nursing Times*, *96*(16): 49–52.

Haissaguerre M., Vigmond E., Stuyvers B., Hocini M. and Bernus O. (2016) Ventricular arrhythmias and the His – Purkinje system. *Nature Reviews Cardiology*, *13*: 155–166. http://doi.org/10.1038/nrcardio.2015.193

Hampton J. and Hampton J. (2019) *The ECG Made Easy* (9th edition). Elsevier, Edinburgh, London, New York.

Hill-Smith I. and Johnson G. (2021) *Little Book of Red Flags*. National Minor Illness Centre, Bedfordshire.

Levick J.R. (2010) *An Introduction to Cardiovascular Physiology* (5th edition). Oxford University Press, New York.

Shiels K. and Brugha R. (2020) *Paediatric Clinical Examination* (2nd edition). Jaypee Brothers Medical Publishers, New Delhi, India.

# 3 Cardiovascular observations (II)

## Blood pressure

### Introduction

The fact that the brain is placed higher than the heart requires the heart to sustain sufficient pressure of blood to supply the brain *uphill, against* gravity. Failure to do this would starve the brain of the vital glucose and oxygen needed for consciousness and mental function. Blood pressure is fundamental to the perfusion of blood through *all* the body tissues. The kidneys must have adequate blood pressure to maintain filtration of urine, the lungs need a constant flow of blood for gas exchange and so on. Movement of blood requires pressure, and understanding blood pressure is essential for the accurate determination of physiological processes and disturbances.

### Physiology of blood pressure

The systemic arterial **blood pressure** (**BP**) is caused *partly* by the contraction of the left ventricle. During **systole** (= ventricular contraction), the left ventricular myocardium pushes the **stroke volume** (**SV**) of blood into the aorta, and this surge of blood causes the aorta to stretch wider. The stroke volume, i.e. the amount of blood ejected with each ventricular contraction, is about 70 ml of blood per ventricle. The wave of high pressure generated continues through the arterial system, causing the **systolic pressure** (**SP**), having an average peak of 100–120 mmHg (millimetres of mercury) in the major systemic arteries in adults. This pressure falls as blood is distributed through the remaining arterial

DOI: 10.4324/9781003389118-3

system and capillary bed, reaching its lowest at close to 0 mmHg in the venous return to the heart (Figure 3.1).

During **diastole**, the period between two systoles, the left ventricle is relaxing and filling with blood. There is no output to the aorta, and this creates a lower pressure in the systemic arteries, i.e. a **diastolic pressure** (**DP**) of about 60–80 mmHg. The human adult BP in the major systemic arteries is therefore recorded as 120 mmHg over 80 mmHg (i.e. alternating between the systolic and diastolic pressures). But if the left ventricle has no output during diastole, the diastolic pressure should *theoretically* fall to zero. Zero pressure would mean that blood flow has stopped. Without a blood supply, the brain becomes unconscious (i.e. fainting). The heart goes through about 72 systoles and diastoles per minute, so with a *theoretical* systemic blood pressure of 120 over 0 mmHg, the person would faint 72 times per minute! Clearly, this is not the case; therefore, diastolic pressure must be maintained sufficiently high to supply the brain during this period of zero cardiac output. The surge of blood (the stroke volume) leaving the left side of the heart during systole causes the aorta to stretch wider to accommodate this blood. What stretches during systole must recoil during diastole, and it is this aortic recoil that continues to push blood onward to the tissues during diastole, while the heart relaxes and refills (Figure 3.2). The aorta is effectively a *diastolic pump*, keeping the pressure up during this time. The same occurs with the pulmonary artery from the right side of the heart, where pulmonary recoil continues to push blood through the lungs during right ventricular diastole. Since the pulmonary circulation is entirely contained within the chest cavity, the pressures within this circulation, i.e. normally about 25 mmHg systolic over 12 mmHg diastolic, are not available for standard clinical observation. They are measured only during specialised cardiac procedures.

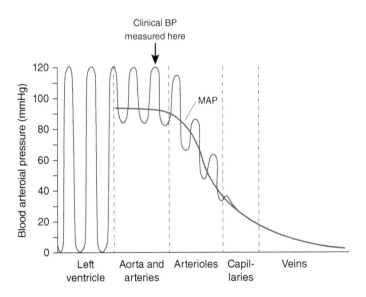

*Figure 3.1* Blood pressure values through the circulatory system. The left ventricle drops to 0 mmHg during diastole while the arterial diastolic pressure is maintained at about 80 mmHg in the arteries. Through the arterioles, the mean arterial pressure (MAP) and both the systolic and the diastolic pressures drop with closure of the pulse pressure, i.e. a loss of the pulsatile nature of the flow by the capillaries. Venous return drops to near zero pressure.

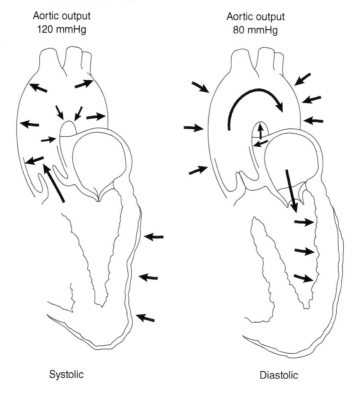

Aortic output
120 mmHg

Aortic output
80 mmHg

Systolic

Diastolic

*Figure 3.2* The left ventricle and the aorta during the cardiac cycle. The short arrows indicate the direction of wall movement; the long arrows show the direction of blood flow. During systole, ventricular contraction occurs, causing a high blood pressure resulting in aortic expansion. The aortic valve is open and the bicuspid valve is closed. In diastole, the events are reversed, with the aortic recoil preventing the blood pressure from falling too low.

At the start of the section *Physiology of blood pressure*, the word *partly* was used because the contraction of the left ventricle is not the entire story. Any pressure of a fluid in a tube is dependent on events taking place at *both* ends of that tube i.e. the volume and force of the fluid entering the tube at one end (e.g. the cardiac output) and resistance to the flow of that fluid at the other end (e.g. the **peripheral resistance** or **PR**). In a garden hose example, the output from the tap is the equivalent to the cardiac output. The flow from the hose at the open end is sufficient to reach the nearby plants, but those at the back may need a higher pressure of water to reach them. This can be achieved by placing a thumb over the end to narrow the opening, and therefore increase the water pressure inside the hose. Water leaving the narrower opening does so at a higher pressure and therefore travels farther. In this garden hose example, the thumb acts as a *peripheral resistance*. In the body the arterial peripheral resistance is achieved first by the reduction in size of the **arterioles** into a network of smaller vessels, and then by the **vasoconstriction** or **vasodilatation** that these smaller arterioles can achieve. In vasodilatation, the arteriole lumen widens and the peripheral resistance is decreased, allowing the blood pressure to fall. In vasoconstriction, the arteriole lumen narrows and the peripheral resistance is increased, forcing the blood pressure up. Involuntary

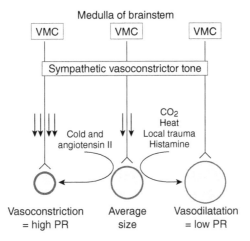

*Figure 3.3* The vasomotor centre (VMC) and the local factors influencing the peripheral resistance (PR). Vasoconstriction is achieved by increasing the vasoconstrictor tone output from the VMC to the arterioles or by the local action of cold or angiotensin II, causing the lumen to narrow and raising the PR. Vasodilatation is achieved by decreasing the sympathetic vasoconstrictor tone from the VMC or by the local action of heat, trauma, carbon dioxide or histamine, causing the lumen to widen and lowering of the PR. The number of arrows represents the strength of sympathetic stimulation.

smooth muscle in the arteriole wall makes the changes to the lumen in response to the **sympathetic nervous system**. This system is influenced by the **vasomotor centre** (**VMC**), a series of diffuse nuclei in the medulla, part of the brain stem, that has a profound effect on blood pressure (Figure 3.3).

The VMC can initiate variations in the peripheral resistance by adjusting the **sympathetic vasoconstrictor tone**,[1] the state of constriction of the smooth muscle wall affecting the lumen of the arterioles. Changes are made in this tone in response to fluctuations in the blood pressure, thereby keeping the BP within normal limits for that individual. To do this, the VMC must have feedback on what the pressure is, and this is achieved via **baroreceptors**, pressure-sensitive receptors found in the aortic arch and carotid arteries that directly measure the arterial BP and send this information to the VMC (Figure 3.4).

When the BP is high, increased baroreceptor activity reduces VMC output (i.e. VMC **inhibition**), causing vasodilatation of the arterioles to lower the pressure. When the BP is low, decreased baroreceptor activity causes increased VMC output, which constricts the arterioles to raise the pressure. The VMC also responds to other factors and adjusts the BP accordingly. A lack of oxygen, an increase in carbon dioxide, mild pain, stress and increased **chemoreceptor** activity all cause more VMC activity and therefore vasoconstriction, raising the BP. Low carbon dioxide, severe pain and emotional shock all cause less VMC activity and therefore vasodilatation, lowering the BP (Figure 3.5).

Chemoreceptors detect levels of carbon dioxide in the blood and feed this information back to the brain for blood pressure and respiratory purposes. A sudden drop in the blood pressure is a common cause of fainting after a sudden emotional shock, such as bad news. Normal BP is maintained by average vasoconstrictor tone stimulation from

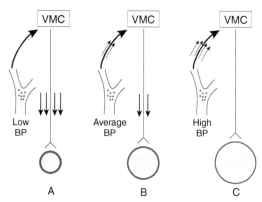

*Figure 3.4* The effect of the baroreceptors on the VMC. (A) In low blood pressure situations, a lack of baroreceptor stimulation allows the VMC to cause vasoconstriction and this raises the blood pressure. (B) Average baroreceptor stimulation allows for normal peripheral resistance. (C) High blood pressure causes considerable baroreceptor stimulation, which inhibits the VMC output and causes vasodilatation to lower the blood pressure. The number of arrows in each case represents the degree of stimulation.

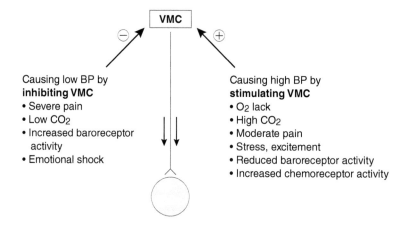

*Figure 3.5* The factors affecting the VMC. Severe pain, low carbon dioxide, increased baroreceptor stimulation and emotional shock all inhibit the VMC and cause low blood pressure by vasodilatation. A lack of oxygen, high carbon dioxide, moderate pain, stress and excitement, reduced baroreceptor stimulation and increased chemoreceptor stimulation all stimulate the VMC, causing higher blood pressure by vasoconstriction.

the VMC. Local factors influencing the peripheral resistance include cold, causing local vasoconstriction in the affected part, and heat, which will dilate the vessels. **Angiotensin II** is a vasoconstrictive hormone converted originally from **angiotensinogen** (from the liver) via **angiotensin I** (Figure 3.6). Angiotensin II has much wider effects on increasing the peripheral resistance and therefore also the blood pressure. Angiotensin II is activated under the emergency situation of low blood pressure to the kidneys, since blood pressure into the kidneys must be maintained to ensure that filtration continues (Figure 3.6). The metabolic wastes (**metabolites**) of muscle activity, such as **carbon dioxide** (Figure 1.3,

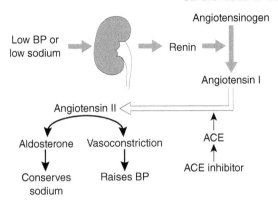

*Figure 3.6* The renin-angiotensin-aldosterone cycle. Low blood pressure or low blood sodium causes the kidney to release renin. Renin activates angiotensinogen to angiotensin I, which is then further converted to angiotensin II by the angiotensin-converting enzyme (ACE). ACE function can be blocked by the ACE inhibitor drugs. Angiotensin II stimulates aldosterone secretion (to conserve sodium) and vasoconstriction (to raise blood pressure), thus correcting the original problem.

p. 4) and other chemical substances associated with **inflammation**, such as **histamine**, cause vasodilatation locally. So also does local **trauma** (injury), especially damage to the skin, as seen in **burns**.

The fundamental pressure is created by the output from the heart (the **cardiac output**, **CO**). The formula that determines cardiac output is:

CO = heart rate (HR) × stroke volume (SV).

Given average HR as 72 beats per minute, and a stroke volume of 70 ml per beat:

CO = 72 × 70 = 5,040 ml per minute (see Chapter 2).

This occurs at the proximal (cardiac) end of the arteries. The other factor is the total **peripheral resistance** (**PR**) at the distal (tissue) end of the arteries. Therefore:

BP = CO × PR or (HR × SV) × PR

However, blood pressure can therefore be seen as a *combination* of many effects. Other effects involved are the **viscosity** (or thickness) of blood, which will vary according to the amount of water obtained from drinking or lost in the urine and the **elasticity** of the vessel wall, which will stretch and recoil with the waves of pressure. Reduced elasticity, as seen with increasing age, will resist the pressure wave, which will then remain at a higher pressure as a result, and if this is a feature throughout the vascular bed, the BP will remain higher than expected.

The difference between the systolic and diastolic pressures is called the **pulse pressure**, and it is about 30–40 mmHg in the aorta:

pulse pressure = systolic pressure – diastolic pressure (e.g. 120–90 = 30 mmHg)

The pulse pressure is measured in the larger arteries where standard BP is measured. The normal rapid narrowing and disappearance of the pulse pressure through the smaller arterioles (Figure 3.1) results in a loss of pulsation in the capillary network within the tissues, and therefore blood flows through the tissues as a continuous flow (known as **tissue perfusion**). A measure of tissue perfusion is possible by applying gentle pressure on the nails so the blood is squeezed out of the nail bed, which then goes white. Release of the pressure should see the return of the blood to the nail bed, which then returns to a normal pink colour. This return of the normal colour is due to the tissue perfusion, and normally this should be instantaneous (or at least take less than two seconds). This is the **capillary refill time**. More than two seconds to restore the nail bed colour indicates a poor tissue perfusion, which suggests a low BP. This could be due to anything that has caused a drop in the blood pressure (e.g. shock), but it may also be due to a local restriction to the blood supply (e.g. a tight plaster cast around a limb to treat a fracture). Always check for restrictions caused by such things as casts or bandages or any other interference to the blood supply in the affected limb if the capillary refill time is delayed while being normal in the other limbs and the patient is not in shock or fainted.

The **mean arterial pressure** (**MAP**) is the main BP driving force of tissue perfusion. The MAP is influenced by both the cardiac output and the total peripheral resistance, which are themselves influenced by other factors (Figure 3.7). MAP is calculated by adding one-third of the pulse pressure to the diastolic pressure:

> MAP = diastolic pressure + one-third pulse pressure or
> MAP = [(systolic pressure – diastolic pressure) ÷ 3] + diastolic pressure.

Given our standard BP of 120 over 90 mmHg, the MAP would be:

> MAP = 90 + [(120 – 90) ÷ 3] or
> 90 + [30 ÷ 3]
> (i.e. 10 + 90 = 100 mmHg).

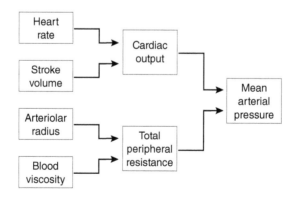

*Figure 3.7* Factors contributing to the mean arterial pressure (MAP). The cardiac output and the total peripheral resistance are themselves influenced by other factors. The heart rate and stroke volume determine the cardiac output, and the arteriolar radius and blood viscosity determine the total peripheral resistance.

Since the heart is in the diastolic period of the cardiac cycle for longer than the systolic period (diastolic = 0.5 seconds, systolic = 0.3 seconds), the mean (= average) arterial pressure must be *closer* to the diastolic pressure (i.e. 100 mmHg MAP in our example earlier is closer to the diastolic pressure [90 mmHg] than it is to the systolic pressure [120 mmHg]). The MAP must be closely regulated because if it is too low, the tissues would be deprived of blood supply, and if it is too high it may cause vascular damage, thereby increasing the workload of the heart.

## Observations of blood pressure

### Blood pressure measurement

The standard clinical blood pressure is measured in systemic arteries (i.e. those coming from the left ventricle), usually the **brachial artery** running down the upper arm, using a **sphygmomanometer** (sphygmo = pulse, manometer = pressure measure: the pulse pressure measure). The older sphygmomanometers are used in conjunction with the **stethoscope**, through which the nurse will hear the sounds (= **auscultation**) associated with pressure changes as they occur in the artery. The modern electronic machines do not require a stethoscope.

Nothing is heard if a stethoscope is simply placed over an artery. This is because blood normally passes down arteries in a straight flow without any disturbance, and this movement is silent. It is generally considered that to create sounds that are audible through a stethoscope, some disturbance to this blood flow is necessary, causing turbulence. Disturbance causes extra currents, so-called **eddy currents**, and these disrupt the straightforward flow and cause sounds. To do this, the artery has to be compressed sufficiently to reduce the lumen; this is a job for the sphygmomanometer.

It is important to carry out the procedure accurately to avoid false high or low readings, as indicated in Table 3.1.

The patient should be lying or seated comfortably with legs uncrossed and should not have changed position for five minutes before the procedure. The brachial artery at the point of the **antecubital fossa** (i.e. the *inside* of the elbow) of the patient's right arm

*Table 3.1* Blood pressure measurement errors

| Error in technique | False high reading | False low reading |
|---|---|---|
| Artery below heart level | ✓ | |
| Artery above heart level | | ✓ |
| Cuff too long | | ✓ |
| Cuff too short | ✓ | |
| Cuff too narrow | ✓ | |
| No systolic estimation | | ✓ |
| Overinflation of cuff | ✓ | |
| Deflation too slow | ✓ | |
| Deflation too fast | | ✓ |
| Reinflation without rest | ✓ | |
| Crossed legs | ✓ | |
| Unsupported arm | ✓ | |
| Tight clothing on upper arm | ✓ | |

should be level with the heart, supported on pillows on a firm surface to relax muscle tension, which may cause a false reading. The left arm should only be used if the right is unavailable, as would be the case if the right had been injured or had been used for an intravenous infusion. A small difference of 5–10 mmHg often exists between the left and right arms of the same individual, and choosing the right arm whenever possible ensures consistency each time the BP is taken. The brachial region above the elbow is exposed with no clothing restrictions above this. A cuff of the correct dimensions is placed around the upper arm *over* the brachial artery. The air bladder of the cuff should cover about two-thirds of the length of the upper arm and at least 80% of the arm circumference (recommended adult width of the bladder is 12–14 cm and the length is 35 cm). Too short an air bladder is more problematic than too long. The centre of the bladder should be in line with the brachial artery, which would be located by palpation (= felt with finger pads, not thumb) at the antecubital fossa (Figure 3.8; see also Figure 2.4, page 27). As the cuff fills with air, it compresses the arm and therefore the artery, and the normal flow is disrupted as blood tries to pass the restriction. Sufficient cuff compression causes eddy currents to begin and the sound of blood flow can be heard in five phases (known as **Korotkoff sounds**; Table 3.2) through a stethoscope placed on the brachial artery below the cuff (Figure 3.8B).

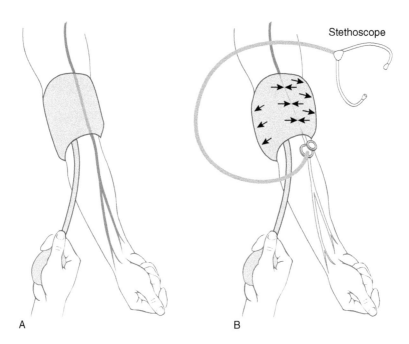

*Figure 3.8* Right arm with sphygmomanometer cuff in place. (A) Before inflation of the cuff, the artery is fully open and filled with blood (solid red). (B) After inflation of the cuff, the artery is compressed and empty of blood below the compression (i.e. the cuff is inflated above systolic pressure). At this point, no sounds are heard through the stethoscope.

*Table 3.2* Korotkoff sounds and phases

| Phase | Sounds |
| --- | --- |
| I | The appearance of faint, clear tapping sounds that gradually increase in intensity |
| II | The softening of sounds that may become swishing (possible auscultatory gap here) |
| III | The return of sharper sounds that become crisper but never fully regain the intensity of phase I |
| IV | The distinct abrupt muffling of sounds that become soft and blowing |
| V | The point at which all sounds cease |

The procedure for the older style sphygmomanometer is as follows:

- *Step 1*: The systolic pressure should first be *estimated*, which is achieved by palpation of the brachial pulse during the *rapid* inflation of the cuff until the pulse can no longer be felt. Then, the *slow* deflation of the cuff allows the point to be noted where the brachial pulse returns, followed by rapid complete cuff deflation. Estimation of the systolic pressure prevents overinflation of the cuff and allows the nurse to miss the **auscultatory gap**, a quiet period (Korotkoff phase II, Table 3.2) occurring between the systolic and diastolic points. If the cuff were inflated to an arbitrary point on the scale, the nurse may then be listening to this gap, which could then be mistaken to be *above* the systolic, and a grossly false systolic pressure would be recorded.
- *Step 2*: One minute is allowed before the full procedure continues; during this time, the arm should be momentarily raised above the head to allow maximum drainage of the venous blood.
- *Step 3*: Inflate the cuff to about 30 mmHg above the estimated systolic pressure; the inflation should be rapid to avoid excessive venous congestion.
- *Step 4*: Deflate the cuff slowly (i.e. the recommended deflation rate is about 3 mmHg per second, or per heartbeat if the pulse rate is 60 beats per minute). This rate accommodates most heart rates and prevents venous congestion in the distal vascular bed. During deflation, the nurse is listening for the sounds through the stethoscope placed over the brachial artery just distal to (i.e. below) the cuff constriction. Above the systolic, there is silence since the artery is fully compressed and all blood flow has stopped. Between the systolic down to the diastolic, the sounds of 'thud, thud . . .' with each beat of the heart can be heard. From the diastolic down to 0 mmHg, there is silence again (Figure 3.9).
- While deflating the cuff, identify the start of the sounds (the upper point where sound begins, i.e. Korotkoff phase I) and mentally note this point as the systolic pressure. Continue to deflate slowly until the sounds disappear (in adults, this is Korotkoff phase V) and mentally note this point as the diastolic pressure, then fully deflate the cuff. Obviously, do not keep the cuff inflated too long, especially above systolic pressure, since this cuts off all blood supply to the arm.
- *Step 5*: If the procedure is to be repeated, a brief pause between attempts is necessary to allow blood to flow to and from the arm. Never reinflate the cuff during or immediately after an attempt as this causes venous congestion and gives a false reading.

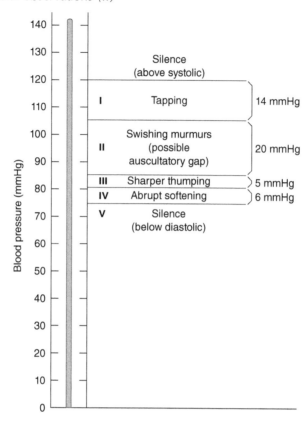

*Figure 3.9* Korotkoff phases and sounds set against the blood pressure column (left) with the pressure differences between the phases shown (right).

It is important to perfect the correct technique, including keeping the arm straight and supported, to maintain accuracy (Campbell *et al.* 1994). Although the sphygmomanometer is measuring the blood pressure, the process is *indirect*. The sphygmomanometer actually measures the pressure of the air in the cuff, but the nurse has skilfully arranged for this air pressure to exactly equal the blood pressure in the artery, first at systolic pressure and then at diastolic pressure.

### A different approach to blood pressure technique

The question concerning accuracy of blood pressure arises because of the possible variability that occurs within the same individual at different times and circumstances. One study (Powers *et al.* 2011) suggested that five to six separate measurements of blood pressure, taken over several days, should be averaged to provide a more accurate reading upon which to make a diagnosis and to base drug prescription. Now, 24-hour monitoring by a portable machine worn by the patient gives similar results.

Another approach to taking blood pressure was developed that still employed a cuff around the upper arm (i.e. to compress the brachial artery), but there is a second wrist strap that measures the pulse wave. Attachment to a monitor allows a computer to calculate the **central aortic systolic pressure** (**CASP**), close to the heart, with an accuracy of 99% when compared to aortic pressures measured though an in situ arterial catheter. There are clear advantages to measuring this pressure via a non-invasive way rather than the invasive method of catheter insertion. The blood pressure in the central aorta, close to the left ventricle of the heart, is a more relevant pressure to measure than in the brachial artery (Hickson *et al.* 2009). However, this approach is of little value to monitoring blood pressure at home or throughout daily activities.

Electronic sphygmomanometers are now in regular clinical practice. They do not have the need for a stethoscope, making the procedure easier. In addition, they give a digital read-out of the systolic and diastolic pressures along with a pulse rate. Some models still require the need to apply a cuff correctly to the upper arm and to follow the procedures regarding patient position and arm support noted earlier. The cuff is plugged into the machine and then it's simply a matter of pushing the start button. The machine then inflates and deflates the cuff before calculating the blood pressure and showing it on a screen. These machines are quick to use and considered to be accurate, and they would normally remove the need for repeating the procedure. Being battery-operated, they are more easily portable than the old machines since they have no mercury column and do not require a stethoscope.

Digital machines are getting smaller and can be used on the wrist and even built into a watch. They use different technology that no longer needs an inflatable cuff and provides the ability to monitor the blood pressure through skin contact continuously for 24 hours on the device or connected to a mobile phone. This is a valuable way to check how the blood pressure varies over the period of one day's activity. The main issues are:

1   Accuracy, a vital issue which must be addressed and maintained since diagnosis – and therefore treatment – may be based on these readings
2   Suitability for everyday use outside of the clinical area and throughout all daily activities. Some devices are small enough to be worn on the wrist and become part of a watch.

There is always a need to keep accuracy in mind. Research followed by approval by health authorities becomes a necessity before any readings from these portable devices can be relied upon and used for clinical purposes.

## Abnormal blood pressure

Abnormalities of systemic blood pressure means either the pressure is too high (**hypertension**) or too low (**hypotension**). In general, a guide to what is high or low is the pressure 90 mmHg. If the *diastolic* consistently reaches 90 mmHg or above and the systolic reaches 140mmHg or above, this suggests the presence of hypertension. The NHS (2022) states high blood pressure as 140mmHg over 90 mmHg or higher or 150mmHg over 90mmHg for the over 80s. If the *systolic* consistently falls to 90 mmHg (*diastolic* 60mmHg) or lower, this indicates hypotension. Hypertension tends to be a chronic, slowly progressing condition with insidious symptoms, while hypotension is often (but not always) a sudden onset acute condition with the obvious symptoms of dizziness, fainting, collapse and weak, rapid pulse.

Blood pressure rises gradually with age normally, but hypertension at any age produces symptoms resulting from damage to organs and tissues, especially the heart itself and the blood vessels. **Essential hypertension** appears to have no identifiable cause, but whatever the cause, the result is sodium and water retention which drives the BP up. **Secondary hypertension** follows on from another pathology, particularly chronic renal disease, which may be accompanied by renin release (see renin–angiotensin–aldosterone cycle, p. 47) or from tumours of the adrenal or pituitary glands. **Malignant hypertension** is regarded as a diastolic pressure exceeding 130 mmHg. It may be irreversible and can cause renal injury,[2] leading to kidney failure and death within a few years. The result of persistent hypertension can be any combination of three **complications**:

1 **Cardiac hypertrophy**, or enlargement of the heart, leading ultimately to heart failure (**congestive cardiac failure**, or **CCF**)
2 **Arteriosclerosis**, or *hardening of the arteries* due to blood vessel wall changes (which themselves will aggravate the high BP problem)
3 Cerebrovascular accidents (CVAs) (see strokes, page 234).

The risk of developing hypertension is increased as a result of:

1 Being male (women suffer less)
2 Increasing age
3 Obesity
4 High levels of salt in the diet
5 Smoking (nicotine is a vasoconstrictor)
6 Sometimes a family history of high blood pressure.

It is interesting that 50% of these risk factors are controllable by the individual, meaning that everyone has the opportunity to significantly reduce their risk of hypertension by losing weight, not smoking and reducing salt intake.

   **Low blood pressure** is strongly resisted in the body by **compensatory mechanisms** that drive up the BP. Rapid compensation to increase BP quickly involves the vasoconstriction of distal arterioles to increase the total peripheral resistance, mediated through the sympathetic vasomotor tone and local factors (Figure 3.5), plus increases in heart rate and stroke volume to improve the cardiac output, mediated through sympathetic influences and some hormones, notably **adrenaline** (from the adrenal medulla) and **thyroid hormone** (from the thyroid gland). **Noradrenaline** has the action of selective vasoconstriction (e.g. in the skin), which will increase the PR and also acts by increasing the **venomotor tone**, which causes a tightening of the veins to improve the venous return of blood to the heart. **Cortisol** is another important hormone that helps in the compensatory mechanisms by preventing water from leaving the circulation into the tissues, thus helping to stabilise the blood volume. Cortisol reduces the permeability of the capillary wall to water and is secreted in higher volumes than normal from the adrenal cortex during stress. In the slightly longer term, water conservation to boost blood volume – and therefore increase BP – can be achieved through greater secretion of **antidiuretic hormone** (**ADH**, from the hypothalamus via the posterior pituitary). ADH conserves water directly by acting on the distal half of the renal tubule. In addition, sodium conservation by **aldosterone** (from the adrenal cortex), also acting on the distal renal tubule, has the effect of conserving water indirectly (see chapters on Fluid balance, page 121 and Elimination (1) page 155).

   **Postural hypotension,** a drop in blood pressure on changing position from lying or bending over to sitting up or standing, is expected in everyone to some extent, but rapid compensatory adjustments ensure that for most people, particularly the young, it is not a problem. It can become a difficulty experienced with increasing age, and nurses should be aware of this when moving elderly people from one position to another. Getting them up from the bed into a chair, or from the chair to standing, should be done *slowly* and in stages, allowing time for the BP to adjust after each stage. A drop in BP when *standing up* (often specifically referred to as **orthostatic hypotension**) is of particular concern when standing up elderly people (McCance *et al.* 2014). Communication with the patient is of key importance, allowing the patient to decide the pace of the move and when to rest and to give the patient the chance to signal any symptoms of low BP that may be experienced, such as feeling faint or dizzy.

**Post-operative observations** are critical to the patient's full recovery, and BP checks are paramount among these. Low or a falling blood pressure after surgery may indicate blood loss is occurring – either internally or externally – and should be reported and acted on quickly.

The ultimate profound hypotension occurs as a feature of **shock**, and this represents a stage where the compensatory mechanisms have failed to maintain the BP. Both the stroke volume and the cardiac output fall, and therefore so does the blood pressure. **Hypovolaemic shock** results from **haemorrhage** (haemo = blood, rrhage = bursts forth), which may be *internal* (within body cavities, or as **bruising** into tissues) or *external* (into the outside environment, such as blood-soaked dressings and bandages). It is difficult to think of bruising as a potential cause of shock, but on an extensive scale it constitutes a considerable amount of blood lost from circulation. Elderly people are at considerable risk of severe shock from bruising (e.g. after a fall downstairs or a brutal assault). Bleeding can be arterial, venous or capillary. Arterial is far more serious as blood is lost quickly from a high-pressure system in pulses, resulting in a massive and rapid loss from circulation, and speed is essential to control this before the person dies from **exsanguination** (i.e. bleeds to death). Shock, especially hypovolaemic shock, is a major cause of a *narrowing* pulse pressure (i.e. the systolic pressure is falling faster than the diastolic pressure and the two pressures appear to be converging). If the systolic pressure should fall below 50 mmHg, the kidneys are at serious risk of failure (see note 2).

Other forms of shock occur even when the blood volume remains normal. These are:

1 **Cardiogenic shock** (i.e. caused by the heart), when the heart as a pump fails to sustain a normal stroke volume.
2 **Vasogenic shock**, where the cause is the vascular (circulatory) system itself.

A common cause of cardiogenic shock is **myocardial infarction** (**MI**), where an area of *dead or dying myocardium* (known as the **infarct**) results from occlusion of the coronary arteries. If this occurs in the ventricular myocardium, the force of contraction – and therefore the stroke volume and blood pressure – is greatly and often suddenly reduced.

Vasogenic shock includes several forms depending on the cause. **Neurogenic shock** occurs when the sympathetic nervous system supply to the cardiovascular system is blocked, causing a low cardiac output, reduced peripheral resistance (page 47) and venous blood pooling. Venous pooling is an important cause of lost circulating blood volume since the veins carry the majority of the blood volume in circulation at any given time, and when this fails to return to the heart (due to pooling in the veins) it produces a poor cardiac output. **Anaphylactic shock** is due to a severe allergic reaction, resulting in massive release of the inflammatory chemical **histamine**, which causes a rapid body-wide vasodilation with profound loss of peripheral resistance and collapse of the blood pressure.

Apart from hypotension and tachycardia, shock, whatever the type, will also cause collapse of the individual affected and an altered state of consciousness (e.g. fainting) as the blood supply to the brain is reduced. Other symptoms include pallor (pale skin colour) and cold skin – caused by diversion of blood away from the skin to the vital organs – and sweating, caused by sympathetic stimulation of the sweat glands, a side effect of the sympathetic compensatory mechanism (see noradrenaline, page 54).

### Central venous pressure (CVP)

The CVP is a measure of the pressure in the major veins returning the blood from the body to the right side of the heart. The bulk of the blood in circulation at any given time is in the venous system. The total circulatory volume is 5,000 ml, and the percentage of this volume for each blood vessel type at any given time are approximately:

- arterial blood = 10% of total volume (500 ml)
- venous blood = between 60 and 80% of total volume (3,000–4,000 ml)
- capillary blood = 5% of total blood volume (250 ml).

The remaining blood volume is in the heart and lungs. It is therefore very useful to know the pressure (which is related to volume) in the venous return to the heart. Any reduction in volume will cause changes in the CVP before it affects arterial pressures, which are maintained relatively high by the action of the heart. CVP gives the best indication of the filling pressures on the right side of the heart. CVP is measured through a cannula inserted along a vein towards the heart, the tip arriving in the thoracic vena cava, close to the right atrium. The vena cava and the right atrium have almost the same pressures. The cannula is connected to a fluid infusion (e.g. normal saline) and calibrated by aligning the measure with the heart (usually the level of the sternal notch with the patient in a flat supine position). Measurements are taken manually using a **manometer**. In critical care situations, CVP can be taken electronically. The normal value for CVP is 3–10 mmHg (5–12 cmH$_2$O). *Low* CVP indicates **hypovolaemia** or dehydration, and *high* CVP may be caused by **hypervolaemia** (possibly due to excessive intravenous infusion of fluids or blood) or due to cardiac failure.

### Blood pressure in children

The *systolic* blood pressure rises normally with age, averaging at about 90 mmHg at 1 year old to about 100 mmHg at 12 years old, although significant variation occurs according to growth rate and size (Table 3.3).

It is important when taking the child's blood pressure to use a cuff of the correct size for their age (Table 3.4). The wrong size cuff, especially the use of an adult-size cuff with children, will result in inaccurate results. The procedure also varies in children, with the Korotkoff stage IV sounds (Table 3.2) used to determine diastolic pressure. Children tend to have a higher cardiac output for body size than adults, and this causes the fifth-phase Korotkoff sounds, used in adults for determining the diastolic pressure, to be too low for paediatric clinical use.

*Table 3.3* Child blood pressures by age

| Age | Systolic (mmHg) | Diastolic (mmHg) |
|---|---|---|
| Birth | 60–85 | 45–55 |
| 4 days | 67–84 | 35–53 |
| 1–12 months | 80–100 | 55–53 |
| 1–2 years | 90–105 | 55–70 |
| 3–5 years | 95–107 | 60–71 |
| 6–9 years | 95–110 | 60–73 |
| 10+ years | 100–124 | 70–79 |

*Table 3.4* Blood pressure cuff size in children

| Age | Cuff width |
|---|---|
| Neonate | 2–5 cm |
| 1–4 years | 6 cm |
| 4–8 years | 9 cm |

### Drugs affecting the blood pressure

Since many cardiac drugs have an effect on both the pulse and the blood pressure, some are the same drugs that are mentioned in Chapter 2 (page 36). There is a good selection of drugs available to reduce high blood pressure, and these are shown in Tables 3.5 to 3.10 according to their mode of action. Some drugs are also available to raise low blood pressure, as shown in Table 3.11.

*Drugs to treat hypertension*

**Positive inotropic** drugs are those that increase the force of contraction, and by raising the cardiac output they increase the blood pressure. These include the **cardiac glycosides** (e.g. **digoxin**; Chapter 2, Figure 2.14).

Other drugs available to lower the BP as a treatment of hypertension include:

1 Drugs that inhibit components of the **angiotensin-converting enzyme** system (**ACE inhibitors**; Table 3.5), which reduce the blood pressure by blocking the action of angiotensin-converting enzyme (ACE), thereby preventing the formation of angiotensin II, and thus blocking its vasoconstrictive effects (Figure 3.6). The result is a reduction in peripheral resistance and thus a drop in blood pressure.
2 Beta-blocking drugs block the beta-receptor on cardiac muscle causing a decrease in the cardiac output (reduced stroke volume) and a lower blood pressure (Figure 3.10; Table 3.6, see also Chapter 2, page 37).
3 **Vasodilator** anti-hypertension drugs can have a dramatic effect on reducing high blood pressure quickly by dilating the major arteries and reducing the peripheral resistance. These drugs should be used under specialist supervision and close monitoring.
4 The **diuretics** are a group of drugs that can be used to lower the BP (and are therefore used as a treatment in hypertension) by causing a larger urine output to reduce the circulatory volume (see Chapter 8, page 155). The **thiazides** (e.g. **Bendroflumethiazide**, Table 3.8)

*Table 3.5* Drug inhibitors of the ACE system

| Drug | Possible side effects | Use and other notes |
|------|----------------------|---------------------|
| Captopril | Insomnia, peptic ulcer, appetite loss, malaise. | Hypertension. ACE inhibitor. |
| Enalapril maleate | Depression, blurred vision, hypersensitivity, anaemia, reduced appetite. | Hypertension. ACE inhibitor, prescribed with or without hydrochlorothiazide. |
| Fosinopril sodium | Eye disorders, mood changes, oedema, pain, visual changes, pain. | Hypertension. ACE inhibitor. |
| Imidapril hydrochloride | Rare but includes joint swelling, limb pain, oedema. | Essential hypertension. ACE inhibitor. |
| Lisinopril | Postural changes, hallucinations, mood changes. | Hypertension. ACE inhibitor, prescribed with or without hydrochlorothiazide. |
| Perindopril arginine | Muscle cramps, visual changes, risk of falling, hypoglycaemia, malaise, mood changes. | Hypertension. ACE inhibitor, prescribed with or without indapamide. |
| Perindopril erbumine | Muscle cramps, visual changes, risk of falling. | Hypertension. ACE inhibitor. |
| Quinapril | Back pain, insomnia, dry throat, depression, gastrointestinal disorders. | Essential hypertension. ACE inhibitor, prescribed with or without hydrochlorothiazide. |
| Ramipril | Gastrointestinal disorders, muscles spasms, anxiety, appetite decreased. | Hypertension. ACE inhibitor, prescribed with or without felodipine. |
| Trandolapril | Gastrointestinal disorders, hot flushes, insomnia. | Hypertension. ACE inhibitor. |
| Azilsartan medoxomil | Rare but include muscle spasms, peripheral oedema. | Hypertension. Angiotensin II receptor antagonist. |
| Candesartan cilexetil | Increased risk of infections, white blood cell irregularities. | Hypertension. Angiotensin II receptor antagonist. |
| Eprosartan | Gastrointestinal disorders. | Hypertension. Angiotensin II receptor antagonist. |
| Irbesartan | Muscle and bone pain, dyspepsia, flushing, tachycardia. | Hypertension. Angiotensin II receptor antagonist, prescribed with or without hydrochlorothiazide |
| Losartan potassium | Anaemia, hypoglycaemia, postural changes, angina, constipation, palpitations. | Hypertension. Angiotensin II receptor antagonist, prescribed with or without hydrochlorothiazide. |
| Olmesartan medoxomil | Joint and bone pain, chest pain, haematuria, oedema, increase in blood uric acid and triglyceride levels. | Hypertension. Angiotensin II receptor antagonist, prescribed with or without amlodipine and with or without hydrochlorothiazide |
| Telmisartan | Not common but includes anaemia, arrhythmias, depression, gastrointestinal discomfort, muscle spasms. | Hypertension. Angiotensin II receptor antagonist, prescribed with or without hydrochlorothiazide. |
| Valsartan | Not common but includes syncope and low blood neutrophil count. | Hypertension. Angiotensin II receptor antagonist, prescribed with or without hydrochlorothiazide. |
| Aliskiren | Joint pain, diarrhoea, dizziness, electrolyte imbalance (Chapter 6). | Essential hypertension. Renin inhibitor. |

*Table 3.6* Beta-blocking drugs (see also Table 2.4, Chapter 2)

| Drug | Possible side effects | Use and other notes |
|---|---|---|
| Acebutolol | Gastrointestinal disorder, psychosis, cyanosis, breathing disorders. | Hypertension, angina. Selective beta-blocker. Has some intrinsic sympathomimetic activity. |
| Atenolol | Gastrointestinal disorder, dry mouth, skin reactions, postural hypotension. | Hypertension, angina. With or without nifedipine. Selective beta-blocker. |
| Bisoprolol fumarate | Constipation, muscle cramps and weakness, postural hypotension. | Hypertension. Selective beta-blocker. |
| Celiprolol hydrochloride | Drowsiness, blood glucose disturbance, palpitations. | Hypertension. Selective beta-blocker. Has some intrinsic sympathomimetic activity. |
| Co-tenidone | Gastrointestinal and blood glucose disturbance. | Hypertension. Selective beta-blocker. |
| Esmolol hydrochloride | Anxiety, loss of appetite, dry mouth, poor concentration, drowsiness, fever, chills. | Perioperative hypertension. Selective beta-blocker. |
| Metoprolol tartrate | Constipation, palpitations, postural hypotension. | Hypertension, angina. Selective beta-blocker. |
| Nebivolol | Constipation, oedema, postural hypotension. | Essential hypertension. Selective beta-blocker. |
| Carvedilol | Anaemia, breathlessness, fluid imbalance, blood glucose disturbance. | Hypertension, angina. Alpha and beta-receptor blocker. |
| Labetalol hydrochloride | Hypersensitivity, urinary disturbance. | Hypertension. Alpha and beta-receptor blocker. |
| Nadolol | Rare but may include appetite loss, constipation, cough, dry mouth. | Hypertension, angina. Alpha and beta-receptor blocker. |
| Pindolol | Arrhythmias, white blood cell and blood sugar disturbance, joint pain, constipation, dry mouth. | Hypertension, angina. Alpha and beta-receptor blocker. Has some intrinsic sympathomimetic activity. |
| Propranolol hydrochloride | Rare but may include memory loss, mood changes, postural hypotension, skin reactions. | Hypertension, angina. Alpha and beta-receptor blocker. |
| Timolol maleate | Rare but may include joint pain, skin reactions, vertigo. | Hypertension, angina. Alpha and beta-receptor blocker. |

and two **loop diuretics** (see Chapter 8, Table 8.4) are used to treat hypertension. They inhibit the reabsorption of sodium in the renal nephron. The extra sodium excreted as a result takes with it extra water, and this water loss reduces the blood volume, one of the influencing factors in BP maintenance. Some diuretic drugs may also have a vasodilatory effect *outside* the kidney, which has a part to play in lowering the BP.

5  Centrally acting anti-hypertensive drugs (Table 3.9) work in the central nervous system (brain and cord). They stimulate alpha-2 adrenoceptors (receptors for adrenaline and noradrenaline) i.e. they are alpha-2 receptor *agonists*. Alpha-2 receptors are found in the sympathetic nervous system. Stimulation of these receptors causes reduced sympathetic activity on the heart leading to less force of contraction (i.e. lower stroke volume) (Chapter 2), and lowering the heart rate, thereby reducing blood pressure.

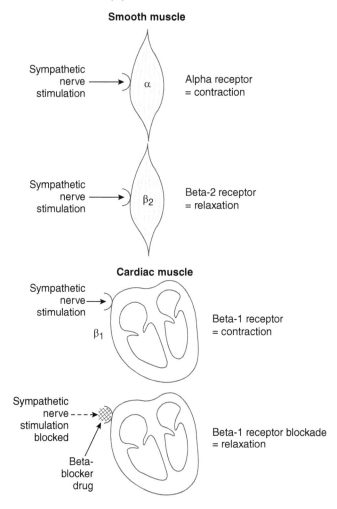

*Figure 3.10* The action of beta-blocker drugs. Sympathetic stimulation of smooth muscles may cause contraction if the alpha (α) receptor is activated or relaxation if the beta-2 ($\beta_2$) receptor is activated. On cardiac muscle, sympathetic stimulation of the beta-1 ($\beta_1$) receptor causes the heart to increase the heart rate and force of contraction, unless the receptor is blocked by drugs that prevent sympathetic stimulation and the heart slows down and decreases the force of contraction. Beta-blocking drugs may cause side effects by blocking beta receptors on smooth muscle (e.g. causing bronchoconstriction).

6  Calcium-channel blockers (Table 3.10) prevent calcium from entering the neuronal cells supplying the heart and blood vessels. Calcium entry promotes cellular activity which then stimulates the heart to work harder. By blocking calcium entry into the cells, these drugs cause the heart rate to slow and the stroke volume to be reduced, thereby lowering the blood pressure.

Eight drugs are available to reduce high blood pressure specifically within the pulmonary artery (i.e. pulmonary hypertension). This pressure is not easily observed or monitored as the pulmonary artery is entirely enclosed within the chest cavity.

*Table 3.7* Vasodilator drugs

| Drug | Possible side effects | Use and other notes |
|---|---|---|
| Sodium nitroprusside | Abdominal pain, arrhythmias, dizziness, headaches, skin rash. | Hypertensive crisis. Given by intravenous infusion (IV). |
| Hydralazine hydrochloride | Angina, diarrhoea, sudden drop in blood pressure, nausea, palpitations. | Severe hypertension and hypertensive crisis |
| Minoxidil | Fluid retention, oedema, tachycardia, pericarditis, skin reactions. | Severe hypertension when other drugs don't work. Potassium channel opener. |
| Prazosin | Constipation, depression, dizziness, headache, nausea, nasal congestion, skin reactions, diarrhoea. | Hypertension. Alpha-blocker with vasodilation activity. |
| Doxazosin | Arrhythmias, cough, dizziness, drowsiness, nausea, dry mouth, skin reactions, breathlessness. | Hypertension. Alpha-blocker with vasodilation activity. |
| Indoramin | Rare, but includes depression, dizziness, drowsiness, dry mouth. | Hypertension. Alpha-blocker with vasodilation activity. |
| Terazosin | Anxiety, arrhythmias, cough, depression, fever, headache, skin reactions. | Hypertension. Alpha-blocker with vasodilation activity. |

*Table 3.8* Thiazide diuretic drugs

| Drug | Possible side effects | Use and other notes |
|---|---|---|
| Bendroflumethiazide | Blood disorder, gout, gastrointestinal disorders, pulmonary oedema. | Hypertension and oedema. |
| Hydrochlorothiazide | Rare but may include appetite loss, gastrointestinal discomfort, muscle cramps. | Used in combination with various other drugs. |
| Co-amilozide | Angina, appetite loss, postural hypotension, joint pain, confusion, headache, gout, fainting, vomiting. | Hypertension and congestive cardiac failure. |
| Indapamide | Hypersensitivity. | Essential hypertension. |

*Table 3.9* Centrally acting anti-hypertensive drugs

| Drug | Possible side effects | Use and other notes |
|---|---|---|
| Clonidine hydrochloride | Constipation, depression, dizziness, fatigue, headache, sleep disturbance, vomiting, postural hypotension. | Hypertension. Rapid withdrawal may cause sudden rebound hypertension. |
| Methyldopa | Abdominal distention, angina, joint pain, and a range of other side effects. | Hypertension. Appears to be safe to use in pregnancy. |
| Moxonidine | Loss of energy, diarrhoea, dizziness, headache, insomnia, nausea, vomiting. | Essential hypertension. Useful if other drugs fail to control the blood pressure. |

*Table 3.10* Calcium-channel blocking drugs

| Drug | Possible side effects | Use and other notes |
|---|---|---|
| Amlodipine | Loss of energy, bowel disturbance, breathlessness, joint pain, muscle cramps. | Hypertension and angina. With or without Valsartan. |
| Diltiazem hydrochloride | Constipation, malaise, heart conduction disorders. | Hypertension and angina. |
| Felodipine | Not common, but includes fatigue and joint pain. | Hypertension and angina. |
| Lacidipine | Abdominal discomfort, loss of energy, polyuria. | Hypertension. |
| Lercanidipine hydrochloride | Rare, but includes angina, loss of energy, diarrhoea. | Hypertension. |
| Nicardipine hydrochloride | Hypotension. | Hypertension and angina. |
| Nifedipine | Constipation, malaise, oedema, sleep disturbance. | Hypertension and angina. |
| Verapamil hydrochloride | Hypotension, vertigo. | Hypertension, angina, and arrhythmias (Table 2.6). |

*Table 3.11* Anti-hypotensive drugs

| Drug | Possible side effects | Use and other notes |
|---|---|---|
| Dopamine hydrochloride | Angina, anxiety, arrhythmias, dyspnoea, headache, hypertension, nausea, palpitations. | Cardiogenic shock. Acts on beta-1 receptors on cardiac muscle. Increases force of contraction. |
| Ephedrine hydrochloride | Anxiety, headache, nausea, insomnia, tremor. | Given by slow intravenous injection. It is also a bronchodilator (Chapter 5). |
| Metaraminol | Headache, hypertension, arrhythmias, nausea, palpitations. | Acute hypotension. Sympathomimetic vasoconstrictor. |
| Midodrine hydrochloride | Cills, flushing, headache, nausea, gastrointestinal disturbance, skin reactions, urinary problems. | Acute orthostatic hypotension. It is a pro-drug converted in the body to desglymidodrine, a sympathomimetic vasoconstrictor. |
| Noradrenaline (Norepinephrine) | Acute glaucoma, anxiety, arrhythmias, confusion, headache, nausea, palpitations. | Acute hypotension. |
| Phenylephrine hydrochloride | Angina, arrhythmias, dizziness, flushing, headache, nausea. | Acute hypotension. |

*Drugs to treat hypotension*

Some drugs act to raise the blood pressure when it is low, i.e. hypotension and in shock (Waller and Sampson 2017). Most are sympathomimetic drugs, i.e. those that mimic the sympathetic nervous system by acting on alpha-adrenergic receptors causing venous vasoconstriction, preventing venous pooling of blood and constriction of peripheral vessels resulting in an increase in the peripheral resistance. These drugs are highlighted in Table 3.11. These drugs should be used in combination with blood replacement treatment

*Table 3.12* Red flag warnings of deteriorating condition

⚑ **Red Flag = serious situation which needs urgent medical attention.**

| Flag warning | Details |
|---|---|
| ⚑ **Red Flag** | **Rapid drop in blood pressure due to severe blood loss from an injury or from an internal source.** **Rapid drop in blood pressure due to severe fluid loss from extensive burns.** |

(After Hill-Smith and Johnson 2021)

where low blood volume is the cause and preferably used in critical care units where BP can be closely monitored.

## Key points

- Blood pressure = cardiac output × peripheral resistance (BP = CO × PR), where the CO = heart rate × stroke volume (CO = HR × SV).
- The average adult arterial BP is 120 systolic over 80 diastolic measured in mmHg (millimetres of mercury).
- The difference between the systolic and diastolic pressures is the pulse pressure.
- The mean arterial pressure (MAP) is the driving force that maintains tissue perfusion of blood.
- The mean arterial pressure is calculated by adding one-third of the pulse pressure to the diastolic pressure (i.e. MAP = diastolic pressure + one-third pulse pressure).
- The systolic blood pressure rises normally with age, about 90 mmHg at 1 year old to about 100 mmHg at 12 years old; variation occurs according to growth rate and size.
- It is important to use a cuff that is the correct size for adults and correct for a child's age; the wrong size cuff will give inaccurate results.
- The new digital portable blood pressure devices that can be worn on the wrist should be assessed and approved for accuracy before being used for clinical purposes.
- Fifty per cent of the risk factors for high blood pressure are preventable by losing weight, not smoking and reducing salt intake.
- Nurses should be aware of the risk of postural hypotension in the elderly before moving them.
- Shock is a major cause of low blood pressure and narrowing pulse pressure.
- Systolic blood pressure below 50 mmHg may result in kidney failure.

## Notes

1 Tone is the state of tension in a muscle. Increased tone results in contraction, which in this case would constrict the arteries. Decreased tone results in no contraction, which in this case would dilate the arteries.
2 The kidneys work on blood pressure and therefore they are sensitive to blood pressure changes.

## References

Campbell N.R., McKay D.W., Chockalingam A. and Fodor J.G. (1994) Errors in assessment of blood pressure: Blood pressure measuring technique. *Canadian Journal of Public Health*, *85*(Suppl. 2): S18–21.

Hickson S.S., Butlin M., Mir F., Graggaber J., Cheriyan J., Yasmin M., Cockcroft J.R., Wilkinson I.B. and McEniery C.M. (2009) The accuracy of central systolic blood pressure determined from the second systolic peak of the peripheral pressure waveform. *Artery Research*, 3(4): 162.

Hill-Smith I. and Johnson G. (2021) *Little Book of Red Flags*. National Minor Illness Centre, Bedfordshire.

McCance K.L., Huether S.E., Brashers V.L. and Rote N.S. (2014) *Pathophysiology: The Biological Basis for Disease in Adults and Children* (7th edition). Mosby, Elsevier, Maryland Heights, MO.

National Health Service (NHS) (2022) *High Blood Pressure (Hypertension)*. www.nhs.uk/common-health-questions/lifestyle/what-is-blood-pressure/ (accessed 23rd December 2022).

Powers B.J., Olsen M.K., Smith V.A., Woolson R.F., Bosworth H.B. and Oddone E.Z. (2011) Measuring blood pressure for decision making and quality reporting: Where and how many measures? *Annals of Internal Medicine*, 154(12): 781–788.

Waller D.G. and Sampson A.P. (2017) *Medical Pharmacology and Therapeutics* (5th edition). Elsevier Health Sciences, Philadelphia, PA.

# 4 Cardiovascular observations (III)

Blood tests

## Introduction

Blood is composed of cells embedded in a fluid matrix (**plasma**) which is water plus other substances. It is the major transport system of the body closely linked to the lymphatic system. Lymph is derived from blood plasma and returns to the blood.

There are approximately 5 L of blood in the adult circulation. Like all tissues, blood replaces itself continually. The plasma is replaced by oral intake of water. The old blood cells die off and are replaced by new cells from bone marrow.

The blood has the task of transporting:

- water and nutrients from the digestive system to the cells
- oxygen from the lungs to the cells
- carbon dioxide from the cells to the lungs
- wastes from the cells to the kidneys
- defensive cells from the bone marrow to sites of infection
- hormones from the glands to the cells
- antibodies from lymphocytes to antigens
- proteins from the liver to all parts of the circulatory system
- heat (see Chapter 1) and much more.

For this reason and because it can be easily accessed, blood becomes a vital medium for assessing the current state of the body. The blood test table results given here are not

DOI: 10.4324/9781003389118-4

*Table 4.1* Abbreviations and symbols used in the tables

| Abbreviation | Full meaning | Explanation (where applicable) |
| --- | --- | --- |
| dL | decilitre | One-tenth of a litre |
| g/dL | grams per decilitre | Gram is one-thousandth of a kilogram |
| g/L | grams per litre | |
| mL | millilitre | One-thousandth of a litre |
| mcg, μg or ug | microgram | One-millionth of a gram |
| μg/dL | micrograms per decilitre | |
| μg/L | micrograms per litre | |
| mg/L | milligrams per litre | Milligram is one-thousandth of a gram |
| μkat/L | microkatals per litre | Katal is the standard international (SI) unit for enzymic catalytic activity; microkatals are one-thousandth of a katal |
| mEq/L | milliequivalent per litre | mEq = one-thousandth [$10^{-3}$] of a chemical *equivalent weight*; the equivalent weight is the amount of a substance that combines with 8.0 g of oxygen or 1.008 g of hydrogen |
| mm³ | cubic millimetre | |
| mmol/L | millimoles per litre | One-thousandth of a mole per litre |
| mole | | SI unit for the amount of a substance that contains as many atoms as in 12 grams of carbon-12 |
| nmol/L | nanomoles per litre | Nanomole is one-billionth of a mole |
| μmol/L | micromoles per litre | Micromole is one-thousandth of a mole |
| ng/mL | nanograms per millilitre | Nanogram is one-billionth of a gram (i.e. 1/1000,000,000 of a gram) |
| pg/mL | picograms per millimetre | Pico is one-trillionth ($10^{-12}$) part of a substance; picogram is one-trillionth of a gram; picomole is one-trillionth of a mole |
| pmol/L | picomoles per litre | |
| < | less than | |
| > | more than | |
| U/L | units per litre | Units are agreed and accepted amounts of a substance |
| IU/L | International units per litre | International units are internationally accepted amounts of a substance |
| kIU | kilo International Units | One thousand IUs ($10^3$) |
| mIU | milli International Units | One-thousandth of an IU ($10^{-3}$) |
| μIU | micro International Units | One-millionth of an IU ($10^{-6}$) |
| secs | seconds | |

inclusive, but they do indicate the most important tests available (Basten 2013). The normal values and units given may vary from one laboratory to another. The figures given in the tables are standard average values. Abbreviations and explanations for the symbols used in the tables are given in Table 4.1.

## Blood plasma

Oxygen and carbon dioxide are mostly carried by the haemoglobin of the red blood cells (RBCs). All the remaining substances are carried in the **plasma**, some dissolved and some in suspension. Plasma consists of 92% water with 7% plasma proteins and 1% dissolved solutes. The end products of digestion and inhaled oxygen are transported to the

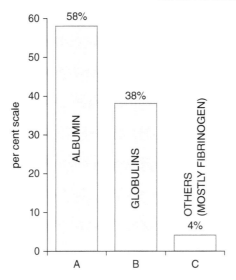

*Figure 4.1* Proportions of protein in blood.

tissues, while the waste products and carbon dioxide are carried to the excretory organs for elimination. Whole proteins, called **plasma proteins**, remain in the blood. **Albumin** is the most common protein in plasma (58% of all the proteins present), with **globulins** (which includes antibodies) being the next common (38%). The remaining 4% include the clotting factor **fibrinogen**, various hormones and others. Plasma proteins have many functions, as noted under each separate protein (Figure 4.1) (Blann and Ahmed 2014).

### Plasma blood tests

There are many plasma tests available, and those that are included here are proteins, vitamins, fats and cholesterol, chemistry, enzymes, hormones, clotting factors, immunity, blood gases and toxins.

### Proteins (Figure 4.1 and Table 4.2)

Plasma transports the *amino acids* derived from the diet and *whole proteins* that are produced by the body, usually the liver. The two major proteins in blood plasma are **albumin** and the **globulins**.

   **Test: Albumin.** This is made in the liver with amino acids from the diet. There are a wide range of functions of albumin (Caironi and Gattinoni 2009) including:

1  Attracting water back into the blood from the tissues and retaining water in circulation, thus maintaining the **intravascular colloid osmotic pressure** (**COP**) and preventing **oedema** (see Chapter 6).
2  Prevention of blood leakage from the vessels.
3  Binding and transporting substances in circulation, including calcium, bilirubin (see Chapter 8), some hormones and drugs.

*Table 4.2* Blood protein tests

| Plasma protein component | Normal test result | Normal test result (SI units) | Notes where applicable |
|---|---|---|---|
| Albumin | 3.5–5.0 g/dL | 35–50 g/L | |
| Alpha-1-globulin | 0.1–0.3 g/dL | 1–3 g/L | |
| Alpha-2-globulin | 0.6–1.0 g/dL | 6–10 g/L | |
| A/G ratio | 1–2 | | < 1.0 is clinically significant |
| Beta-globulin | 0.7–1.1 g/dL | 7–11 g/L | |
| Gamma-globulin | 0.5–1.6 g/dL | 5–16 g/L | |
| Globulin (total) | 1.5–3.5g/dL | 15–35 g/L | |
| Protein (total) | 6.3–8.0 g/dL | 63–80 g/L | |
| B-type natriuretic peptide (BNP) | <100 pg/mL | <100 ng/L | |
| C-peptide | 0.50–3.5 ng/mL | 0.17–1.17 nmol/L | |
| C-reactive protein | < 1 mg/L | < 9.52 nmol/L | < 1 mg/L = low risk of heart disease > 3 mg/L = high risk of heart disease |
| Cardiac-specific troponins | TnI very low (0–0.4 ng/mL) TnT 0–0.1 ng/mL | 0–0.4 µg/L 0–0.1 µg/L | Often undetectable |
| Creatine-kinase (CK) | 50–200 U/L | 0.85–3.40 µkat/L | |
| Alpha-fetoprotein | < 10 ng/mL | < 10 µg/L | |
| Myoglobin | 19–92 µg/L | 1.0–5.3 nmol/L | Males higher than females |

Low albumin in the blood is associated with liver disease, protein malnutrition, chronic inflammation, nephrotic syndrome and diabetes (see Chapter 8). Dehydration is often caused by raised albumin level.

   ***Test: Globulins.*** There are three main types of globulins: alpha ($\alpha$), beta ($\beta$) and gamma ($\gamma$). Alpha is divided into alpha-1 ($\alpha$-1) and alpha-2 ($\alpha$-2) globulins. Similarly, beta is divided into beta-1 ($\beta$-1) and beta-2 ($\beta$-2) globulins. The alpha and beta globulins are made in the liver. The specialised gamma globulins, called **immunoglobulins** or **antibodies**, are made in **B-cell lymphocytes** (called **plasma cells**) as part of the immune system. The functions of the globulins include binding and transportation of elements such as iron (see haemoglobin, Hb, page 92) and to fight infection (see immunoglobulins, Ig, page 86). Raised globulin levels in the blood may be due to various autoimmune diseases (e.g. rheumatoid arthritis) or a number of blood disorders such as leukaemia and haemolytic anaemia. Low levels can be present in liver, kidney or autoimmune diseases. Albumin and globulin tests are done as a part of a collection of tests.

   ***Test: Total protein and A/G ratio.*** This is the sum total of all the major proteins in the blood, notably albumin and globulin. High levels of protein indicate a possible infection or inflammation, or it can be linked to bone marrow disease. Low levels are seen in malnutrition, especially a lack of protein in the diet, and it can be seen in liver or kidney disorders. The normal ratio of albumin to globulin (i.e. the **A/G ratio**) is calculated by the formula:

**Albumin/(total protein – albumin)** (i.e. with an albumin value of 4g/dL and a total protein of 7g/dL, the A/G ratio would be 4/(7 − 4), or 4/3, which is 1.33)

The value varies depending on different laboratories. Generally, the normal value is considered to be between 1.0 and 2.0, with some laboratories accepting 1.7 as the optimum value. The test serves as an index for a state of disease but cannot be used for diagnosis. A low A/G ratio (often quoted as < 1.0) suggests an overproduction of globulins or low albumin production. This can be the case in autoimmune disease or multiple myeloma, but further investigation is required. A high A/G ratio may indicate an underproduction of antibodies (immunoglobulins), and this may be present in leukaemia or some genetic disorders.

   **Test: B-type natriuretic peptide (BNP).** This is a hormone produced by the ventricles of the heart in response to excessive stretching of the **cardiomyocytes** (heart muscle cells). This stretching follows changes in the internal blood pressure within the ventricles; blood pressure changes consistent with heart failure. In ventricular failure, levels of BNP rise, returning to normal when the heart muscle improves. Heart failure causes levels to rise in excess of 450 pg/ml in the under-50 age group and to rise in excess of 900 pg/ml in the over-50 age group. A diagnostic 'grey area' occurs between 100 and 500 pg/ml, when the test results are often inconclusive. As a hormone, BNP binds to receptors, causing a drop in blood pressure via several mechanisms, including reducing systemic peripheral vascular resistance (see Chapter 3) and **natriuresis** (the loss of sodium through the kidney in urine). This lowering of the blood pressure (especially the central venous pressure) reduces the cardiac output.

   **Test: C-peptide.** Connecting peptide (C-peptide) (Figure 4.2) connects the two chains (A-chain and B-chain) of insulin together at the **proinsulin** stage. It is removed, leaving the two chains connected by two **disulphide** (sulphur to sulphur) **bonds** to form the insulin molecule. The remaining C-peptide is secreted into the blood in approximately the same amounts as insulin, so blood C-protein levels correlate with insulin levels. It can be useful in distinguishing between type 1 and type 2 diabetes (Chapter 8), where different levels of insulin are produced. High levels of C-peptide are seen in type 2 diabetes or **insulinoma** (pancreatic tumour producing too much insulin). Too little C-peptide is found in type 1

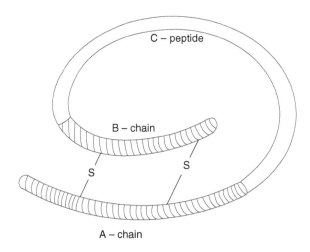

*Figure 4.2* The C-peptide incorporated as part of the proinsulin molecule prior to its separation. Once the C-peptide is removed the A and B chains will be joined by two disulphide bonds (S).

diabetes, liver disease, severe infections and **Addison disease**, i.e. inadequate cortisol produced from the adrenal cortex.

*Test: C-reactive protein.* This is produced by the liver in response to inflammation. It therefore becomes a marker for inflammation somewhere in the body (i.e. not specific to any organ). Some evidence suggests that raised C-reactive protein (above 3 mg/L) is a sign of higher-than-average risk of cardiovascular disease or stroke, although this may not be universally accepted. A level greater than 10 mg/L should be investigated further.

*Test: Cardiac-specific troponins I and II.* **Troponins** are highly specialised proteins found in skeletal and cardiac muscle. They constitute a complex made from three different subunits named according to function:

1 Troponin I (TnI) *inhibits* the enzyme actomyosin adenosine triphosphatase; normal value in blood is < 0.35 ng/ml
2 Troponin T (TnT) binds to *tropomyosin*; normal value in blood is < 0.20 g/L
3 Troponin C (TnC) binds *calcium* to the complex (Figure 4.3).

cTnT means that it is an isoform of TnT that is specific to cardiac muscle (sTnT and fTnT are specific to different forms of skeletal muscle). Similarly, cTnI is also specific to cardiac muscle, but TnC is not specific to cardiac muscle (it is found in all muscles), and therefore it is not used as a test for myocardial damage. The troponin complex (TnI, TnT and TnC) attaches to the actin filament within muscle cells (Figure 4.3). The function of the complex is to regulate muscle contraction, which requires calcium.

In the event of a **myocardial infarction** (**MI**), muscle damage occurs within the myocardium. This damage varies from very minor, which may produce few or no symptoms, to very severe, which may threaten life. Damaged and dying muscle tissue releases troponins into the general circulation. Large areas of damage will release greater quantities of troponins than small, minor areas. Detecting significant levels of TnT and TnI in circulation, in association with other symptoms such as chest pain, strongly indicates the presence of a myocardial infarction. In this situation, concentrations of both TnT and TnI

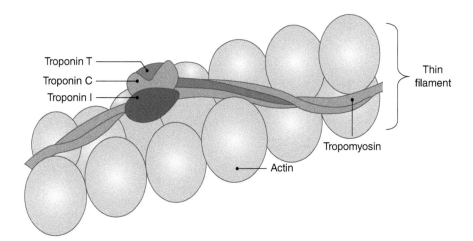

*Figure 4.3* The troponin complex in muscle. Troponins T and I are released into the blood when muscle is damaged.

are elevated within 4 to 8 hours after the muscle injury, and the levels peak about 12 to 24 hours after the event. TnT may remain high for 2 weeks or more, while TnI may remain elevated for 5 to 7 days. The test is usually repeated 3 hours after the first test to confirm the diagnosis, and this usually requires hospital admissions for those with suspect myocardial infarction (see also *blood tests in development*, page 94). The use of troponins is more sensitive and more specific for cardiac muscle, therefore more reliable than the previous test for the cardiac enzyme **creatine-kinase-MB** (**CK-MB**). This is also released from damaged muscle. There are two variants of creatine-kinase, CKM and CKB, and the test is for the combined form CK-MB.

 **Test: Alpha-fetoprotein (AFP)**. In a foetus, AFP is the most abundant plasma protein present. It is produced by the foetal liver. Newborn infants have high AFP, but this falls to a low level by the end of the first year and remains low for life. Therefore, a high adult level of AFP (> 500 ng/ml) acts as a marker for some malignancies, which could be a liver tumour, specific germ-cell testicular or ovarian tumours, lymphomas, lung, breast or colon tumours. Pregnant women with AFP levels higher than expected could be carrying a foetus with a **neural tube defect**. This disorder is an abnormal development of the foetal brain and spinal cord, and it may be associated with a lack of folic acid (vitamin $B_9$) in the maternal diet and blood. However, an unexpected AFP result detected during pregnancy may be due to a multiple pregnancy, foetal death, a foetal chromosomal defect or simply inaccurate dating of the pregnancy.

 **Test: Myoglobin.** This protein binds and stores oxygen in skeletal and cardiac muscle. It can release this oxygen to the mitochondria for energy production when oxygen is low. Blood plasma levels are normally very low (6–85 ng/ml) because it is normally restricted to muscle tissue. Raised levels indicate muscle trauma, which causes release of myoglobin into circulation. It is not specific to cardiac muscle, and blood levels can rise following intramuscular injection, exhaustive exercise, electrical shock cardioversion, skeletal muscle disease and muscle trauma. A medical history can help to exclude the non-cardiac causes. The myoglobin test is most accurate in assessing acute myocardial infarction if done within 6 hours of the onset of symptoms.

*Vitamins (Table 4.3 and Figure 4.4)*

The word 'vitamins' comes from 'vital amines'. Being vital means that they are required in the diet since most cannot be synthesised in the body, although some are stored in the liver. Blood tests for B complex or specific B vitamins are usually done when the symptoms suggest a possible lack of that vitamin in the diet (i.e. vitamin malnutrition) or less often when the symptoms indicate vitamin excess. Further details of each of the major vitamins can be found in Table 7.3 (page 142).

 **Test: Vitamin A (retinol) and retinal-binding protein (RBP).** Being fat-soluble, vitamin A is stored in the liver and can be recovered from the liver when required for use. It is necessary for cell reproduction, embryonic development and vision. If the blood levels of retinol are too low, this could be the result of inadequate dietary supply or inability to absorb the vitamin from the bowel. Low blood levels cause night blindness (difficulty seeing in the dark, i.e. the eyes do not adjust well to low light), regular infections, hair loss, skin rashes and dry, inflamed eyes. **Hypervitaminosis A** (or **vitamin A toxicity**) is caused by excess of retinol caused by excessive intake of high-dose supplements. This causes visual and skin changes, bone pain, and liver damage. Retinol is carried in the circulation by a protein called **retinol-binding protein** (**RBP**), and therefore the amount of retinol

*Table 4.3* Blood tests for vitamins

| Vitamin | Normal test result | Normal test result (SI units) | Notes |
|---|---|---|---|
| A (retinol) | 30–80 µg/dL | 1.05–2.80 µmol/L | Fat-soluble vitamin stored in the liver |
| Retinol-binding protein (RBP) | 40–60 µg/mL | 264.8–397.2 µmol/L | |
| $B_1$ (thiamine) | 2.5–7.5 µg/dL | 74–222 nmol/L | Water-soluble vitamin requires daily intake |
| $B_2$ (riboflavin) | 4–24 µg/L | 106–638 nmol/L | Water-soluble vitamin requires daily intake |
| $B_3$ (niacin or nicotinic acid) | 0.2–1.8 µg/mL | 0.9–8.2 µmol/L | Water-soluble vitamin requires daily intake |
| $B_5$ (pantothenic acid) | 0.2–1.8 µg/mL | 0.9–8.2 µmol/L | Water-soluble vitamin requires daily intake |
| $B_6$ (pyridoxine) | 5–30 ng/mL | 20–121 nmol/L | Water-soluble vitamin requires daily intake |
| $B_7$ (biotin) | 200–500 pg/mL | 0.82–2.05 nmol/L | Water-soluble vitamin requires daily intake |
| $B_9$ (folate, folic acid) | Adult 5–25 ng/mL  Child 5–21 ng/mL | 11–57 nmol/L  11–47.6 nmol/L | Water-soluble vitamin requires daily intake  The synthetic form of B9 is folic acid found in supplements; folate occurs naturally in foods |
| RBC folate | Adult 166–640 ng/mL  Child > 160 ng/mL | 376–1450 nmol/L | Water-soluble vitamin requires daily intake |
| B12 (cyanocobalamin) | 160–950 pg/mL | 118–701 pmol/L | Water-soluble vitamin requires daily intake |
| C (ascorbic acid) | 0.4–1.5 mg/dL | 23–85 µmol/L | Water-soluble vitamin requires daily intake |
| 25-hydroxy-vitamin D (calcifediol) | 30–100 ng/mL | 75–250 nmol/L | Fat-soluble vitamin stored in the liver |
| E (tocopherol) | Adult 5.5–17 µg/mL  Child 4–18.4 µg/mL | 127.7–394.7 µmol/L  92.9–427.3 µmol/L | Fat-soluble vitamin stored in the liver |
| $K_1$ (phylloquinone) | 0.13–1.9 ng/mL | 0.29–2.64 nmol/L | Fat-soluble vitamin stored in the liver |

transported in the blood depends on the liver's ability to produce adequate RBP. Retinol levels in circulation correlates well with the levels of RBP, and the test for RBP is easier and cheaper than the retinol test, therefore, the RBP test is often used instead.

**Test: Vitamin $B_1$ (thiamine).** Thiamine is essential for energy production. Low levels of thiamine cause a disease called **beriberi**.[1] It would be caused by malnutrition due to alcoholism, which is often associated with a poor diet, anorexia, starvation or malabsorption. A lack can result in fatigue, headache, nausea and depression.

**Test: Vitamin $B_2$ (riboflavin).** A low riboflavin may be due to poor intake in the diet, alcoholism, diarrhoea or malabsorption.

**Test: Vitamin $B_3$ (niacin or nicotinic acid).** Deficiency of niacin in the diet can result in fatigue, vomiting, insomnia and **pellagra**,[2] the symptoms including memory loss, glossitis, skin rash and mental disturbances.

**Test: Vitamin $B_5$ (pantothenic acid).** Pantothenic acid deficiency may cause rashes, sore tongue, tingling or burning of the hands or feet (called **peripheral neuropathy**), anaemia, depression and memory loss.

**Test: Vitamin B$_6$ (pyridoxine).** Lack of pyridoxine can cause fatigue, muscle pains, confusion, depression and anaemia.

**Test: Vitamin B$_9$ (folic acid).** Folic acid deficiency during early pregnancy has been linked to foetal neural tube defects (e.g. spina bifida).

**Test: Vitamin B$_{12}$ (cyanocobalamin).** Cyanocobalamin deficiency causes **pernicious anaemia**, i.e. fatigue, glossitis and nerve damage.

**Test: Vitamin C (ascorbic acid).** Vitamin C intake creates a total body pool of about 1,500 g. Daily intake is necessary to top up this pool. Vitamin C is required for tissue health and repair, in particular the maturity of collagen. Lack of vitamin C causes **scurvy**.[3]

**Test: Vitamin D (calcifediol).** The synthesis of vitamin D is shown in Figure 4.4. The final stage is the production of **calcitriol**, the biologically active form. The main role of calcitriol is to regulate the concentration of calcium and phosphates (both components of bone), thus promoting bone development. It also acts to promote cell growth and is

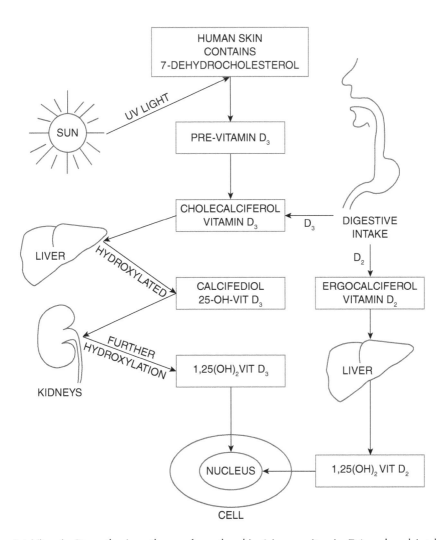

*Figure 4.4* Vitamin D synthesis pathways from the skin (via pre-vitamin D$_3$) and oral intake (via vitamin D$_2$).

involved in healthy neuromuscular and immune functions. A blood level less than 30 ng/mL indicates vitamin D deficiency, and less than 12 ng/mL is a serious deficiency. This may lead to **rickets** in children and **osteomalacia** in adults.[4]

*Test: Vitamin E (tocopherols).* Vitamin E is a group of related compounds that act as important **antioxidants**, preventing the potential cell damage caused by **free radicals**. Other functions include promoting the immune system and red blood cell development. Deficiency is considered to be below 3.0 µg/mL in children aged 3 months and below 4.0 µg/mL in children aged 2 years.

*Test: Vitamin K$_1$ (phylloquinone).* This vitamin exists in various forms, K$_1$ (**phylloquinone**) being the naturally occurring form, found in vegetables and dairy products. K$_2$ is a group of closely related compounds called **menaquinones** that are manufactured by the bacteria in the bowel, known as the **intestinal flora**. This intestinal source supplements the body's needs but a dietary source is still required. Vitamin K$_1$ is essential for blood clotting. Deficiency causes bleeding, bruising, heavy menstrual periods and blood in the stools and urine (Table 7.3, page 142).

*Fats and cholesterol (Figure 4.5 and Table 4.4)*

**Triglycerides** (Figure 1.7, page 6) are the main fats carried in blood plasma, but since fat and water cannot mix, the triglycerides must be transported in one of several types of **lipoproteins**, a combination of fat with protein. Lipoproteins includes **chylomicrons**, which carry fats from the digestive tract to the liver. They are formed in the wall of the small intestine during absorption. A chylomicron consists of 84% triglycerides, 7% phospholipids, 8% cholesterol and 1% protein. Other types of lipoproteins found in general circulation are as follows (the values given for contents are averaged over multiple studies; Figure 4.5):

- **Very low-density lipoprotein** (**VLDL**), which is made by the liver, contains 50% triglycerides, 18% phospholipids, 22% cholesterol and 10% protein.
- **Intermediate-density lipoprotein** (**IDL**), which is formed from the degradation of VLDL contains 31% triglycerides, 22% phospholipids, 29% cholesterol and 18% protein.
- **Low-density lipoprotein** (**LDL**) contains 8% triglycerides, 21% phospholipids, 50% cholesterol and 25% protein.
- **High-density lipoprotein** (**HDL**) contains 4% triglycerides, 29% phospholipids, 30% cholesterol and 33% protein.

LDL is sometimes called '*bad cholesterol*' because these particles can transport lipid into arterial walls, causing a build-up of fatty plaques that often precedes coronary artery disease.

*Table 4.4* Blood fats and cholesterol tests

| Plasma component | Normal test result | Normal test result (SI units) |
| --- | --- | --- |
| Triglycerides | 10–190 mg/dL | 0.11–2.15 mmol/L |
| **Cholesterol** | | |
| HDL cholesterol | 40–60 mg/dL | 1.03–1.55 mmol/L |
| LDL cholesterol | < 100 mg/dL | < 2.59 mmol/L |
| Total cholesterol | Adult < 200 mg/dL | < 5.17 mmol/L |
| | Child < 170 mg/dL | < 4.4 mmol/L |
| Total cholesterol: HDL ratio | < 5.0 | |

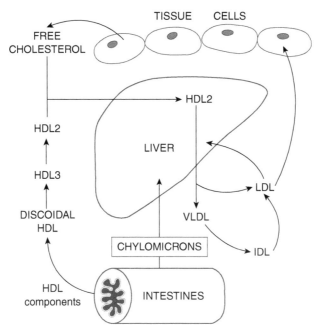

*Figure 4.5* The cholesterol cycle.

*Table 4.5* Statins

| Drug | Possible side effects | Use and other notes |
| --- | --- | --- |
| Atorvastatin | Epistaxis, hypersensitivity, muscle or joint pain, hyperglycaemia. | Hypercholesterolaemia. |
| Fluvastatin | Rare but could include muscle weakness, facial oedema, abnormal sensations. | Hypercholesterolaemia. |
| Pravastatin sodium | Rare but could include hair and scalp problems, vision and urinary impairment. | Hypercholesterolaemia. |
| Rosuvastatin | Rare but could include joint pain, haematuria, cough. | Hypercholesterolaemia. |
| Simvastatin | Rare, but could include renal damage, muscle cramps, anaemia. | Hypercholesterolaemia. With or without ezetimibe or fenofibrate. |

HDL is sometimes called '*good cholesterol*' because these particles can collect fat that has been removed from cells of the artery wall, reducing plaque formation.

The **cholesterol ratio** is calculated by dividing the total cholesterol by the HDL value (e.g. if the total cholesterol is 150, and the HDL cholesterol is 50, the ratio is 150 divided by 50, i.e. 3). This helps to predict the risk of heart attack. High risk is associated with a ratio greater than 5.

For those with high cholesterol, drugs called **statins** are often prescribed for long term oral use. These are inhibitors of the enzyme **3-hydroxy-3-methylglutaryl coenzyme A** (**HMG CoA**) which is involved in cholesterol synthesis, notably in the liver (Table 4.5).

*Blood chemistry (Table 4.6)*

**Test: Ammonia**. Ammonia ($NH_3$) is produced by bacteria in the digestive tract from protein and amino acids. It is transported to the liver where it is mostly converted to urea and glutamine. Liver efficiency can be assessed by measuring the blood ammonia level since levels will rise if the liver fails to do this conversion. Ammonia is toxic and can enter the brain across the blood-brain barrier. In the brain, ammonia causes oedema and impaired neuronal transmission. Increased blood ammonia has many other causes, including acute leukaemia, blood transfusion, bleeding into the digestive tract, smoking and renal failure.

   **Test: Bicarbonate**. Bicarbonate ($HCO_3{}^-$) is a negatively charged electrolyte found in the blood. It is essential to buffer the blood pH value to within 7.3–7.4. Bicarbonate prevents the blood from becoming acidic (i.e. pH below 7); therefore, it is part of the acid-base balance of the blood. Acidity occurs when excess free hydrogen ions ($H^+$) are released in the blood. This happens as the result of several chemical reactions. Bicarbonate reacts with

*Table 4.6* Blood chemistry tests

| Plasma component | Normal test result | Normal test result (SI units) | Notes where applicable |
|---|---|---|---|
| Ammonia (as $NH_3$) | Adult 15–50 µg/dL | 11–35 µmol/L | |
| | Child 40–80 µg/dL | 29–57 µmol/L | |
| | Newborn 90–150 µg/dL | 64–107 µmol/L | |
| Bicarbonate ($HCO_3$) | 21–28 mEq/L | 21–28 mmol/L | |
| Bilirubin (total) | 0.3–1.2 mg/dL | 2–18 µmol/L | |
| Blood urea nitrogen (BUN) | 8–23 mg/dL | 2.9–8.2 mmol/L | |
| Calcium (Ca) | 8.2–10.2 mg/dL | 2.05–2.55 mmol/L | |
| Chloride | 96–106 mEq/L | 96–106 mmol/L | |
| Copper (Cu) (total) | 70–140 µg/dL | 11.0–22.0 µmol/L | |
| Copper (free) | 10–15 µg/dL | 1.57–2.35 µmol/L | |
| Ceruloplasmin | 20–40 mg/dL | 200–400 mg/L | |
| Creatinine | 0.6–1.2 mg/dL | 53–106 µmol/L | |
| Cystatin C | 0.52–0.98 µg/mL | 0.52–0.98 mg/L | |
| Ferritin | Male 15–200 ng/mL | 15–200 µg/L | Transferrin normal saturation: 20–50% |
| | Female 12–150 ng/mL | 12–150 µg/L | |
| Transferrin | 200–380 mg/dL | 2.0–3.8 g/L | |
| Glucose | 70–99 mg/dL | 3.9–5.4 mmol/L | |
| Iron (Fe) | 60–150 µg/dL | 10.7–26.9 µmol/L | |
| Iron-binding capacity (total) | 250–400 µg/dL | 44.8–71.6 µmol/L | |
| Ketones | < 10 mg/dL | < 1.72 mmol/L | |
| Lactic acid | 4.5–19.8 mg/dL | 0.5–2.2 mmol/L | Venous blood (arterial blood is lower: 3.0–11.3 mg/dL) |
| Magnesium (Mg) | 1.5–2.5 mg/dL | 0.62–1.03 mmol/L | |
| Phosphorus | 2.3–4.7 mg/dL | 0.74–1.52 mmol/L | |
| Potassium (K) | 3.5–5.0 mEq/L | 3.5–5.0 mmol/L | |
| Selenium | 58–234 µg/L | 0.74–2.97 µmol/L | |
| Sodium (Na) | 136–142 mEq/L | 136–142 mmol/L | |
| Uric acid | 4.0–8.5 mg/dL | 0.24–0.51 mmol/L | |
| Zinc (Zn) | 50–150 µg/dL | 7.7–23.0 µmol/L | |

these hydrogen ions so they are no longer free and therefore can no longer contribute towards the pH. The reaction is:

$$H^+ + HCO_3 - \rightarrow H_2CO_3 \text{ (carbonic acid)}$$

The previously free hydrogen ions are now bound up in the carbonic acid. This can then break into carbon dioxide ($CO_2$) and water ($H_2O$):

$$H_2CO_3 \rightarrow CO_2 + H_2O$$

The carbon dioxide can be exhaled through the lungs and water excreted through the skin or the kidneys, and blood pH is maintained at 7.3–7.4.

Bicarbonate measurement is done as part of electrolyte balance assessment, during excessive diarrhoea or vomiting, breathing difficulties, fever and anaemia.

*Test: Bilirubin*. Bilirubin is a product of haemoglobin breakdown (Chapter 8). High blood levels may be due to excessive haemoglobin destruction (e.g. **haemolytic anaemia**), obstructed bile drainage from the liver (Figure 8.11, page 166) or liver disease that prevents the normal breakdown. The test forms part of the investigations of **jaundice**, which includes yellow discolouration of the skin and dark urine (page 173).

*Test: Blood urea nitrogen (BUN)*. This measures of the amount of nitrogen in urea present in the blood. Urea is produced from ammonia (see *ammonia*, page 76). The nitrogen in both ammonia and urea is toxic, but urea nitrogen is safer to transport than ammonia. Very high blood levels of urea are dangerous (**uraemia**) and may be the result of liver disease or kidney failure.

*Test: Calcium (Ca)*. This is a mineral nutrient obtained from the diet and is required for healthy bone and dentine production, nerve impulse conduction, muscle contraction and the blood clotting mechanism (Figure 4.7, page 86). Excess calcium in the blood may lead to urinary stones (renal or bladder **calculi**) since the kidneys try to remove this unwanted calcium through the urine. Blood calcium levels may also be disturbed in bone disease, parathyroid gland overactivity (**hyperparathyroidism**), various cancers and drug side effects.

*Test: Chloride (Cl)*. This is a negatively charged electrolyte ($Cl^-$). It helps to maintain the normal blood volume and pressure and the normal pH of body fluids, and it stabilises fluid balance within the tissues and cells (Chapter 6 and Chapter 7, Table 7.4). Excessive chloride in the blood (**hyperchloraemia**) is due to a lack of fluid, either inadequate intake (dehydration) or excessive loss (e.g. vomiting or diarrhoea). It is also seen in kidney disease because normal kidneys regulate electrolyte balance (Chapter 6). Low levels (**hypochloraemia**) may be due to heart failure, excessive and prolonged vomiting (where electrolytes are depleted), and conditions that cause excessive fluid build-up

*Test: Total copper (Cu), free copper and ceruloplasmin*. Copper is another mineral nutrient required in small quantities from the diet (Table 7.4, page 144). Some copper is held in the liver (20–50 μg/g of liver tissue) and muscles, but copper in the blood is largely transported bound to a protein called **ceruloplasmin**. The small portion of copper not bound to ceruloplasmin is the 'free' copper. The total copper test measures all the copper in the blood, both free and bound. The test for ceruloplasmin assesses the blood's ability to transport copper. **Wilson disease** is a genetically inherited disturbance of copper metabolism where there is a lack of ceruloplasmin. Copper is lacking in the brain (causing neurological deficits) and an excess is deposited in the liver causing liver damage (Blows 2022: 364–366).

***Test: Creatinine.*** Creatinine is a waste product from the breakdown of **creatine**, a muscle-based compound necessary for energy recycling. Approximately 2% of the creatine in the body is converted to creatinine each day. Creatinine in the blood is filtered out by the kidneys into the urine. Measuring the blood creatinine levels is an indication of how well the kidneys are working to remove it, i.e. high blood levels indicate poor renal excretion of creatinine. It can also be assessed from the urine, called a **creatinine clearance test** (Chapter 8).

***Test: Cystatin C.*** **Cysteine proteases** are enzymes that degrade proteins. Cystatin C is a cysteine protease inhibitor produced by all nucleated cells in the body and found in all body fluids. It is produced at a constant rate and excreted in the urine. Blood test measurement of cystatin C has become a test of kidney function by making it possible to assess the **glomerular filtration rate** (**GFR**) (Chapter 8). If levels of cystatin C are high, the GFR is functioning less than it should.

***Tests: Ferritin and transferrin.*** Ferritin is an iron-storage protein stored in the body's cells, notably the liver and immune system. The blood levels are relatively low. When required, ferritin combines with another protein called **transferrin**, which carries it into circulation and to the bone marrow where the iron is used in haemoglobin. Low blood ferritin suggests iron deficiency, and high ferritin may indicate an iron-storage disorder, such as **haemochromatosis**, also known as *iron overload* (too much iron in the body). This may be familial – i.e. occurs in families due to genetic error – or from other non-genetic causes.

***Test: Glucose.*** Glucose is the sugar normally found in blood as the main source of cellular energy (Chapter 1). All other sugars are converted to glucose before passing into general circulation. High blood glucose (**hyperglycaemia**) is seen in **diabetes** (Chapter 8). Low blood glucose (**hypoglycaemia**) is also seen in diabetes if too much insulin is taken or from a low sugar intake (e.g. starvation) (Chapters 7 and 8). Laboratory tests for glucose are accurate but take time for the results, and blood glucose can change quickly. A quick and simple blood test for glucose estimation is available, i.e. blood monitoring sticks, e.g. **BM-stix**. It involves a small finger prick to obtain a drop of capillary blood. This blood is placed on the reactive pad at the end of a plastic strip. The pad with the blood is slotted into a small electronic meter that measures the blood glucose content in seconds and provides a digital read-out display. The advantages are the portability of the system, making it available at any time and any place, plus the speed of obtaining a result. The disadvantage could be the accuracy, which may be affected by several factors, including not enough blood being placed on the pad. It is useful for diabetics to have an estimate of their blood glucose level so they can manage the disorder. These sticks are not suitable for monitoring blood glucose levels in neonates due to the potential for poor accuracy in these children (Rennie and Kendall 2013).

***Test: Iron (Fe).*** Iron is a natural nutrient in the diet and is required for the production of haemoglobin. It is stored in the liver. Low iron levels lead to **iron-deficiency anaemia** (Chapter 7, Table 7.4).

***Test: Iron-binding capacity (total).*** This test measures the amount of iron that can be carried in the blood. High iron-binding capacity indicates iron deficiency, and low iron-binding capacity occurs in iron overload (**haemochromatosis**; see also *test: ferritin*, page 78).

***Test: Ketones.*** These are by-products of fat metabolism (see *ketones in urine*, Chapter 8). Excessive ketones in the blood causes **ketoacidosis** due to their acidic nature, and this causes a drop in blood pH that can occur when diabetes gets out of control (Chapter 8).

***Test: Lactic acid.*** Energy for muscle activity, as in exercise, comes from glucose metabolism, resulting in **lactic acid** (also called **lactate**). The body then processes this using oxygen (*aerobic* exercise). When exercise is strenuous enough, lactic acid may accumulate in muscles because it is produced faster than the body can deliver the oxygen to process it (*anaerobic* exercise). The muscles then become acidic and this reduces the glucose to pyruvate energy pathway (Chapter 1), and the muscle becomes inefficient. The blood test measures the amount of lactic acid in circulation. Its acidic nature may cause a lowering of the blood pH (called **lactic acidosis**).

***Test: Magnesium (Mg).*** This is a natural nutrient necessary for bones, nerves and muscle function (Table 7.4, page 144), and low blood levels may occur in some diets or as part of malnutrition.

***Test: Phosphorus.*** This is also a natural nutrient required for bones and energy metabolism. Low levels are likely to occur in malnutrition (Table 7.4, page 144).

***Test: Potassium (K).*** This is an electrolyte ($K^+$) in the diet, often as the compound KCl (**potassium chloride**; Chapter 6 and Chapter 7; Table 7.4). Potassium is mostly kept within the body cells, and the low level of potassium in the blood must be kept within strict limits by renal excretion since high levels are dangerous.

***Test: Selenium (Se).*** Selenium is a nutrient within the diet required in only trace amounts (Table 7.4, page 144). Excess in the blood can be toxic (**selenosis**), and deficiency may cause no symptoms initially but can seriously affect the immune system and the heart.

***Test: Sodium (Na).*** This is an electrolyte present in the diet, often as the compound NaCl (**sodium chloride**, used as common table salt). In solution, sodium separates from the chlorine to become positively charged electrolytes ($Na^+$; see *electrolyte balance*, Chapter 6, and Table 7.4, page 144). Sodium loss from the blood through the kidneys is controlled by the hormone **aldosterone** (from the adrenal cortex; Chapter 8), and excessive sodium in the blood may be due to disturbance of this hormone.

***Test: Uric acid.*** This is derived from foods containing **purines**, which is one of the two nucleotide bases found in **DNA** (**deoxyribonucleic acid**) and **RNA** (**ribonucleic acid**; Chapter 8). Excessive uric acid in the blood can result in **gout**, where uric acid crystals form in the joint, often the toes, causing swollen and painful joints. It mostly arises from the kidneys' inability to excrete uric acid sufficiently.

***Test: Zinc.*** This is a mineral from the diet needed in small quantities (Table 7.4, page 144). Zinc deficiency is a much bigger problem than zinc excess, which has little effect on the body except maybe to affect iron and copper absorption. Deficiency can affect the skin (acne and rashes), the immune system and brain function, and it causes diarrhoea, allergies and hair loss.

*Blood enzymes (Table 4.7)*

Enzymes are usually proteins that facilitate and accelerate the function of **metabolism**, either breaking down chemical compounds (**catabolism**, e.g. in the digestive tract) or building compounds (**anabolism**, e.g. growth and muscle building). Many act within cells, while others are produced by glands and pass down ducts, acting within body

*Table 4.7* Blood enzyme tests

| Plasma component | Normal test result | Normal test result (SI units) | Notes where applicable |
|---|---|---|---|
| Alanine aminotransferase (ALT) | 10–40 U/L | 10–40 U/L | |
| Alkaline phosphatase (ALP) | 50–120 U/L | 50–120 U/L | |
| Amylase | 27–130 U/L | 0.46–2.21 µkat/L | |
| Angiotensin converting enzyme (ACE) *and related tests*: | 8–52 U/L | 0.14–0.88 µkat/L | The renin-angiotensin-aldosterone cycle is shown in Figure 3.6 (page 47) |
| Aldosterone | 7–30 ng/dL | 0.19–0.83 nmol/L | |
| Renin | 30–40 pg/mL | 0.7–1.0 pmol/L | |
| Aspartate aminotransferase (AST) | 20–48 U/L | 0.34–0.82 µkat/L | |
| Lactate dehydrogenase (LDH) | 50–200 U/L | 50–200 U/L | |
| Lipase | 0–160 U/L | 0–2.72 µkat/L | |

cavities (i.e. they are *exocrine*) such as the digestive enzymes. The amount present in the blood is usually very low (Table 4.7).

**Test: Alanine aminotransferase (ALT).** This enzyme is largely found in the liver, with small amounts in other organs and low levels found in the blood. Any rise in the blood level indicates a potential liver disorder or injury, causing ALT to be released into circulation. ALT is a transaminase enzyme that switches an amine group ($NH_3$) from the amino acid alanine to alpha-ketoglutarate to form pyruvate (Chapter 1). The test is a good indicator of liver damage along with the test aspartate aminotransferase (AST) (see page 81) and is part of the investigation of jaundice.

**Test: Alkaline phosphatase (ALP).** This enzyme is concentrated in the liver, bile duct, kidney, intestines and bone, with less in other organs. It removes a phosphate group ($PO_4^{3-}$; called **dephosphorylation**) from enzymes that is part of the phosphorylation-dephosphorylation cycle of enzymes. This cycle deactivates enzymes (phosphorylation) by adding phosphates and reactivates enzymes (dephosphorylation) by removing phosphates. High or low levels of ALP in circulation indicates the presence of several pathologies somewhere in the body, but further investigations needed to localise the source.

**Test: Amylase.** This enzyme acts to reduce carbohydrates to sugars. It is present in saliva (active in the mouth) and pancreatic juice (active in the intestines). Very little should be in the blood, but if the blood level should rise it suggests a possible pancreatic disorder (e.g. pancreatitis) or blockage of the pancreatic duct. This may cause leakage of the enzyme into circulation.

**Test: Angiotensin Converting Enzyme (ACE).** This enzyme converts the hormone **angiotensin I** (from the adrenal cortex) to **angiotensin II**. **Renin** is a hormone released from the kidney when the blood passing through the kidney is at low volume or contains low salt levels. Renin activates **angiotensinogen** from the liver, creating **angiotensin I**. This is further converted to **angiotensin II** by ACE. Angiotensin II increases antidiuretic hormone (ADH; see ADH test, page 81) and promotes **aldosterone** release from the adrenal cortex (Figure 3.6, page 47). Aldosterone regulates sodium balance by acting in the kidney to conserve sodium in the body. Low aldosterone results in sodium loss in the urine. Sodium balance is important for many reasons, not least for helping to control blood pressure (see Chapters 3, 6 and 8). Angiotensin II raises blood pressure by vasoconstriction. The ACE blood test estimates the amount of ACE present in circulation because raised levels may be an indication of **sarcoidosis**, an inflammatory **granulomatous** disease of multiple organs. **Granulomas** are abnormal clumps of cells that can produce excessive ACE. The aldosterone test looks for abnormally high or low levels of aldosterone, which may be due to diseases causing malfunction of the adrenal cortex, cardiac or renal disease or consumption of very high or zero salt levels.

*Test: Aspartate aminotransferase (AST).* This is another transaminase enzyme similar to ALT (see page 80) that moves an amine ($NH_3$) from aspartate and attaches it to alpha-ketoglutarate to form glutamate. This is important in the **tricarboxylic cycle** for energy production (Figure 1.3, page 4). AST is found in the liver, but significant levels are also found in other organs, which means it is less specific to liver disorders than ALT.

*Test: Lactate dehydrogenase (LDH).* LDH is an enzyme that is involved in energy production by converting lactate (lactic acid) to pyruvate (see *lactic acid test*, page 79). This enzyme is normally low in blood plasma, but since it is present in every cell in the body it can leak into circulation when tissue is inflamed or otherwise damaged.

*Test: Lipase.* This enzyme breaks down dietary fats within the digestive system. It is produced by the pancreas and it drains into the intestines. Normally, it is at a low level in the blood. High blood levels indicate that the enzyme is leaking into circulation from a pancreatic disorder or obstructed pancreatic duct.

*Hormones (Table 4.8)*

Hormones (Table 4.8) are either protein- or fat-based compounds (**steroids**) produced by glands in the body. They pass directly into the blood (i.e. they are *endocrine* products). Their purpose is to influence the function of other tissues.

*Test: Adrenocorticotropic hormone (ACTH).* This hormone is produced by the anterior pituitary gland. It regulates the production of cortisol from the adrenal cortex. Above or below normal levels of ACTH in the blood suggests a problem with the anterior pituitary or the adrenal cortex.

*Test: Adrenaline.* This hormone is produced by the adrenal medulla at times of excitement or fear. Adrenaline, along with the other **catecholamines** (noradrenaline and dopamine), prepares the body for 'fight or flight' by enhancing the sympathetic response. High adrenaline in the blood may be due to a persistent state of stress, or it could be a rare, adrenaline-producing tumour of the adrenal medulla called a **pheochromocytoma**.

*Test: Antidiuretic hormone (ADH).* This hormone is produced by the hypothalamus and released into circulation from the posterior pituitary gland. It aids with water balance in the body by preventing water loss from the kidneys (Chapter 8). Abnormal levels of ADH in the blood may indicate a problem with either the hypothalamus or pituitary gland (e.g. a head injury or tumour).

*Test: Calcitonin.* Calcitonin is a hormone produced by C-cells in the thyroid gland and is involved in regulating the blood calcium level. It is important in bone metabolism. There are several causes for high calcitonin levels in the blood, including smoking, overweight, renal disease, lung and thyroid cancers.

*Test: Cortisol.* This is another adrenal cortex hormone (Chapter 3). It is stimulated by the adrenocorticotrophic hormone (ACTH; see *ACTH blood test*). Cortisol has several functions, especially in relation to anti-stress, and higher levels are produced during

*Table 4.8* Blood hormone tests

| Plasma component | Normal test result | Normal test result (SI units) | Notes where applicable |
|---|---|---|---|
| Adrenocorticotropic hormone (ACTH) | < 120 pg/mL | < 26 pmol/L | There is some diurnal variation |
| Adrenaline | < 60 pg/dL | < 330 pmol/L | |
| Antidiuretic hormone (ADH) | 1–5 pg/mL | 0.9–4.6 pmol/L | |
| Calcitonin | < 19 pg/mL | < 19 ng/L | |
| Cortisol | 5–25 µg/dL (8 a.m.) | 138–690 nmol/L | There is some diurnal variation |
| | 3–16 µg/dL (4 p.m.) | 83–442 nmol/L | |
| Erythropoietin (EPO) | 5–36 mIU/mL | 5–36 IU/L | |
| Follicle-stimulating hormone (FSH) | Male 1.42–15.4 mIU/L | 1.4–15.4 IU/L | Variations according to gender and female ovarian cycle |
| | Female 1.37–9.9 mIU/L (follicular) | 1.3–9.9 IU/L | |
| | 1.09–9.2 mIU/L (luteal) | 1.0–9.2 IU/L | |
| | 6.17–17.2 mIU/L (ovulation) | 6.1–17.2 IU/L | |
| | 19.3–100.6 mIU/L (postmenopausal) | 19.3–100.6 IU/L | |
| Growth hormone | < 10 ng/mL | < 10 µg/L | Fasting |
| Insulin | 5.0–20 µU/mL | 34.7–138.9 pmol/L | Fasting |
| Insulin-like growth factor | 130–450 ng/mL | 130–450 µg/L | |
| Luteinising hormone (LH) | Male 2.0–12.0 mIU/L | 2.0–12.0 IU/L | |
| | Female 2.0–15.0 mIU/L (follicular) | 2.0–15.0 IU/L | |
| | 22.0–105.0 mIU/L (ovulation) | 22.0–105.0 IU/L | |
| | 0.6–19.0 mIU/L (luteal) | 0.6–19.0 IU/L | |
| | 16.0–64.0 mIU/L (postmenopausal) | 16.0–64.0 IU/L | |
| Noradrenaline | 110–410 pg/mL | 650–2,423 nmol/L | |
| Oestradiol (E2) | Male < 20 pg/mL | < 184 pmol/L | |
| | Female 20–350 pg/mL (follicular) | 73–1,285 pmol/L | |
| | 150–750 pg/mL (ovulation) | 551–2,753 pmol/L | |
| | 30–450 pg/mL (luteal) | 110–1,652 pmol/L | |
| | < 59 pg/mL (postmenopausal) | < 218 pmol/L | |
| Parathyroid hormone | 10–50 pg/mL | 10–50 ng/L | |
| Progesterone | Male 0.13–0.97 ng/mL | 0.4–3.1 nmol/L | |
| | Female 0.1–0.7 ng/mL (follicular) | 0.5–2.2 nmol/L | |
| | 2–25 ng/mL (luteal) | 6.4–79.5 nmol/L | |
| Prolactin | 1–25 ng/mL | 1–25 µg/L | Non-lactating |
| Testosterone | Male 300–1,200 ng/dL | 10.4–41.6 nmol/L | |
| | Female < 85 ng/dL | < 2.95 nmol/L | |
| ***Thyroid tests*** | | | |
| Thyroid-stimulating hormone (TSH) | 0.5–5.0 µIU/mL | 0.5–5.0 mIU/L | |
| $T_3$ total | 80–200 ng/dL | 0.9–2.8 nmol/L | |
| $T_4$ free (FT4) | 0.9–2.3 ng/dL | 12–30 pmol/L | |
| $T_4$ total | 5.5–12.5 µg/dL | 71–160 nmol/L | |
| Thyroxin-binding globulin | 10–26 µg/dL | 129–335 nmol/L | |

stressful situations. High levels may be due to a pituitary gland tumour producing too much ACTH or an adrenal cortex tumour producing too much cortisol. Low levels occur in **Addison disease** or a pituitary disorder producing inadequate ACTH.

*Test: Erythropoietin (EPO).* This hormone stimulates red blood cell production from the bone marrow. It is produced by the kidneys when blood oxygen levels are low. The release of EPO promotes new erythrocyte production – and therefore additional haemoglobin in circulation – to improve oxygen-carrying capability. The test would help to determine the reasons for the presence of **polycythaemia** (excessive red cells in circulation) or **anaemia** (low haemoglobin level in the blood possibly due to low red cell numbers).

*Test: Follicle-stimulating hormone (FSH).* This is a hormone produced by the anterior pituitary gland. It stimulates the development of ova in ovaries and sperm in testes. FSH blood levels drop naturally in women during pregnancy and may be raised normally after menopause. Abnormal levels have to be seen in the context of age, gender and stage of life (e.g. puberty and menopause). Levels may become abnormal due to poor diet, pituitary tumours, alcohol or drug abuse and for genetic reasons.

*Test: Growth hormone.* This is another anterior pituitary hormone. The test is not routine but may be requested to help assess poor growth and development in children and adolescents or problems concerning muscle bulk or bone density in adults. It may help to assess pituitary activity.

*Test: Insulin.* This hormone is produced by the beta-cells of the Islets of Langerhans in the pancreas. Its role is to lower blood glucose levels (**glucagon** is the hormone that raises blood glucose levels). Insulin promotes glucose uptake into cells. Low insulin blood levels are seen in type 1 diabetes and may also be present in some patients with type 2 diabetes (Chapter 8). Blood insulin levels are tested when blood glucose levels are abnormal (e.g. **hyperglycaemia**, high blood glucose, or **hypoglycaemia**, low blood glucose). The test for C-peptide may also be requested when investigating blood glucose levels (Figure 4.2 and Table 4.2, and see *C-peptide test,* page 69).

*Test: Insulin-like growth factor-1.* This hormone regulates the function of growth hormone in children and continues to have an anabolic function in adults (see *growth hormone,* earlier). It has a similar structure to insulin, and blood levels relate closely with the levels of growth hormone, making it a useful additional test for growth problems.

*Test: Luteinising hormone (LH).* This is a hormone produced by the anterior pituitary gland and acts on the ovaries, causing **ovulation** and acts on the testes to produce testosterone. Measurement of the blood level is done when problems occur with the reproductive system, e.g. investigating the causes of early or late puberty, low testosterone or potential infertility.

*Test: Noradrenaline.* Like adrenaline, this hormone is produced by the adrenal medulla during stress and has similar functions (see *adrenaline blood test,* page 81).

*Test: Oestradiol (E2).* This is the most potent of several oestrogen hormones produced by the ovaries. There is a natural variation in oestrogen level across the 24 hours (i.e. a **diurnal** variation). Oestrogen has several functions, many of which relate to the female reproductive system and secondary sexual characteristics (e.g. breast formation). Blood oestrogen is tested as part of assessment of the female reproductive system, especially for ovarian function.

*Test: Parathyroid hormone (PTH).* This hormone is produced by the parathyroid gland. It regulates blood calcium levels. Low PTH allows calcium to be stored in bone and raised PTH causes a release of calcium from bone. It can be done at the same time as the calcium and phosphorous blood tests (see page 76) as part of an assessment of bone calcium density or to investigate parathyroid function.

**Test: Progesterone.** This hormone is produced by the ovaries, mostly over the second half (days 15 to 28) of the ovarian cycle (i.e. after ovulation). One week after ovulation, progesterone levels should peak, and this is usually the time when the test is done. Progesterone prepares the uterus for pregnancy should the ovum become fertilised. It is likely to be part of a group of tests that will assess ovarian function.

**Test: Prolactin.** This is a hormone from the anterior pituitary gland that promotes breast milk production during lactation. The blood levels are low during the time when women are not breastfeeding and also in males. High levels at inappropriate times may indicate a benign tumour of the pituitary gland called a **prolactinoma** that produces too much prolactin.

**Test: Testosterone.** This is mostly produced by the testes and is the main **androgen** hormone. It is essential for sperm production and the secondary sexual characteristics, including muscle- and bone-building and male libido. Testosterone peaks during the teens and early twenties and gradually declines with age. Low testosterone production (**hypogonadism**) may cause low sperm count, erectile dysfunction, low libido and many other physical problems concerning body growth and sexual development.

**Test: Thyroid-stimulating hormone (TSH).** This is another hormone produced by the anterior pituitary gland. It stimulates the **thyroid gland** to produce thyroid hormone, a combination of two hormones: $T_3$ (**triiodothyronine**) and $T_4$ (**tetraiodothyronine**; Figure 4.6). Thyroid hormone is mostly transported in the blood by a globulin protein.

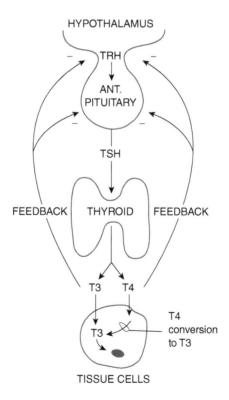

*Figure 4.6* Thyroid hormone circulation and feedback.

Together, $T_3$ and $T_4$ promote metabolism and are very important for growth and development. The related tests are for $T_3$ ***total*** (the full amount of $T_3$ in circulation), $T_4$ ***free*** (***FT4***; the amount of $T_4$ in circulation that is not bound to protein) and $T_4$ ***total*** (the full amount of $T_4$, bound and unbound, in circulation). The test for ***thyroxin-binding globulin*** is to measure the amount of globulin available for transporting thyroid hormone in circulation. The combination of these tests is used to assess for possible **thyrotoxicosis** (also called **hyperthyroidism**), which is excessive thyroid hormone in circulation. It may be primary (i.e. caused by the thyroid gland itself producing too much thyroid hormone) or secondary (caused by an anterior pituitary problem producing too much TSH). It is vital to distinguish between these two causes of hyperthyroidisms so that treatment can be targeted at the correct gland. **Hypothyroidsim** (also called **myxoedema**) is low thyroid hormone levels in circulation.

*Clotting factors (Figure 4.7 and Table 4.9)*

Blood needs to clot to prevent bleeding to death (called **exsanguination**) at the time of injury.

There is a clotting mechanism involving the chemical interactions between a number of proteins and other factors, which ultimately results in a solid clot (called a **thrombus**; Table 4.9, Figure 4.7).

Some of these factors may be in low quantity or even missing in some conditions, and this makes the clotting mechanism fail, causing a haemorrhage that is difficult to control. Blood tests are available to check the levels of these factors (Table 4.9). Also shown are the results of some coagulation times (**partial thromboplastin time, PTT, activated partial thromboplastin time, aPTT**, and **prothrombin time, PT**). They are an indication of how fast blood will clot (shown in seconds). PTT over 100 seconds and aPTT over 70 seconds suggest a high risk of bleeding.

As prophylaxis in some cardiac disorders (e.g. rheumatic heart disease) or following heart surgery, drugs are often used to prevent thrombus formation. Anticoagulants are

*Table 4.9* Blood clotting factors

| Clotting factor | Normal test result | Normal test result (SI units) | Notes where applicable |
|---|---|---|---|
| Activated coagulation time (ACT) | 80–160 secs | | |
| Antithrombin | 21–30 mg/dL | 210–300 mg/L | |
| Bleeding time | 2–9 mins | | |
| Coagulation factor I (fibrinogen) | 150–400 mg/dL | 1.5–4.0 g/L | |
| Coagulation factor II (prothrombin) | 70–130% | | |
| Partial thromboplastin time (PTT) | 60–70 secs | | |
| Activated partial thromboplastin time (aPTT) | 30–40 secs | | PTT with added activator to speed the reaction and results in a narrow time range |
| Prothrombin time (PT) | 10–20 secs | | |

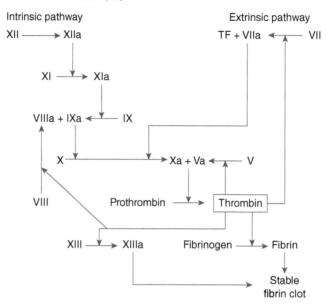

*Figure 4.7* Blood clotting mechanism via the intrinsic (caused by internal damage to blood vessels) and extrinsic (caused by external injury to tissues) pathways. The factors are numbered in Roman numerals (e.g. X, etc.) where 'a' is the activated form (e.g. Xa). Thrombin is a key component that activates VII to VIIa, XIII to XIIIa and fibrinogen to fibrin, the main substance of the clot.

mostly given by mouth on a long-time basis and work best on the venous side of the circulation where the blood is moving slowly. Included are the vitamin K antagonists (Table 4.10). Vitamin K is essential for blood clotting and vitamin K antagonists prevent this from acting.

Other anticoagulant drugs (e.g. the heparins) are given by subcutaneous or intravenous injection when required to act quickly. The heparins are divided into **heparin** (**unfractionated**) and the **low molecular weight** heparins (Table 4.10). Unfractionated heparin acts rapidly but has a shorter duration of action than the low molecular weight heparins.

*Immunity (Table 4.11)*

The immune system involves specialised blood cells and their protein products, plus chemical agents, all dedicated to protecting the body against foreign organisms (called **antigens**) such as bacteria and viruses. The system involves killing any agents that have gained entry to the body. The cells are **leukocytes** (white blood cells), of which the **lymphocytes** are shown in Table 4.11 (other leukocytes are in Table 4.14). Lymphocytes bearing receptors called CD4 and CD8 (CD = cluster differentiation) are important regarding the **human immunodeficiency virus** (**HIV**). Tests for CD4 and CD8 lymphocytes are used to assess and monitor the immune system in response to HIV infection and treatment.

Other immune system elements are listed in Table 4.11. These include the **immunoglobulins** (Ig; **antibodies**). There are five classes of antibodies IgA, IgG, IgM, IgD and IgE. They are proteins that are specifically against certain antigens. The last two (IgD and IgE) are naturally low in quantity, but the levels would rise if their specific antigens entered the

*Table 4.10* Anticoagulant drugs

| Drug | Possible side effects | Use and other notes |
|---|---|---|
| Acenocoumarol | Rare but could include liver damage, loss of appetite. | Vitamin K antagonists. |
| Phenindione | Urine discolouration, kidney damage, reduce white cell count, hepatitis. | Vitamin K antagonists. |
| Warfarin sodium | Liver malfunction. | Vitamin K antagonists. |
| Heparin (unfractionated) | Adrenal malfunction, hypokalaemia, thrombocytopenia. | Venous thrombosis and pulmonary emboli. For injection or infusion. |
| Bemiparin sodium | Epidural haematoma. | Deep vein thrombosis. Low molecular weight heparin. |
| Dalteparin sodium | Haemorrhage. | Deep vein thrombosis. Low molecular weight heparin. |
| Enoxaparin sodium | Haemorrhagic anaemia, headache, hypersensitivity. | Deep vein thrombosis. Low molecular weight heparin. |
| Tinzaparin sodium | Anaemia. | Deep vein thrombosis. Low molecular weight heparin. |

*Table 4.11* Blood immunity tests

| Plasma component | Normal test result | Normal test result (SI units) | Notes where applicable |
|---|---|---|---|
| CD4 lymphocyte count | 500–1,500/mm$^3$ | | |
| CD4/CD8 ratio | 0.9–2.0 | | |
| CD8 lymphocyte count | 150–1,000/mm$^3$ | | |
| Complement component C3 | 1,200–1,500 µg/dL | 1.2–1.5 g/L | |
| Complement component C4 | 350–600 µg/dL | 0.35–0.60 g/L | |
| Hepatitis A | Negative | | Antiviral hepatitis A antibodies |
| Hepatitis B | HBsAg negative = no current infection; immune status depends on HBsAb (anti-HBs) being positive | | Three tests needed to confirm status: HBsAg (surface antigen); HBsAb (anti-HBs); HBcAb (anti-HBc) |
| Hepatitis C | Negative (non-reactive) | | Antiviral hepatitis C antibodies; further tests are available to search for the viral antigen |
| Human immunodeficiency virus (HIV) test | Negative | | HIV antibodies |
| IgA | 0–83 mg/dL (< 1 year), then rises with age until 50–350 mg/dL (adult) | 0–0.83 g/L  0.5–3.5 g/L | 15% of all antibodies in blood |
| IgG | 231–1,411 mg/dL (< 1 year), then rises with age until 600–1,560 mg/dL (adult) | 2.31–14.11 g/L  6.0–15.6 g/L | 80% of all antibodies in blood |

*(Continued)*

*Table 4.11* (Continued)

| Plasma component | Normal test result | Normal test result (SI units) | Notes where applicable |
|---|---|---|---|
| IgM | 0–145 mg/dL (< 1 year), then varies with age until 54–222 mg/L (adult) | 0–1.45 g/L

0.5–2.2 g/L | 5% of all antibodies in blood |
| IgD | 0.5–3.0 mg/dL | 5–30 mg/L | 0.2% of all antibodies in blood |
| IgE | 0–1,500 µg/L | 0–1.5 mg/L | Trace quantity in blood |
| Prostate-specific antigen (PSA) | 0–4 ng/mL | 0–4 µg/L | Figure given for males |
| Rheumatoid factor | < 30 IU/mL | < 30 kIU/L | |

body. The **complement system** (**C3** and **C4** are shown) is a blood-based chemical cascade that, if activated, results in killing antigens (see *type II reaction*, Chapter 15, page 330).

Blood tests for specific diseases look for either antibodies created to fight that disease (e.g. **hepatitis A** and **HIV**) or a combination of both antibodies and viral antigen (e.g. **hepatitis B**, **hepatitis C**).

*Test: Prostate-specific antigen (PSA).* This protein is produced by the cells of the **prostate gland**. The test may show raised levels in males with **benign prostate hyperplasia** (**BPH**) and those with **prostate cancer**. These are two different disorders. In BPH, the word *benign* indicates that it is not cancer, and *hyperplasia* is an enlargement of the gland due to extra cell growth. Because PSA is raised in both conditions, additional assessment is required, including physical examination and taking into account the risk factors, to exclude or confirm the presence of prostate cancer.

*Test: Rheumatoid factor (RF).* This antibody is found in the blood of about 80% of those with **rheumatoid arthritis**. It is not normally found in blood. About 20% of people without rheumatoid arthritis are RF-positive (false positives), so it is not 100% reliable. The antibody attacks the body's own tissues, causing inflammation, particularly in the smaller joints of the fingers in older people.

### Blood gases (Table 4.12)

Blood carries the gases **oxygen** to the tissues and **carbon dioxide** to the lungs (Chapter 5). $PO_2$ is the partial pressure of oxygen and $PCO_2$ is the partial pressure of carbon dioxide (Chapter 5). The letter 'a' indicates in arterial blood (Table 4.12). Venous blood gives different values that are of little clinical significance.

*Test: $PaO_2$* is the partial pressure of oxygen in arterial blood.

*Test: $PaCO_2$* is the partial pressure of carbon dioxide in arterial blood.

*Test: $O_2$ saturation.* This means the amount of oxygen carried by the haemoglobin inside the red blood cells. Arterial blood should be close to 100%.

*Test: pH.*[5] This is the acid-base scale for indicating the acidity or alkalinity of a fluid. The scale runs from strong acidity at pH 1, neutral at pH 7 and strong alkaline at pH 14 (Chapter 8, Figure 8.14, page 173). Blood pH is stabilised at pH 7.4, with very little tolerated movement up or down. Carbon dioxide concentrations in circulation have a significant impact on blood pH values (see *respiratory acidosis*, Chapter 5).

*Table 4.12* Blood gases

| Blood gas | Normal result | Notes |
|---|---|---|
| PaO$_2$ | 80–100 mmHg | Arterial blood |
| PaCO$_2$ | 35–42 mmHg | Arterial blood |
| O$_2$ saturation of Hb | 94–100% | |
| pH | 7.35–7.45 | Arterial blood |

*Table 4.13* Blood toxin tests

| Toxin | Normal result | Notes where applicable |
|---|---|---|
| Arsenic (As) | Negative | |
| Cadmium (Cd) | Negative | |
| Chromium (Cr) | Negative | |
| Drugs (e.g. alcohol, barbiturates, opiates, amphetamines etc.) | Negative | Time limits apply to all drug screening since they are eliminated by the kidneys, thus reducing the blood level; this also makes urine a useful means of screening |
| Lead (Pb) | Negative | |
| Mercury (Hg) | Negative | |

*Blood tests for toxic substances (Table 4.13)*

Toxic substances (Table 4.13) will be eliminated as quickly as possible to minimise the damage they could do. Elimination may include processing by the liver and removal from the blood by the kidneys, making these organs the most susceptible to toxic damage. The brain is also susceptible to those toxins capable of crossing the blood-brain barrier. Screening for toxins must be done as soon as possible before the blood level falls (Table 4.13). Urine is also a useful substance to screen for toxins (Chapter 8).

**Test: Arsenic.** This is most toxic in its inorganic form (i.e. not chemically bound to an organic substance). Exposure may be through ingestion or during industrial processes using arsenic. Severe exposure can cause red cell destruction (**haemolysis**), shock and rapid death.

**Test: Cadmium.** This is used in several industrial processes. It is highly toxic and inhaled cadmium dust is dangerous to the lungs and kidneys, causing renal failure. Cadmium compounds are also carcinogenic.

**Test: Chromium.** Concentration of chromium inside cells damages DNA and inhaled chromium dust is carcinogenic. Especially dangerous is **hexavalent chromium** (chromium 6) as part of a larger compound. This damages multiple organs and body systems and can be carcinogenic. The use of chromium in several industrial processes may mean that workers in this environment could be exposed if not properly protected.

**Test: Lead.** Lead poisoning is now established and can be prevented in industries using the metal. Lead is toxic in two ways: (1) it binds to enzymes and mimics other metals, becoming substituted for other metals in metabolic processes, e.g. during haemoglobin production leading to anaemia; (2) the brain is particularly susceptible to lead poisoning by passing through the blood-brain barrier which disturbs neuronal development in children. It also disrupts the normal release of the neurotransmitters dopamine and glutamate in the brain.

**Test: Mercury.** Mercury is a metal that is liquid at room temperature. It is poorly absorbed through the digestive tract and skin, but mercury vapour is easily absorbed through the lungs when inhaled. It is quickly transported to the brain and affects multiple cognitive functions, particularly in children. It inhibits brain development by preventing myelin sheath formation and causes neurological birth defects in foetuses.

### Blood cells

The cells in blood are:

- **red blood cells** (**RBCs**, also called **erythrocytes**)
- **white blood cells** (**WBCs**, also called **leucocytes**)
- **platelets** (or **thrombocytes**; Figure 4.8; Bain 2017).

Erythrocytes carry **haemoglobin** (**Hb**), which accounts for about 33% of the cell weight and gives blood its red colour. Haemoglobin binds the gases oxygen and carbon dioxide (Chapter 5). Like all blood cells, erythrocytes are developed in bone marrow, but as

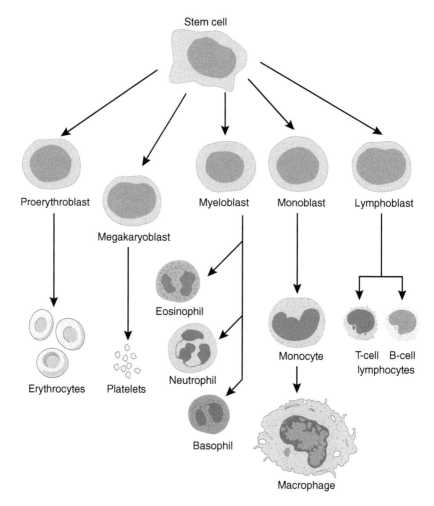

*Figure 4.8* Blood cells derived from bone marrow stem cells.

mature cells they have no nucleus, and therefore their survival in circulation is limited to about 120 days. They are continually being replaced by new ones.

White cells are nucleated and last longer. Their role is to fight infection, part of the body's defence strategy. Several kinds of WBCs exist: **lymphocytes**, which use various mechanisms to kill invading organisms (**antigens** are foreign organisms, i.e. anything that provokes an immune reaction), and **monocytes**, which are **phagocytic** (i.e. they engulf and destroy antigens). Lymphocytes and monocytes are **agranulocytes**, i.e. there are no granules in their cytoplasm. There are various types of **granulocytes**, i.e. they do have granules in their cytoplasm. The types of granulocytes are **neutrophils**, **eosinophils** and **basophils**, and these release important chemicals as part of the defensive role. **Platelets** are cell fragments, being the breakdown product of larger cells called **megakaryocytes** (Figure 4.8). They help to control blood loss following injury to blood vessels either by blocking small holes in the vessel wall if the injury is microscopic or by triggering the blood-clotting mechanism.

### *Blood tests (cells, Table 4.14)*

The normal numbers of blood cells (red, white and platelets) are shown Table 4.14.

*Table 4.14* Blood cell tests. The normal average number of blood cells varies between the different types

| Blood cell | Normal test result | Normal test result (SI units) | Notes where applicable |
|---|---|---|---|
| Basophils | 0–200 per µL | 0–0.2 × 10$^9$ per L | |
| Eosinophils | 0–450 per µL | 0–0.45 × 10$^9$ per L | |
| Erythrocyte (red blood cells) count | Male 4.6–6.0 × 10$^6$ per µL<br>Female 3.9–5.5 × 10$^6$ per µL | 4.6–6.0 × 10$^{12}$ per L<br>3.9–5.5 × 10$^{12}$ per L | |
| Erythrocyte sedimentation rate (ESR) | Male 0–22 mm/hour<br>Female 0–29 mm/hour | | Under 50-year-old female < 20 mm/hour<br>Under 50-year-old male < 15 mm/hour |
| Glycosylated haemoglobin or HbA1c | 4.0–5.6% | | |
| Glucose-6-phosphate dehydrogenase (G-6-PD) | 10.0–14.0 U/g Hb | 0.65–0.9 U/mol Hb | |
| Haematocrit (packed cell volume, PCV) | Male 41–50%<br>Female 35–45% | 0.41–0.50<br>0.35–0.45<br>Fraction of 1 | |
| Haemoglobin (Hb) | Male 13.5–17.5 g/dL<br>Female 12.0–15.5 g/dL<br>Child 12–14 g/dL<br>Newborn 14.5–24.5 g/dL | 135–175 g/L<br>120–155 g/L<br>120–140 g/L<br>145–245 g/L | |
| Haemoglobin-binding protein, haptoglobin (HPT) | 40–180 mg/dL | 0.4–1.8 g/L | |
| Lymphocytes | 1,000–4,800/µL | 1.0–4.8 × 10$^9$/L | |

*(Continued)*

*Table 4.14* (Continued)

| Blood cell | Normal test result | Normal test result (SI units) | Notes where applicable |
|---|---|---|---|
| Mean corpuscular volume (MCV) | 80–100 µm³ | 80–100 fL | |
| Mean corpuscular Hb (MCH) | 27–33 pg/cell | 1.70–2.05 fmol/cell | |
| Mean corpuscular Hb concentration (MCHC) | 33–37 g Hb/cell | 330–370 g/L | |
| Monocytes | 0–800/µL | $0–0.8 \times 10^9$/L | |
| Neutrophils | 1,800–7,800/µL | $1.8–7.8 \times 10^9$/L | |
| Platelet count | $150–450 \times 10^3$/µL | $150–450 \times 10^9$/L | |
| Reticulocyte count | 1–1.5% of total RBC | | |
| White cell count (WBC) | 4,500–11,000/µL | $4.5–11.0 \times 10^9$/L | |

**Test: Erythrocyte sedimentation rate (ESR).** This measures the rate at which red cells form a sediment over one hour. It is an observation of those factors *promoting* versus those factors *resisting* sedimentation. The ERS increases due to inflammation, rheumatoid arthritis, pregnancy, anaemia, infections and some cancers. A reduced ERS occurs in polycythaemia, leukaemia and sickle-cell anaemia, low plasma protein and congestive cardiac failure (CCF).

**Test: Glycosylated haemoglobin (HbA1c).** This measures the average haemoglobin blood glucose level for the three-month period prior to the test. Haemoglobin can become *glycosylated* (bound to glucose). The more glucose there is in circulation, the greater the degree of glycosylation. Because of the limited lifespan of red blood cells and the fact that they are replaced daily, the test only shows what blood glucose levels were over the previous three months. It is a useful test for diagnosing diabetes or monitoring blood glucose levels as part of diabetic control.

**Test: Glucose-6-phosphate dehydrogenase (G-6-PD).** This is an enzyme present in the blood that protects red blood cells from the damaging effects of **reactive oxygen species** (**ROS**). These chemicals attack red cells and can cause **haemolysis** (red cell breakdown), leading to anaemia (**haemolytic anaemia**). Sudden onset anaemia or jaundice will probably require this test in order to detect any deficiency in G-6-PD. Deficiency could be due to a genetic mutation in the G-6-PG gene that can run in families.

**Test: Haematocrit (or packed cell volume, PCV).** This measures the red cell volume relative to the total blood volume. This is a guide to assessing anaemia, where the volume of red cells is likely to decrease due to lower numbers or smaller cells. The haematocrit will also decrease if the plasma increases. An increase in the red cell volume may occur in severe dehydration, causing the plasma volume to reduce.

**Test: Haemoglobin (Hb)** This protein inside red blood cells carries oxygen. Low haemoglobin in circulation carries inadequate oxygen causing anaemia, and this may be due to low red cell numbers or normal numbers carrying reduced haemoglobin. It is a common test used to assess risk of anaemia, e.g. tiredness, breathless and pallor.

**Test: Haemoglobin-binding protein (haptoglobin, HPT).** This protein is produced by the liver and binds with free haemoglobin, i.e. haemoglobin released from the red blood cell during red cell breakdown. It prevents haemoglobin destruction while still in circulation, preventing iron loss and protecting the kidneys from free haemoglobin damage. A large release of haemoglobin, as in haemolytic anaemia, uses up much of the haptoglobin and the level in the blood becomes low.

*Test: Mean corpuscular volume (MCV).* This is a calculation of the average volume of a red blood cell. The formula for this is:

MCV = haematocrit ÷ [RBC]

That is, MCV equals the haematocrit (see *haematocrit*, earlier) divided by the concentration of red blood cells.

The volume of red cells can be measured directly. Red cells with high volume are seen in **pernicious anaemia** (see *vitamin* $B_{12}$ *deficiency*, page 73), causing **macrocytic** (large red cell) anaemia. A low volume of red cells (**microcytic**) is seen in **iron deficiency anaemia**.

*Test: Mean corpuscular Hb (MCH).* This is the average amount of haemoglobin found in each red blood cell. The formula for this is:

MCH = (10 × haemoglobin) ÷ (red blood cell count)

Low MCH is due to various types of anaemia and iron deficiency in the diet. High MCH may be due to liver disease, some cancers and infections.

*Test: Mean corpuscular Hb concentration (MCHC).* This is the average concentration of haemoglobin in a given volume of packed red blood cells. The formula is:

MCHC = (haemoglobin × 100) ÷ (haematocrit)

The haemoglobin is divided by the haematocrit (see *haematocrit*, page 92). High MCHC may be due to the presence of **spherocytosis** (red cells with exceptionally high amounts of haemoglobin) in circulation. Unstable Hb or deficiency of vitamin $B_{12}$ and folic acid may be other causes.

*Test: Reticulocyte count.* Reticulocytes are immature erythrocytes. They would not usually be released into circulation (from bone marrow) until fully mature. A raised reticulocyte level in circulation indicates that the bone marrow is producing these cells quickly and releasing them to compensate for low or high levels of red cells, due to anaemia or bone marrow disorders.

## Blood groups (Tables 4.15, 4.16)

There are at least 14 different blood grouping systems known. The only two used in clinical practice are the ABO system (discovered in 1901) and the rhesus (Rh) system (discovered in 1940) (Daniels and Bromilow 2013). The other systems cause mild and transient reactions. The reactions caused by the ABO and rhesus systems are potentially fatal.

The ABO system is based on the fact that red cells have a combination of two **antigens** on their surface: **antigens A** and **B**. If the red cells have only antigen A, this is **blood group A**; red cells with only antigen B produce **blood group B**; red cells with antigens A and B together create **blood group AB** and those with no A or B antigen present is **blood group O**. **Antibodies** are present in the plasma (see *antibodies*, page 86), but individuals cannot

*Table 4.15* Blood groups and antigens. The table shows which antigen exists on the red blood cell (RBC) and which antibody exists in the plasma of each of the four blood types

| Blood group | Antigen on RBC | Antibodies in plasma |
| --- | --- | --- |
| A | A | Anti-B (reacts with B antigen) |
| B | B | Anti-A (reacts with A antigen) |
| AB | A+B | No antibodies |
| O | No antigens | Anti-A and anti-B (reacts with both A and B) |

*Table 4.16* The ABO blood groups compatibility grid. The donor's red cells (A and B antigens) are matched with the recipient's plasma (anti-A and anti-B antibodies) to identify any dangerous reaction ( ✗ ) or no reaction ( ✓ ). Recipient AB can take blood from any group (universal recipient) provided the rhesus factor (not shown) is positive (AB Rh+), and donor O can give blood to any group (universal donor) provided the rhesus factor (not shown) is negative (O Rh−)

| Donor blood | Recipient blood | | | |
| --- | --- | --- | --- | --- |
| | A<br>Anti-B antibody | B<br>Anti-A antibody | AB<br>None | O<br>Anti-A + anti-B antibodies |
| A | ✓ | ✗ | ✓ | ✗ |
| B | ✗ | ✓ | ✓ | ✗ |
| AB | ✗ | ✗ | ✓ | ✗ |
| O | ✓ | ✓ | ✓ | ✓ |

have the antibodies that react with their own antigen. Instead, they have antibodies that react with *other* antigens (Tables 4.15 and 4.16).

The **rhesus system** involves the RBC surface antigen called the **D-factor** (the **rhesus factor**). If the D-factor is present, the blood is **rhesus-positive** (**Rh+**), and the plasma has no **anti-D antibody**. If the D-factor is absent, the blood is **rhesus-negative** (**Rh−**), and the plasma has got **anti-D antibody**. Any of the four ABO groups can be either Rh+ or Rh− (i.e. a total of 8 blood groups). The plasma antibodies cannot react with their own red cells, but **transfusion** of blood from one person to another creates the conditions that could cause a reaction, and this must be avoided. **Haemolysis** (haemo = blood; lysis = break down) is one type of reaction where red cells are destroyed, haemoglobin is released and the patient can suffer severe **anaemia** with **jaundice**. **Agglutination** is another type of reaction where red cells clump together in large lumps that can block smaller vessels, such as the arterioles within the kidneys, causing kidney failure. These reactions happen due to **mismatched** transfusions, and careful checking is required to prevent this (Table 4.16).

### Blood tests in development

• A blood test that can determine the presence or not of a myocardial infarction (MI) quicker than the current troponin tests (see page 70) could be available. The test gives results in about 20 minutes, and unlike troponins it does not need repeating some hours later. It rapidly excludes a lot of patients who present with non-cardiac chest pain and who could then be sent home. It identifies the presence of any **cardiac myosin-binding**

**protein C** (**cMyC**), which is raised earlier and higher in the blood following a myocardial infarction than the troponins (see *troponin tests*, page 70).

- Several blood tests are based on the detection of **cell-free DNA** (**cfDNA**) in blood plasma. DNA fragments from these dead cells are constantly being discharged into the blood. It is now possible to collect these fragments in a sample of blood and analyse this DNA. Several examples are:

  1 cfDNA in the maternal blood from the unborn foetus during the early stages of pregnancy can be checked for the presence of **Down's syndrome** (**trisomy-21**)
  2 cfDNA from tumours or foreign organisms can be found and analysed to detect new growths or infections
  3 cfDNA from transplanted organs can be checked in the recipient blood to identify any signs of organ rejection, when the cfDNA would rise
  4 cfDNA in the blood may soon be able to detect the death of pancreatic islet cells before symptoms of diabetes occur.

These tests are now available. One of the problems has been identifying what organ or tissue the cfDNA comes from, but already a system identifying the methylation of DNA (the attachment of methyl groups to the DNA) has been devised since methylation varies for different organs.

Tests to detect the presence of biomarkers for brain-derived proteins in circulation that are released in brain injury or diseases such as **Alzheimer disease** (**AD**). **Neurofilament light** (**NFL**) rises sharply in blood plasma after brain injury and be a blood biomarker for the presence of several chronic neurodegeneration disorders, including AD, in those with a history of head injury. In a separate test, the relative amounts of the various beta-amyloid proteins present in the brain can now be assessed from the beta-amyloid found in the blood. The blood results correlate well with beta-amyloid found in brain scans.

## Key points

- The total blood volume in circulation is 5,000 ml (5 L).
- The blood cells are erythrocytes (red blood cells), leucocytes (white blood cells) and thrombocytes (platelets).
- Blood cells have a limited lifespan and are replaced by new cells from bone marrow.
- Plasma transports many substances and a lot of these can be tested for.
- Plasma proteins are mostly albumin and globulin, with others in smaller quantities, including some hormones, enzymes, clotting factors and antibodies.
- Plasma proteins are mostly produced in the liver.
- Blood group A has antigen A on the RBCs and anti-B antibodies in the plasma. Blood group B has antigen B with anti-A antibodies in the plasma. Blood group AB has antigens A and B and no anti-A or anti-B antibodies, and blood group O has no A or B antigen and anti-A and anti-B antibodies in the plasma.
- The rhesus factor (D-factor) is present in rhesus-positive (Rh+), the plasma having no anti-D antibody. The D-factor is absent in rhesus-negative (Rh−), the plasma having anti-D antibody.

## Notes

1 The symptoms of beriberi are fatigue, poor appetite, weight loss, diarrhoea, muscle wasting, oedema, paralysis and heart failure (Table 7.3, page 142).

2 The four D's of pellagra are diarrhoea, dermatitis, dementia and death (Table 7.3, page 142).
3 Early symptoms of scurvy are weakness and tiredness, and later sore gums, bleeding and anaemia (Table 7.3, page 142).
4 Rickets causes soft, bent bones in children with vitamin D deficiency. Osteomalacia is the adult equivalent, causing easy fractures and bone pain. The difference is due to the fact that rickets is the disease in bone that is still growing, while osteomalacia is the disease in fully mature bones.
5 Note that the capital *H* is the chemical symbol for hydrogen (since acidity is all about hydrogen ion concentration), so it becomes meaningless to write a small *h*. Because hydrogen is *H* and not *PH*, it important to write a small *p* (*p* stands for *potential*). So, PH, Ph and ph are all wrong and meaningless. It must always be *pH* (potential hydrogen), even at the start of a sentence (see also *acid-base measurement of urine*, Chapter 8, and Figure 8.14).

## References

Bain B. (2017) *A Beginner's Guide to Blood Cells* (3rd edition). Wiley-Blackwell, Hoboken, NJ.

Basten G. (2013) *Blood Results in Clinical Practice*. M&K Update, Keswick.

Blann A. and Ahmed N. (2014) *Blood Science: Principles and Pathology*. Wiley-Blackwell, Hoboken, NJ.

Blows W.T. (2022) *The Biological Basis of Mental Health* (4th edition). Routledge, Abingdon, UK and New York.

Caironi P. and Gattinoni L. (2009) The clinical use of albumin: The point of view of a specialist in intensive care. *Blood Transfusion*, *7*(4): 259–267. http://doi.org/10.2450/2009.0002-09

Daniels G. and Bromilow I. (2013) *Essential Guide to Blood Groups* (3rd edition). Wiley-Blackwell, Hoboken, NJ.

Rennie J.M. and Kendall G.S. (2013) *A Manual of Neonatal Intensive Care* (5th edition). CRC Press, Boca Raton, FL.

# 5 Respiratory observations

## Introduction

Although we need oxygen ($O_2$) from the air, oxygen is not the main driving force of breathing. The need to remove carbon (C) from the body is the primary drive. Oxygen is required for this process, by combining with waste carbon ($CO_2$) and removing it from the body. $CO_2$ (carbon dioxide) is the by-product of tissue energy production (Chapter 1, Figure 1.3, page 4). It is excreted via the lungs, having been transported there by the blood. Observations of respiration are a means of assessing the efficiency of this process and detecting any abnormalities. Carbon dioxide is both beneficial and harmful, depending on the quantity present. Constant volumes of this gas in both the tissues and the blood are essential to maintain the driving force for breathing. Too much carbon dioxide in the cells would cause life threatening problems with energy production. Oxygen has a smaller role in maintaining the respiratory drive. Its main role is to combine with the two waste products of cellular metabolism, hydrogen and carbon and remove these from the body:

- Two hydrogens (2H) combine with oxygen (O) to form water ($H_2O$), which is excreted through the lungs and skin.
- One carbon (C) combines with oxygen ($O_2$) to form $CO_2$, which is excreted through the lungs.

DOI: 10.4324/9781003389118-5

Air passes from the atmosphere into the lungs through the **airway**, which consists of the nasal and oral openings, the **pharynx**, the **larynx** (often called the *voice box*), the **trachea** (sometimes called the *windpipe*), both left and right **bronchi**, multiple **bronchioles** and the tiny air sacs (called **alveoli**) at the end (Figure 5.1). Most of the airway is lined with mucous membrane that produces **mucin** (mucous). Mucous membrane warms incoming air to body temperature, particularly within the nose, adds moisture to it so it will not dry out the alveoli, and traps unwanted pollutants which stick to the mucous. Tiny hairlike cellular extensions (called **cilia**) then beat in an upward motion to 'sweep' the mucous and pollutants out of the lungs towards the throat, where they will be swallowed. This is called the **muco-ciliary escalator**. Beneath the mucous membrane, in most of the airway, is a smooth muscle layer. In the bronchi, this smooth muscle can *contract* (causing a narrowing of the airway, called **bronchoconstriction**) or *relax* (causing a widening of the airway, called **bronchodilation**). The narrowest part of the upper airway, the **glottis**, is within the larynx. This is where the vocal cords are stretched across the airway to produce sound. Some parts of the upper airway wall, especially the trachea and bronchi, are reinforced with stiff cartilage rings to prevent airway collapse.

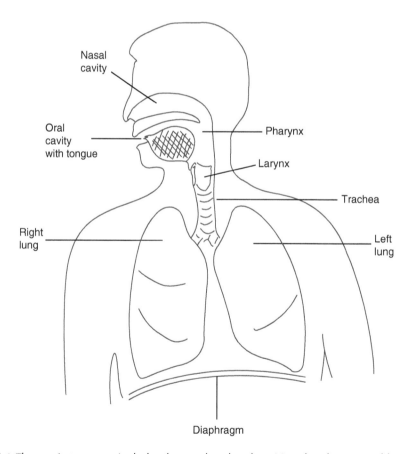

*Figure 5.1* The respiratory tract includes the nasal and oral cavities, the pharynx and larynx (voice box) and the trachea which divides at the lower end into left and right bronchi, one for each lung.

## Respiratory physiology

Respiration means the exchange of the gases oxygen and carbon dioxide. There are two places where these gases are exchanged with the blood, i.e. in the lungs (**external respiration**) and in the tissues (**internal respiration**). Breathing is the act of getting air into and out of the lungs.

**The alveoli** are minute air sacs that make up the bulk of lung tissue and provide the location for gas exchange (external respiration). There are three gas exchange compartments: (1) the *air* within the alveoli (called **alveolar air**); (2) the *blood* and (3) the *tissues* of the alveolar wall (Figure 5.2).

While the air and blood are constantly being changed, the tissues provide a constant close yet distinct barrier between the two. Gases move across this barrier, driven by the **concentration gradient**. Substances will flow from a high concentration to a low concentration, a movement referred to as **diffusion**. This is defined as the movement of substances such as gases or liquids from the point of greatest concentration to areas of lower concentration. This equals out the concentration so no gradient exists and movement stops. In respiration, diffusion refers to the movement of oxygen and carbon dioxide during external and internal respiration.

In the lungs, the gradient – and therefore gas flow – is maintained, i.e. equalisation of concentration is prevented. During breathing, oxygen is moving into the blood but is kept in a higher concentration in the alveoli than in the blood by the continued addition of new oxygen from the air. Carbon dioxide is moving into the lungs from the blood, but the concentration of this gas in the alveoli is kept lower than in the blood by the continued

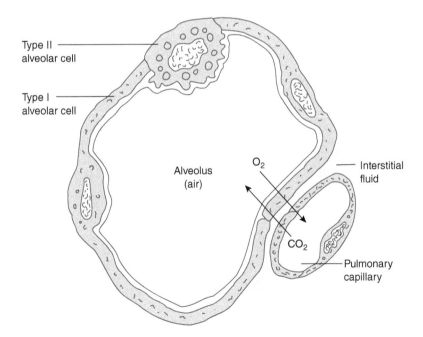

*Figure 5.2* Microscopic view of the lung showing an alveolus containing air, with walls of type I and type II cells, a pulmonary capillary containing blood and interstitial fluid between the capillary and the alveolus. The direction of gas movement is shown.

removal of $CO_2$ from the alveoli by breathing. The act of breathing itself ensures that these concentration gradients are maintained, and therefore these gases will continue to flow in and out of the lungs and blood (Figure 5.2).

### Mechanics of breathing

Breathing is a mechanical process that involves the movement of muscles within the chest wall and diaphragm. These movements control lung expansion and contraction because the lungs are held tightly against the chest wall by a slight negative pressure (or vacuum, i.e. −4 mmHg). This vacuum exists between the membrane attached to the outer surface of the lungs (the **visceral layer** of the **pleura**) and the membrane attached to the inner surface of the chest wall (the **parietal layer** of the pleura), causing these two surfaces to stick close together (Figure 5.3).

The negative *intrapleural pressure* is 4 mmHg *lower* than the atmospheric pressure outside the chest wall and inside the lungs. As the chest wall moves the lungs must go along with it. If this vacuum is compromised the lungs and chest wall will separate, i.e. complete or partial lung collapse, or **atelectasis**. It could be air that gets into this space (a **pneumothorax**) or water from blood plasma (a **hydrothorax**) or whole blood (a **haemo-thorax**) or any combination of these, e.g. a **haemopneumothorax**. The lungs would fail to respond to chest wall movements, making breathing very difficult and painful.

The muscle of the chest wall operates the ribs, which during inspiration are moved upwards and outwards, expanding the volume (or space) within the chest two-dimensionally from front to back and side to side. Contraction of the diaphragm at the same time causes it to flatten (at rest it is normally slightly dome-shaped), increasing the chest volume in the third dimension (i.e. from top to bottom). The lungs are stretched outwards in all directions, causing the air pressure inside the lungs to drop below atmospheric

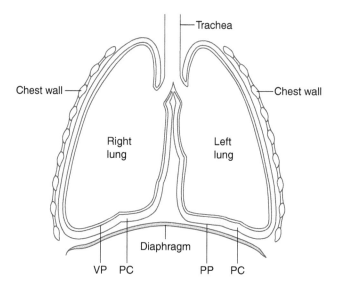

*Figure 5.3* The lungs and the pleural membrane. PC: pleural cavity containing the negative (suction) pressure; PP: parietal layer of the pleural membrane attached to the chest wall and diaphragm; VP: visceral layer of the pleural membrane attached to the lung surface.

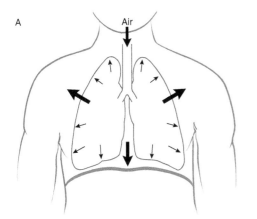
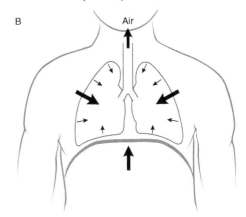

*Figure 5.4* Inspiration and expiration. (A) During inspiration, the chest wall moves upwards and outwards, and the diaphragm flattens, causing the lungs to be stretched in all directions. The resulting increase in the volume inside the lungs causes the pressure to fall, and air is drawn in to fill the space. (B) During expiration, the return of the lungs and diaphragm decreases the lung space, forcing the pressure up, and air is blown out.

pressure, thus creating a partial vacuum within the lungs that must be instantly filled by air taken in from the atmosphere (**inhalation** or **inspiration**). The reverse is also true, when the respiratory muscles relax, allowing the ribs and diaphragm to return to their previous normal position. This squeezes the lungs, increasing the pressure inside the lungs above atmospheric pressure, which then forces the air back out into the atmosphere (**exhalation** or **expiration**; Figure 5.4).

The cycle of diaphragmatic movements starts with contraction of its muscle component, which flattens the normal dome shape. This pushes down the abdominal contents, notably the liver which lies immediately below the diaphragm. Relaxation of the diaphragm results in its return to a domed shape, aided by the liver and other abdominal contents pushing back. Pressure from within the abdomen aids expiration, and this is the reason why, in some positions, abdominal movements can be seen during breathing.

The relationship between volume and pressure seen in the lungs is expressed in **Boyle's law**, where the pressure inside the lungs falls if the volume increases at a constant temperature (as in inhalation), or the pressure rises if the volume decreases at a constant temperature (as in exhalation). The muscles used during normal breathing are **primary**, since they act all the time. Sometimes additional effort must be made to breathe, e.g. immediately after exercise, and **secondary** (or **accessory**) muscles are used to assist in chest wall movement. These standby muscles of breathing include some of the muscles of the neck and shoulders. The most efficient position for the use of these muscles is upright, leaning slightly forward, with arms raised to a horizontal position. Severely breathless patients will adopt this position to aid their breathing if they are able to do so.

*Air volumes*

The volume of air we take in with each breath is the **tidal volume**, i.e. the air moving in and out of the lungs. This volume is about 500 ml in adults (Figure 5.5). The 500 ml can

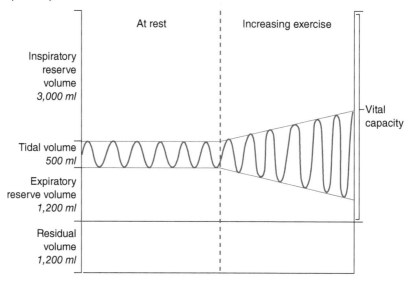

*Figure 5.5* Breathing volumes at rest and during exercise. The tidal volume (TV) is approximately 500 ml at rest. As exercise begins, the TV increases by incorporating part of the lungs' inspiratory reserve volume (IRV) and expiratory reserve volume (ERV). The residual volume remains in the lungs, preventing lung collapse. The vital capacity (VC) represents the entire movable air in or out of the lungs and is the sum of IRV+ERV+TV.

be subdivided into two volumes, i.e. the volume that *will* reach the alveoli and exchange gas with the blood, the **alveolar air** (about 350 ml) and the volume that *will not* reach the alveoli and thus does not exchange gas, the **dead space**. Dead space air fills the air passages, the **trachea**, the **bronchi** and the **bronchioles**. Exhaled dead space air contains the same gas mixture as inhaled air, whereas alveolar air has more carbon dioxide and less oxygen in it due to gas exchange with the blood. The tidal volume formula is:

tidal volume (TV) = alveolar air + dead space air

The dead space remains relatively constant, averaging about 150 ml unless there is any change in the diameter of the bronchi or the bronchioles known as **bronchoconstriction** if the diameter narrows or **bronchodilation** if the diameter widens. These changes can be mostly ignored and calculations involving tidal volume assume a constant dead space. Therefore the formula for alveolar air is:

500 ml (TV) – 150 ml (dead space) = 350 ml of alveolar air at rest

These values change during exercise when breathing is faster and deeper. Exercise increases tidal volume by stretching the lungs farther than at rest. A bigger tidal volume means a bigger alveolar air volume rather than the dead space volume which will increase very little. Increases in the alveolar air volume provide more air available for gas exchange with the blood, and respiration becomes more efficient. But respiration also speeds up with exercise, and this can reduce the efficiency if the respiratory rate increases too much. This is because by squeezing more tidal volumes in per minute, i.e. increasing the respiration rate, each tidal volume has less time to get in and out, and this reduces the tidal volume. Assuming a relatively constant dead space, the largest reduction must occur in the alveolar air, making less air available for gas exchange and therefore reducing lung efficiency. Slow, *deep* breathing is more efficient than rapid, *shallow* breathing. Here, the words deep and shallow reflect the size of the tidal volume: deep is a *large* tidal volume (mostly alveolar air = efficient) and shallow is a *small* tidal volume (mostly dead space = not efficient). The tidal volume is taken in and out about 18 times per minute at rest (the **respiratory rate**, or **RR**). Multiplying the tidal volume with the respiratory rate will give the total volume of air moved in and out of the lungs per minute: the **pulmonary ventilation rate (PVR**; thus TV × RR = PVR). It may be important to calculate how much of the PVR is alveolar air (i.e. how much air is exchanging gases with the blood per minute, called the **alveolar ventilation rate** or **AVR**). This is worked out by deducting the dead space from the tidal volume *before* multiplying that answer by the respiratory rate:

(TV – dead space) × RR = AVR
(Remember to do the bracketed calculation first)

Some patients require a surgical procedure that shortens the airway, a **tracheostomy**, where they breathe through an opening in the throat, directly into the trachea below the larynx (Figure 5.6). A tracheostomy tube is often in place to maintain the opening. This

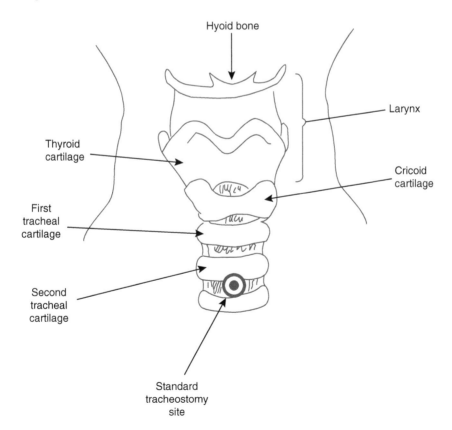

*Figure 5.6* Tracheostomy.

procedure is done either to relieve or bypass an obstruction or to reduce the dead space in those who will be ventilated for some time, making ventilation more efficient. It is vital to check that breathing is normal through a tracheostomy and that no infection or obstruction occurs.

The functional **inspiratory reserve volume** (**IRV**) is the maximum inspiration taken during a deep breath, and a functional **expiratory reserve volume** (**ERV**) is the maximum expiration produced by forced exhalation. The increase in tidal volume during exercise is a widening of the TV to include some of both the IRV and ERV volumes (Figure 5.5).

All the potentially *movable* air volumes in the lungs add up to the **vital capacity** (**VC**):

VC = IRV + ERV + TV

The vital capacity can be measured by the **spirometer** or the **vitalograph**, which is a portable spirometer. Both require the subject to take a maximum inspiration, followed by a forced maximum expiration into a tube attached to the machine. A **forced expiratory volume** in 1 second (**FEV$_1$**) can be directly measured, i.e. the maximum amount of air that can be forcefully expired in 1 second after a maximum inspiration. The use of a constant time period (1 second) enables standardisation between subjects. Most individuals will normally expire about 80% of their vital capacity in 1 second, but reduced patency of the airway (e.g. asthma) will delay this, and the total vital capacity will take several seconds more to expire.

It is not possible to breathe out all the air in the lungs, since to do so would require the lungs to collapse. This remaining volume is called the **residual volume** (Figure 5.5). The residual volume still exchanges gas with the atmosphere and with the blood, i.e. it is a volume that remains constant in the lungs but is being replaced by new air all the time.

### The neurophysiology of respiration

Respiration is controlled by the **respiratory centres**, i.e. several areas in the **medulla** and the **pons**, parts of the **brainstem**. The respiratory centres send nerve impulses to the muscles of the respiration and increase the respiratory rate and depth as required. There are many factors that influence the respiratory centres, the most important being the $CO_2$ level in the blood. Rising $CO_2$ blood level stimulates the centre to increase the rate and depth of breathing to excrete more $CO_2$. Low $CO_2$ blood level reduces the stimulus and breathing becomes slow and shallow. Complete absence of $CO_2$ in the blood would cause **apnoea**, i.e. cessation of breathing. This is a feedback mechanism, part of the body's homeostasis, regulating the internal environment within certain parameters. In this case, the blood gas concentrations (see *blood gases*, Chapter 4, and Table 4.12, page 89). **Chemoreceptors** in the carotid and aortic arteries and in the medulla are sensory nerve endings specialising in detecting the gas composition of the blood and sending this information back to the respiratory centres. Chemoreceptors are sensitive to the pH of the blood, i.e. the acid-base balance (see *blood pH*, Chapter 4, and Table 4.12, page 89). pH is a measure of the **hydrogen ion** concentration ([H$^+$][1]), and a high H$^+$ concentration causes acidic conditions (i.e. a low pH). Blood is about pH 7.4, on the alkaline side of neutral (pH 7.0), and this pH level is critical. $CO_2$ is thought of as an *acid gas* because in combination with water (as in plasma), it forms **carbonic acid** ($CO_2 + H_2O = H_2CO_3$), and carbonic acid can liberate H$^+$ (i.e. $H_2CO_3 \rightarrow HCO_3^- + H^+$). Any $CO_2$ retention creates a **respiratory acidosis** in the blood. High concentrations of H$^+$, i.e. low pH, can be corrected *in the short term* by stimulating respiration to excrete more $CO_2$, thus forming less carbonic acid. An oxygen lack mostly stimulates the carotid chemoreceptors which will increase respiration to improve oxygen intake.

The respiratory centres are separate groups of neurones in the medulla and the pons (Figure 5.7).

The medullary **inspiratory centre**, called the **dorsal respiratory group** (**DRG**), sends nerve impulses to the muscles of respiration in an *on-off cycle*. Switching on the cycle causes inspiration; switching off allows expiration, a passive event that occurs when relaxed muscles allows the chest wall to return to a natural position. The medullary **ventral respiratory group** (**VRG**) helps to maintain the muscle tone of the inspiratory muscles. It also actively assists the chest wall during expiration when passive expiration alone is not fast enough, as in exercise. The pons **pneumotaxic centre** sends inhibitory impulses to the DRG to limit inspiration, fine-tune the rhythm and prevent overinflation of the lungs. The function of the pons **apneustic centre** is less well understood. Impulses from this

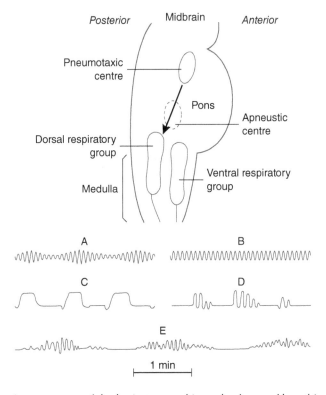

*Figure 5.7* The respiratory centre of the brainstem and irregular forms of breathing. The dorsal respiratory group provides inspiratory signals at all times, and the ventral respiratory group helps to trigger inspiration during times of greater pulmonary need (e.g. exercise). The pneumotaxic centre of the pons influences the cut-off point for inspiration to prevent overinflation of the lungs. This cut-off signal may be itself blocked by the apneustic centre under various conditions, thus allowing increased inspiration. Abnormal forms of breathing are shown. (A) Cheyne-Stokes. (B) Central neurogenic hyperventilation. (C) Apneustic breathing. (D) Cluster breathing. (E) Biot (ataxic) breathing (for explanation, see page 106).

centre stimulate the DRG and would prolong inspiration if the DRG was not inhibited by the pneumotaxic centre. The apneustic centre itself can be directly inhibited by the pneumotaxic centre (Hickey 2013; Figure 5.7). Feedback to the DRG on inspiration comes from the lungs via stretch receptors in the bronchi and bronchioles.

The medullary breathing centre has morphine receptors, called μ-receptors (mu receptors). Mu receptors block pain, but on the respiratory centre they cause respiratory depression, i.e. slow, shallow breathing. Patients receiving morphine for pain should be observed for depressed breathing. It may prove detrimental to the patient, especially elderly people or those with chronic respiratory disease, and the drug should be reduced or replaced.

Abnormalities of the breathing pattern (Figure 5.7) are sometimes due to disturbances affecting the respiratory centre, e.g. after **head injury** or due to **raised intracranial pressure**, **RICP** (see Chapter 11). **Cheyne-Stokes** respiration is a rhythmic coming and going (waxing and waning) of the depth and rate of breathing interspersed by periods of apnoea. The cycle occurs over about 1 minute, within which breathing stops for about 20 seconds. The apnoea causes an increase in $CO_2$ that stimulates a short period of excessive over-breathing. This removes $CO_2$, which then causes the next period of apnoea. Cheyne-Stokes respiration can occur in patients with head injuries, brain tumours, heart failure and strokes and may precede death. **Apneustic breathing** is a prolonged inspiration of 2 or 3 seconds followed by a long expiratory phase. A complete respiratory cycle takes about 50 seconds, during which the patient has breathed once. The lesion responsible is in the pons or upper medulla following a stroke or brain trauma. It is often caused by a blockage (occlusion) of the main arterial blood supply in the area. **Cluster breathing** is the term used to describe a series of rapid breaths (5 or 6 together) that diminish in depth to complete apnoea for 20 seconds or so before starting again. The lesion responsible is in the upper medulla or lower pons. **Biot breathing** are irregular, alternating bouts of shallow then deep inspirations followed by unpredictable periods of pause (10–30 seconds). The lesion is brainstem pressure or trauma involving the medulla. **Central neurogenic hyperventilation** is a continuous pattern of fast, deep breaths (more than 25 breaths per minute). It is especially rare, the dominant cause being expanding tumours of the brain involving the pontine area of the brainstem. Such rapid breathing causes **alkalosis** (blood is above pH 7.4), since excessive $CO_2$ is lost. It indicates that $CO_2$ is no longer stimulating breathing (Hickey 2013).

## Observations of breathing

The respiratory system is a vital part of the patient's oxygen delivery system to the tissues and of carbon dioxide excretion, both important parts of cellular metabolism (Owen 1998).

### Respiratory rate and depth

**Respiratory rate**, the number of breaths per minute, is the usual respiratory observation. Adults breath about 12–18 times per minute, but this can reach 30 or more during exercise when additional oxygen is required or as a result of respiratory and cardiovascular disorders. A breathing cycle consists of inspiration, expiration and a brief pause. Modest increases in respiratory rate and tidal volume improves respiratory efficiency, as seen in exercise. Fast or very slow rates are inefficient. Slow rates, e.g. below 12 breaths per minute, improve efficiency if there is a greater *depth* of breathing, i.e. increased tidal volume.

Fast respiratory rates (**tachypnoea**), i.e. up to 30 breaths per minute, can be seen in infections involving fever, especially respiratory infections. Fever involves increased breathing rates, probably to supply additional oxygen for the raised tissue metabolism. Faster
breathing may also help to cool the body (see Chapter 1), as panting does in dogs. **Hyperventilation** is over-breathing, which may be due to physical or psychological causes.
Pain and stress can cause hyperventilation, and it is a feature of emotional reactions such
as panic. Hyperventilation can severely reduce the carbon dioxide levels in the blood,
which would normally slow breathing down by taking away the main respiratory drive.
However, the higher centres of the brain (i.e. those involved in the stress reaction) over-
ride this chemical stimulus and drive respiration independently of carbon dioxide levels.
The low carbon dioxide causes an **alkalosis**, i.e. raised blood pH, and this reduces the
amount of freely available calcium in circulation. This free calcium reduction causes
peripheral tingling and numbness, stiff contractions of the hands and fingers, and a feeling
of unreality, all of which may add to the patient's stress.

Oxygen and carbon dioxide in the blood create between them a gas pressure called
**blood gas tension** (Figure 5.8), similar to the pressure created by the dissolved gas in an
unopened fizzy drink bottle.

Each gas contributes part of this total pressure, known as the **partial pressure** of oxygen
(**$PO_2$**) or the partial pressure of carbon dioxide (**$PCO_2$**). They depend on the volume of
each gas carried by the blood. The $PO_2$ of *arterial* blood ($PaO_2$) is 13.3 kPa (kilopascals)
or 100 mmHg, whereas the $PaCO_2$ is 5.3 kPa or 40 mmHg. The values for *venous* blood

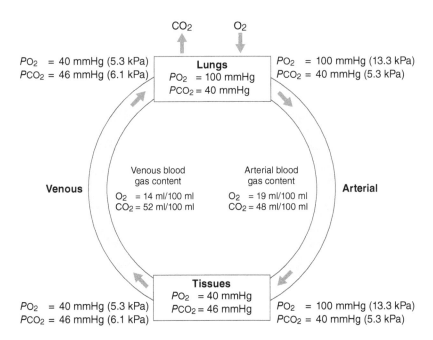

*Figure 5.8* The blood gas tensions in arterial and venous blood compared with the gas tensions of
the lungs and tissues. Notice that the arterial blood gas tensions adopt the same values
as the lungs, and the venous blood gas tensions adopt the same values as the tissues
(measured in mmHg and kPa). Blood gas contents are also shown for arterial and venous
blood.

reflect the loss of oxygen to the tissues (venous $PO_2$ = 5.3 kPa or 40 mmHg) and the gain of carbon dioxide from the tissues (venous $PCO_2$ = 6.1 kPa or 46 mmHg[2]) (Figure 5.8; see Figure 4.12, page 89). Respiratory rate increases would result from increased $PCO_2$ or decreased $PO_2$ in arterial blood. Measurement of these values requires an *arterial* blood sample since arterial blood records the results of gas exchange taking place in the lungs, i.e. one of several *lung function tests*. A venous blood sample would only reflect gas exchange in the tissues, and this is not useful for the diagnosis of lung disease.

**Dyspnoea** means difficulty in breathing and is recognised by the patient becoming very anxious and struggling to breathe (called **air hunger**). They attempt to sit upright and forward if possible (see page 101). There is a rapid respiratory rate, cyanosis (see page 111) and possibly abnormal respiratory sounds (see page 111) (Grey 1995). Fast intervention is needed to relieve the lack of oxygen and the distress caused by dyspnoea. Difficulty in breathing occurs in air containing less oxygen than the body requires (called **rarefied air**), e.g. at high altitudes if not acclimatised to the situation. High altitude also involves lower atmospheric air pressure, which exacerbates the problem. Deep-sea diving causes problems because the increased water pressure on the body with depth allows more gas to be carried in the blood. Additional gas must be removed *slowly* by gradual decompression as the diver comes to the surface. Failure to do this results in rapid release of the extra gas into the circulation forming gas bubbles in the blood (**gas emboli**). This is known as **the bends**, **caisson disease** or **decompression sickness** (**DCS**). It can cause the death of the diver.

Patients may often experience difficulty in breathing while lying flat (known as **orthopnoea**), which necessitates that they sleep in an upright position. The sitting-up position improves breathing because there is no restriction of chest wall movement caused by the bed. It also improves the flattening of the diaphragm as gravity removes the pressure caused by the abdominal contents below the diaphragm. Any fluids in the lungs drain by gravity towards the **base** while sitting up, freeing the **apical** (top) areas of the lungs for a better air supply and more efficient gas exchange. Sitting upright also allows for more efficient use of the secondary muscles of respiration (see page 101).

In respiratory and heart diseases, the cause of an increased respiratory rate is a lack of oxygen (low $PO_2$), which the increased rate attempts to rectify. These diseases include **obstructive respiratory** (or **pulmonary**) **diseases**, including **asthma**, where bronchoconstriction and mucosal swelling narrow the airway; **bronchitis**, where chronic swollen mucous membrane with excessive secretions obstruct the airway and **emphysema**, where breakdown of the alveolar wall reduces the surface area available for gas exchange. **Chronic bronchitis** is a disease associated with a cold, wet climate and smoking. Over many years, the reduced gas exchange causes persistently reduced oxygen (low $PO_2$) in the blood. The respiratory centre normally responds to **hypoxia** (low $O_2$) by stimulating breathing. In diseased and inefficient lungs, $CO_2$ can be retained in the blood (increased $PCO_2$), and the patient becomes reliant on the hypoxia to maintain breathing. Consequently, when the patient is admitted, oxygen therapy should not be started without medical advice, since the correction of the hypoxia may decrease the respiratory drive, worsen the lung efficiency and increase the retained $CO_2$. The result could be a respiratory acidosis. Oxygen may seem the obvious treatment for the breathless, cyanosed patient, but under these circumstances it may bring reality to the phrase *killing with kindness*. Oxygen is useful in acute respiratory problems, but for the chronic sufferer it must be used with great caution. This will mean that $O_2$ would be prescribed by a doctor in low dosage and the patient monitored closely for respiratory deterioration (Forbes-Faulkner 1998).

Heart diseases can be a cause of increased respiratory rate, including **heart** (or **cardiac**) **failure**. **Left heart failure** (or **left ventricular failure**, **LVF**) causes blood to accumulate in the pulmonary veins awaiting the opportunity to get into the left side of the heart. This 'traffic jam' of blood gets back to the lungs, where fluid from the plasma can leak into the alveolar spaces causing **pulmonary oedema** (see Chapter 6). This prevents gas exchange across any alveolar spaces that are involved in collecting this fluid. This is sometimes referred to as the **backward problem** (see Chapter 2). **Right heart failure** (**RHF**, or **congestive cardiac failure**, **CCF**) can cause increased respiratory rates by reducing the amount of blood being pumped to the lungs, whilst slowing down circulation in the tissues. The tissues become starved of $O_2$ and cannot pass their $CO_2$ quickly to the blood, and the resulting changes in the $PO_2$ and $PCO_2$ affect the respiratory centre. In acidosis, low blood pH (i.e. below the normal of pH 7.4) causes increased respiration in an attempt to remove $CO_2$ gas from the blood.

Increased respiration also occurs as a result of lung collapse (**atelectasis**), which can be due to chest trauma or occur spontaneously. Atelectasis is the result of a loss of the negative pressure between the two layers of the pleura which then separate (page 100). A **tension pneumothorax** occurs where air is sucked in through a chest wound and builds up in the pleura, progressively collapsing the lungs. A **pneumothorax** is air in the pleura from a burst **bulla**, or air blister, within the visceral layer of the pleura. A simple fractured rib can increase respiration rates because the pain prevents taking deep breaths. Faster but shallow breathing reduces respiratory efficiency (see page 106). Respiratory changes due to the pain of fractured ribs could be life-threatening to an elderly patient, especially with other respiratory problems such as chronic bronchitis.

Since blood tends to reach all the alveoli, the efficiency of gas exchange also depends on air reaching all the alveoli as well. This varies slightly, with more air than blood occurring in the **apex** (top) of the lung and more blood than air occurring in the basal areas. The best 'blood-air' flow ratio occurs in the central regions of the lungs, although fine-tuning of the airflow to match the blood flow throughout the lungs means that small variations make little difference. Big differences occur when serious 'air-blood' flow disturbances take place, e.g. in **shunting**, where blood passes through areas of unventilated alveoli, returning from the lungs without any gas exchange. This *high $PCO_2$/low $PO_2$* blood then mixes with blood that has exchanged gases, altering the blood gas tensions of arterial blood. This is an example of how arterial blood gas measurements record lung function efficiency. If shunting is severe enough, it will affect oxygenation of the tissues causing respiratory increases, cyanosis and dyspnoea. Shunting occurs in atelectasis, fluid accumulating in the alveoli e.g. in **lobar pneumonia** or pulmonary oedema or in tension pneumothorax. Lobar pneumonia is a lung infection characterised by **exudate**, i.e. leaked fluid accumulating in the alveoli and preventing air from entering. **Bronchial pneumonia** is similar, where the fluid collects in the bronchus. A tidal volume that is too low, i.e. very shallow breathing, is also an estimate of respiratory efficiency. Low inhaled volumes will be mostly dead space with little alveolar air. The dead space is the first part of the airway to exchange gas with the atmosphere but *not* with the blood. In shallow breathing the dead space gas exchange has little or no change to the alveolar air lower down. A slow respiratory rate with deep breathing can be a feature of some periods of sleep. Slow rates accompanied by shallow breaths, i.e. low tidal volume, is an indication of poor respiratory efficiency. This kind of breathing pattern is often seen when the patient is close to death. **Sleep apnoea** is cessation of breathing during sleep and requires further investigation (Strohl 1996).

*Peak flow*

**Peak flow** measures air *speed* or the maximum speed (peak) of air leaving the lungs (flow) during a *forced* expiration, lasting about one second. Vehicle speed is a measure of distance *compared with a time*, e.g. miles or kilometres *per hour*. Similarly, peak flow compares an air volume *with time* (litres *per minute*). The adult peak flow variation is large, owing to differences in sex, age, build, fitness and smoking habits. The average adult peak flow is about 400 L per minute, with male values slightly higher than female. The peak flow meter is an *assumption* that 400 L *would be* expelled from the lungs if the current maximum speed *had been* maintained for 60 seconds. The meter actually measures a fraction of this volume over a period of about one second. The value is dependent on healthy **lung compliance** – i.e. the lungs' ability to stretch to accommodate incoming air – and on the patency of the air passages. Reduced lung compliance, which limits the lungs' air capacity or partial airway obstruction, i.e. airway narrowing as in an asthma attack, will reduce the peak flow. Peak flow is achieved by blowing as hard and as fast as possible into a peak flow meter, after taking the greatest possible deep breath (inspiratory reserve volume). The full peak flow involves expelling as much of the vital capacity as quickly as possible. The accepted result is the best of three attempts. Severely breathless patients may not be able to perform this test.

*Cough*

Coughing and sneezing are respiratory phenomena with a purpose, i.e. clearing the airway of obstructions or irritants. The cough reflex centre is in the medulla, in association with the respiratory centre, and it initiates coughing from stimuli received from the upper respiratory tract. Choking is an emergency that may occur after the failure of severe coughing to relieve an acute upper respiratory obstruction, such as food. Coughing can also be chronic and persistent, and it is necessary to look for a pattern that will identify the cause of the cough. Some information needs to be known:

1  Is the cough dry (nothing coughed up) or productive (coughing produces something from the lungs)?
2  Is the cough accompanied by a sore throat or hoarse voice?

A dry cough suggests that a throat irritation is the cause, possibly an **upper respiratory tract infection** (**URTI**) such as the common cold. A sore throat and a hoarse or lost voice may further confirm this. A productive cough recovers some substance, usually mucus, from the lungs, indicating the problem is lower in the respiratory system.

Mucous could be substantial, being coughed up every few minutes throughout the day, as in chronic bronchitis. It may be infected, being mixed with pus, and it may appear green. Blood coughed from the lungs (**haemoptysis**) is potentially very serious because it is blood lost from circulation potentially causing shock, and it fills the airway preventing inhalation and gas exchange. The result can be fatal if there is much bleeding and it is not treated quickly. Haemoptysis has various causes:

• **Lung cancer** that has eroded through a main blood vessel;
• Left ventricular failure, where a backflow of blood creates pulmonary congestion;

- Erosion and enlargement of alveolar lung tissue (cavitations of the lung called **emphysema**) caused by the persistent long-term cough of chronic bronchitis.

Emphysema is a permanent complication of smoking that causes chronic dyspnoea. Since smoking is a lung irritant, it is a major cause of several lung and heart disorders, such as cancer, chronic bronchitis, emphysema and coronary thrombosis. The patient's history of smoking is important in lung assessment as smoking could be the reason for many chronic coughs with mucus production.

### Respiratory sounds

Respiration is almost silent, so observing sounds that occur during breathing is important. **Rales** are crackles or bubbling noises heard mostly on inspiration when air enters parts of the airway with fluid present, as in pulmonary oedema due to heart failure or pneumonia. They are unaffected by coughing. **Rhonchi** are wheezes heard mostly on expiration and often clear after coughing. High-pitched rhonchi (**sibilant rhonchi**) come from the small branches of the respiratory passages and are heard in patients suffering from asthma. Lower-pitched rhonchi (**sonorous rhonchi**) are from the larger bronchi and occur in **bronchitis**. These sounds can be identified using **auscultation**, i.e. listening to the chest through a stethoscope, but severe forms of the sound may be heard while in close proximity to the patient without any listening aids. Urgent intervention may be necessary to improve the patient's breathing. **Stridor** is a loud, harsh, high-pitched and vibrating sound, sometimes called '*crowing*', during mostly inspiration and caused by partial obstruction of the larynx (**laryngeal stridor**) or trachea. Sometimes this can happen in new born babies, called **congenital laryngeal stridor**. The cause in the new born is a congenital defect of the upper opening of the larynx, but the sound usually disappears by around 1 year of age. Stridor can be heard in **croup**, an acute upper-respiratory (larynx and trachea) infection, which is often viral in origin and affects mostly children. It is accompanied by dyspnoea and distress and sometimes sternal and ribcage retraction, when the chest wall is pulled back during inspiration. If inadequate air reaches the lungs, cyanosis may occur.

### Cyanosis

Cyanosis is a grey, blue or mauve discoloration of the skin, depending on the degree of severity. It is caused by a lack of oxygen in the tissues (**tissue hypoxia**), but the skin colour change is due to an accumulation of **reduced haemoglobin** in the tissues. Reduced haemoglobin is haemoglobin without oxygen that takes on a hydrogen ion ($H^+$) in order to buffer these ions and prevent pH changes in the circulation (see page 88). Excess reduced haemoglobin occurs as a result of inadequate oxygenation, when there is an excess of vacant haemoglobin capable of binding hydrogen ions. If the colour change is observed in the periphery (i.e. the hands and feet), it is due to normal adequate arterial blood oxygenation, but the tissues are extracting excess oxygen from this blood, leaving larger than normal quantities of reduced haemoglobin in the very small veins (called **venules**). These tiny veins contribute to the visible colour of the skin. Restriction of blood supply to a part or whole of a limb may cause a degree of peripheral cyanosis in that affected limb. If the cyanosis occurs more centrally, i.e. the trunk or face, it is due to the lack of oxygenation of arterial blood by the lungs. The greater the volume of reduced haemoglobin, the more severe the colour change from grey to deep purple. Central cyanosis can be treated with oxygen, which will occupy larger quantities of haemoglobin and therefore lower the level of reduced haemoglobin in the tissues.

### Oxygen blood saturation (pulse oximetry)

Each haemoglobin molecule in the blood can bind and carry four oxygen molecules to the tissues, and as such haemoglobin would be 100% saturated. A haemoglobin molecule with only three oxygen molecules is 75% saturated; with two oxygen molecules it is 50% saturated and so on. A mixture of millions of haemoglobin molecules, some at 100%, some at 75%, some at 50% etc., results in a saturation value for *whole* blood at figures between those stated, e.g. 95% saturated. The oxygen saturation should normally be close to 100%, i.e. fully saturated. This can be monitored by attaching the patient's finger to a clip-on sensor that gives an instant read-out of both the pulse and oxygen saturation level: the pulse oximeter. Low levels of oxygen saturation, e.g. less than 97%, indicates a problem, often in the lungs, that is preventing full oxygenation. Such problems include chronic bronchitis and pneumonia. The advantage of this on-the-spot method, when compared with repeated arterial blood sampling, becomes obvious. Oxygen saturation of blood is affected by the blood gas tension of oxygen ($PO_2$), and a correlation of oxygen saturations over a range of $PO_2$ is shown by the oxygen saturation curve (Figure 5.9).

   The difference between the two is that saturation involves the *volume* of oxygen carried, whereas the $PO_2$ gas tension is the *pressure* it exerts. The greater the volume carried, the greater is the pressure exerted. The curve shows a high saturation (98.5%) in the lungs giving a $PO_2$ of 100 mmHg, and a lower saturation (74%) in the tissues giving a lower $PO_2$ of 40 mmHg (see *blood gas tensions*, Figure 5.8, page 107). This represents an offloading of oxygen in the *tissues* that desaturates haemoglobin by about 23% and a corresponding on-loading of oxygen in the lungs. Under exercise conditions, oxygen is used faster than usual, which lowers the $PO_2$ in the tissues below 40 mmHg. Because of the shape of the left half of the curve, i.e. the steep section, a drop in the $PO_2$ in the tissues below 40 mmHg causes a steep drop in the oxygen saturation. For example, if the $PO_2$ in the tissues drops to 30 mmHg, i.e. a 10 mmHg drop during exercise, this causes a desaturation of haemoglobin from 74% down to 43%. This desaturation offloads a lot of oxygen to tissues to accommodate for the exercise. Compare this with the same (10 mmHg) drop in $PO_2$ in the tissues in the upper (flatter) part of the curve, i.e. from 100 mmHg down to 90 mmHg, with only a corresponding drop in saturation from 98% to 96%.

   Shifts in this curve (Figure 5.9), either to the right or left, occur as a result of various changes in certain physical parameters. Shifts to the *right* can be caused by an increase in the $PCO_2$, i.e. more haemoglobin will be carrying $CO_2$, less $O_2$. This is the **Bohr effect**. Similarly, low $PCO_2$ causes the curve to shift to the *left*, the **Haldane effect**, allowing more haemoglobin for carrying $O_2$. Blood pH also affects the curve. Increasing acidity (lower pH) shifts the curve to the *right*, while alkalinity (higher pH) shifts the curve to the *left*. Higher blood temperature shifts the curve to the *right*, and lower blood temperature shifts the curve to the *left*. An end product of red blood cell metabolism is **2,3-diphosphoglycerate** (**DPG**). If DPG increases, the curve shifts to the

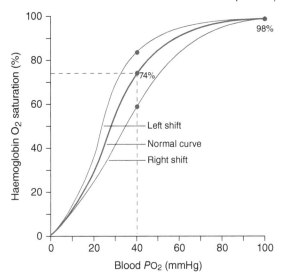

*Figure 5.9* The oxygen saturation curve. The percentage of oxygen saturation of haemoglobin is plotted against the oxygen blood gas tension ($PO_2$). The normal curve (centre) shows an offloading of oxygen to the tissues from 98% down to 74% saturated ($PO_2$ of tissues being approximately 40 mmHg) and a loading of oxygen to the haemoglobin from 74% to 98% saturation in the lungs ($PO_2$ of the lungs being approximately 100 mmHg). So, blood is moving from the lungs at 98% saturation (100 mmHg pressure) to the tissues where oxygen is delivered, reducing saturation to 74% (40 mmHg pressure). The blood then returns to the lungs to restore full saturation again. Shifts of the curve to the left or right can happen (see page 112).

*right,* but it shifts to the *left* if DPG levels drop, as can be the case with stored blood in the blood bank.

### ABCDE assessment

Airway and breathing are the first priorities to assess and manage in any state of cardio-pulmonary emergency where the vital functions have either failed or are failing. Resuscitation always starts with checking to see if the patient is breathing through a clear airway. To ensure the best possible outcome from any resuscitation attempt, a systematic approach that sets out the priorities of management has been established: the **ABCDE assessment** (Table 5.1).

The ABCDE system goes beyond resuscitation and becomes a basis upon which a diagnosis can be determined and urgent care can be administered. Establishing if the patient is conscious (see Chapter 11) is important. This involves the use of the *alert, voice, pain, unresponsive* (AVPU) system (see page 232). A conscious patient will at least be breathing, with or without breathing difficulty. Their response (if any) to the AVPU assessment should give information about their conscious state. Failure of the patient to respond would require further urgent examination of their airway, breathing and circulatory status. The red flag situations, i.e. those which need urgent attention, are stated in Table 5.2.

*Table 5.1* The ABCDE assessment

| | | Notes |
|---|---|---|
| **A** | Airway | Check for any obstruction to the airway and clear these quickly if possible. In unconscious patients, the airway may be obstructed by the tongue, and measures must be taken to correct this. In a first-aid situation, this means putting the head back with the jaw extended forward to lift the tongue clear. In a hospital situation, this will probably be managed by intubation. Cyanosis may be apparent (see page 111). Partial obstruction results in reduced and often noisy ventilation, coupled with choking and serious distress in the conscious patient. |
| **B** | Breathing | Make sure the patient is breathing by observing for chest wall movements and feeling the warmth of exhaled air. Failure of breathing requires immediate ventilation, either by mouth-to-mouth or by mechanical means, once the airway is patent. Respiratory sounds may be present (see page 111) and the patient may be using the accessory muscles for breathing (see page 101). Conscious patients are likely to be in severe distress (i.e. fighting for each breath, known as 'air hunger'). Oxygen should be used if available, although there are limitations for patients with chronic retention of $CO_2$ (see page 109). |
| **C** | Circulation | Check the central pulse (notably the carotid) for any evidence of a pulse that indicates an active circulation. As blood pressure falls, the peripheral pulses (notably the radial pulse at the wrist) become absent first, and central pulses fail afterwards (see page 28). The absence of peripheral pulses indicates failure of circulation to the extremities, as further identified by cold fingers and toes, coupled with severe pallor and cyanosis of hands and feet and a slow or absent capillary refill time (see page 48). In cardiac arrest (i.e. no cardiac output), all pulses will be absent. Central cyanosis (see page 111) will become established quickly. Circulatory resuscitation must begin urgently, with manual chest compressions and, if suitable and if available, defibrillation (depending on the nature of the cardiac arrest; see page 34). In a hospital situation, access to venous blood via cannulation is vital but may not be easily achieved, depending on the extent of the circulatory collapse. |
| **D** | Disability | Information on what may be the cause of the patient's current condition would be gathered at this stage. If time and the situation permit, a full AVPU assessment, i.e. alert, voice, pain, unresponsive (see page 232) would be useful to acquire more information on the patient's conscious level, which may aid a diagnosis. Checking the blood sugar would be of value and glucose administered if the cause was hypoglycaemia. Pupil size and reactions to light may give clues to the cause of any alteration in consciousness. |
| **E** | Exposure and examination | Maintain the body temperature (see page 10) to prevent hypothermia, and keep the patient covered as much as possible. Physical examination should be done in a private, warm environment if possible, while maintaining patient dignity. |

## Childhood breathing

Normal respiration rates vary in childhood according to age. At birth, the rate is from 30 to 55, in early childhood it is from 20 to 30 and in late childhood from 14 to 22 (Table 5.3).

The infant lung volumes are much smaller than the adult, the tidal volume being about 15 ml, with a corresponding smaller dead space. Diaphragmatic breathing is dominant

*Table 5.2* Red flag warnings of deteriorating condition

ϕ **Red Flag = any of the following serious situations which needs urgent medical attention.**

| Flag warning | Details |
|---|---|
| ϕ **Red Flag** | **Not breathing, possible obstructed airway.** |
| | **Sudden onset of severe breathlessness with use of secondary muscles of respiration, inability to talk properly and exhaustion.** |
| | **Inadequate response to medication.** |
| | **Previous hospital admissions for breathing difficulty.** |
| | **O₂ saturation 92% or less.** |
| | **Blue lips, drowsy or confused.** |

(After Hill-Smith and Johnson 2021)

*Table 5.3* Child normal respiratory rates

| Age | Normal respiration rate |
|---|---|
| < 1 year | 30–55 |
| 1–2 years | 20–30 |
| 3–5 years | 20–25 |
| 6–11 years | 14–22 |
| 12–15 years | 12–18 |

| Assessment | Score | | |
|---|---|---|---|
| | 0 | 1 | 2 |
| Heart rate | Absent | Slow (< 100/min) | Over 100/min |
| Respiratory effort | Absent | Slow or irregular | Good crying |
| Muscle tone | Limp | Some flexion of extremities | Action motion |
| Response to stimulation | None | Poor, with grimace | Good crying |
| Colour | Blue or pale | Body pink extremities blue | Completely pink |

Score 0–3 = severe distress of infant
Score 4–7 = moderate distress of infant
Score 8–10 = no difficulty of infant to adjust to extrauterine life

*Figure 5.10* The Apgar score.

over chest wall movements during the early years, and it may be easier to count abdominal movements rather than chest wall movements. Respiratory effort forms part of the **Apgar score** carried out at birth to assess the infant's condition (i.e. 0 = absent breathing, 1 = gasping or irregular breathing, 2 = crying or rhythmic breathing; Figure 5.10; Letko 1996).

Breathing responses to illness, exercise and emotion are greater in children. The most common respiratory symptom in children is coughing, which is usually caused by a throat irritation or a mild **upper respiratory tract infection** (**URTI**), such as the common cold. Just occasionally, it may be more serious (e.g. pneumonia; Kambarami *et al.* 1996).

The child who is born before full term is *premature* and as a result may suffer severe respiratory problems. **Hyaline membrane disease** (**HMD**) is due to a lack of **surfactant** on the alveolar wall. Lungs must switch from being fluid-filled to air-filled at birth as they expand. Surfactant produced in the lungs lowers the resistance of the alveolar wall to stretching, i.e. it lowers the **surface tension**. A lack of surfactant results in lungs that will not expand properly and therefore will not admit enough air. It results in **respiratory distress syndrome** (**RDS**), a complication seen in very preterm babies, i.e. those with immature lungs, but the condition is rare in children born after 37 weeks' gestation. RDS involves respiratory rates over 100 breaths per minute, expiratory **grunting** sounds – due to expiration against a partially closed **glottis** – and chest wall retraction. In severe cases, the baby is cyanosed with gasping respirations and even apnoea and will need resuscitation, oxygen and assisted breathing, possibly ventilation. Hypoxia must be prevented because it can cause brain damage and less surfactant production, but a high oxygen level is also dangerous since it can cause blindness by damaging the retina. Oxygen supplementation should be medically prescribed and strictly monitored.

Young children are more prone than adults to lung infections, mostly because they have an immature immune system that is exposed to infectious agents (**antigens**) that are new to them. Cystic fibrosis is a genetic congenital disorder of exocrine gland secretion that affects mostly the mucus of the lungs and digestive system. Mucous becomes thick and sticky, with repeated infections not only causing malabsorption and malnutrition but also chronic respiratory obstruction with breathing difficulty. The disorder is caused by any of several mutations of the **cystic fibrosis transmembrane conductance regulator** (**CFTR**) gene on chromosome 7 (gene locus 7q31.2).[3] It is a recessive gene error which means that to get the disease the child has inherited the mutation from both parents. Children born with the condition in the past had a limited life expectancy, but this has improved with advances in care and treatment.

### Drugs affecting the respiratory system

Drugs active on the respiratory system include:

**Bronchodilators** (Figure 5.11), which cause widening of the airway to improve airflow in and out of the lungs. They are used to treat asthma, where the airway passages are severely narrowed. There are several groups of bronchodilators:

- The $\beta_2$ **selective agonists**[4] are drugs that stimulate the $\beta_2$ receptors causing smooth muscle cells to relax in the airway wall, thus dilating the airway (Figure 5.11B). $\beta_2$ receptors are one of three classes of receptors, alpha ($\alpha$), beta-1 ($\beta_1$) and beta-2 ($\beta_2$) that are acted on by the **sympathetic nervous system** on muscle tissue (Table 5.4). Bronchodilators are required to treat acute respiratory distress due to bronchoconstriction, as in acute asthma attacks, and as such they are better administered directly into the lungs by inhalation. This route of administration promotes rapid relief of symptoms and reduces side effects because the drug is not as well absorbed

*Table 5.4* $\beta_2$ selective agonist bronchodilators to treat bronchoconstriction

| Drug | Possible side effects | Use and other notes |
| --- | --- | --- |
| Bambuterol hydrochloride | Anxiety, abnormal behaviour, muscle cramps, sleep disturbance. | Long acting $\beta_2$ agonist. |
| Formoterol fumarate | Dizziness, muscle cramps, nausea. | Long acting $\beta_2$ agonist. |
| Indacaterol | Chest pain, cough, dizziness, muscle pain, peripheral oedema. | Long acting $\beta_2$ agonist. |
| Olodaterol | Rare but includes dizziness, rash, joint pain. | Long acting $\beta_2$ agonist. |
| Salmeterol | Muscle cramps, skin reactions, nervousness. | Long acting $\beta_2$ agonist. |
| Salbutamol | Muscle cramps. | Short acting $\beta_2$ agonist. |
| Terbutaline sulfate | Hypokalaemia (low blood potassium), hypotension (Chapter 3), muscle cramps, nausea. | Short acting $\beta_2$ agonist. |

*Table 5.5* Antimuscarinic bronchodilators

| Drug | Possible side effects | Use and other notes |
| --- | --- | --- |
| Aclidinium bromide | Diarrhoea, nasopharyngitis. | Given by inhalation. |
| Glycopyrronium bromide | Increase infection risk, insomnia, pain. | Alone or combined with either formoterol fumarate or indacaterol. |
| Ipratropium bromide | Throat problems, poor gastrointestinal motility. | Alone or combined with salbutamol. |
| Tiotropium | Gastrointestinal disturbance, increase infection risk. | Alone or combined with olodaterol. |
| Umeclidinium | Altered taste, eye pain. | Alone or combined with vilanterol. |

into general circulation from the lungs as it would be from the digestive system. **Ephedrine hydrochloride** is a *mixed action* **sympathomimetic**[5] drug, acting on alpha and beta receptors to cause bronchodilation.

- The **antimuscarinic** bronchodilators cause dilation of the airway by blocking the **muscarinic receptors**, i.e. receptors that normally bind acetylcholine. These receptors are part of the **parasympathetic nervous system** that normally act on smooth muscle in the airway to cause constriction. By blocking these receptors, the airway dilates (Figure 5.11B, Table 5.5).
- **Xanthines** are chemical agents found naturally in body cells and tissues and in some plant products such as caffeine. They are mild stimulants and bronchodilators. The best-known drugs in this group are **theophylline** and **aminophylline**, which is a complex of theophylline with ethylenediamine. Aminophylline is not normally a first-choice drug as it is given by slow intravenous injection.
- **Mast cell stabilisers** – or **cromones** – are drugs that reduce the risk of histamine release from mast cells. Mast cells store histamine, and this is released in an immune reaction to an antigen. Histamine release triggers a number of different effects leading to an inflammatory response, including bronchoconstriction if the mast cells

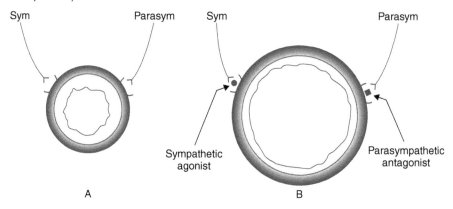

*Figure 5.11* The bronchodilator drugs. Cross sections of the bronchioles showing the darker outer layer (smooth muscle) with the pale pink inner lining (mucous membrane). (A) Bronchoconstriction, where the lumen is narrowed, often due to an imbalance between the sympathetic nervous system (sym) and the parasympathetic nervous system (parasym). (B) Sympathetic agonists drugs can be used to increase (+) sympathetic activity which then dilates the bronchus, or parasympathetic antagonists can be used to block (−) parasympathetic activity, which then does not oppose sympathetic bronchodilation.

*Table 5.6* Corticosteroid drugs used to prevent bronchoconstriction, as in asthma

| Drug | Possible side effects | Use and other notes |
|---|---|---|
| Beclometasone dipropionate | Throat irritation, wheezing. | Alone or combined with formoterol or with formoterol plus glycopyrronium. |
| Budesonide | Excess nasal secretion, sneezing, coughing, nausea. | Alone or combined with formoterol. |
| Ciclesonide | Cushing's syndrome (excess steroid hormone). | Prevention of asthma. |
| Fluticasone | Rare. Possibly indigestion (dyspepsia). | Alone or combined with formoterol or salmeterol or vilanterol or umeclidinium and vilanterol. |
| Mometasone furoate | Candida infections. | Alone or combined with indacaterol or glycopyrronium and indacaterol. |

releasing histamine are in the respiratory tract. This would happen particularly if the antigen was inhaled, such as pollen or pollutants in the air. The drug in this group is **sodium cromoglicate**, usually given by aerosol inhalation.

- **Corticosteroids** are anti-inflammatory drugs, and those used in respiratory disorders are normally delivered as a daily **prophylaxis** (preventative measure) by inhalation (Table 5.6). They reduce or prevent inflammation of the respiratory mucosa, thus reducing the risk of airway obstruction caused by swollen mucus. Some of these drugs can be given, along with the bronchodilators, by intravenous or oral route, in acute asthmatic attacks as an additional treatment.
- **Leukotriene receptor antagonists**, i.e. **montelukast**, is an orally administered drug that blocks the effects of specific leukotrienes within the respiratory tract. Leukotrienes are chemicals produced by mast cells, basophils and macrophages

(see page 90), and they are involved in causing inflammation and bronchoconstriction. This drug blocks the leukotriene receptors (i.e. they are antagonists) and thus prevent leukotriene activity and bronchoconstriction.

## Key points

### Anatomy and Physiology

- The lungs are held tightly against the chest wall by a negative pressure – or vacuum – existing between the visceral and parietal layers of the pleura.
- We need oxygen ($O_2$) from the air, but the primary driving force of breathing is carbon dioxide ($CO_2$).
- Breathing consists of inspiration, expiration and a brief pause.
- The volume of air taken in with each breath is the tidal volume, about 500 ml in adults, subdivided into the alveolar air, which will exchange gas, about 350 ml, and the dead space, which will not exchange gas, about 150 ml.
- Movement of gases across the body membranes uses gas concentration gradients.
- Oxygen and carbon dioxide in the blood create a gas pressure, called the blood gas tensions.
- The average respiratory rate in an adult is about 15–18 times per minute, but the rate can rise to > 30 times per minute during exercise or when there is a respiratory or cardiac disorder.
- Respiration depends on the respiratory centre, which is shared between the medulla and the pons, in the brainstem.

### Investigations

- Peak flow measures the maximum speed of air leaving the lungs during a forced expiration.

### Pathology

- In acidosis, blood below pH 7.4 causes increased respiration in an attempt to remove carbon dioxide, an acid gas, from the circulation.
- Pneumothorax is air in the pleural space.
- Left heart failure (LVF) causes blood to back up into the pulmonary veins, and fluid from the plasma leaks into the alveoli causing pulmonary oedema and dyspnoea.
- Shunting involves blood passing through areas of unventilated alveoli, returning from the lungs without any gas exchange.
- Cyanosis is a grey to mauve discoloration of the skin caused by a lack of oxygen, resulting in an accumulation in the tissues of reduced haemoglobin (i.e. haemoglobin that has a hydrogen ion attached).
- Stridor is a loud, harsh, high-pitched sound during inspiration caused by partial obstruction of the larynx (laryngeal stridor) or trachea.
- Respiration is normally silent; therefore, abnormal breath sounds should be reported.
- Respiratory distress syndrome (RDS) is sometimes seen in very preterm babies.
- Smoking is a lung irritant and a major cause of lung cancer, chronic bronchitis, emphysema and heart diseases.

*Pharmacology*

• The main drugs used in respiratory disorders are the bronchodilators and corticosteroids.

## Notes

1 Square brackets mean 'concentration of', in this case concentration of hydrogen ions [$H^+$].
2 1 kPa = 7.5 mmHg
3 Gene locus means the location of the gene on the chromosome, in this case chromosome number 7, on the long arm (q) at band 31.2 away from the centromere.
4 Agonist is a drug that binds to a receptor and activates (or stimulates) that receptor (see Chapter 15, page 315)
5 Sympathomimetic means to mimic the sympathetic nervous system by stimulation of sympathetic receptors.

## References

Forbes-Faulkner L. (1998) Oxygen therapy: Challenges for nurses. *Kai-Tiaki: Nursing New Zealand*, 4(3): 17–19.

Grey A. (1995) Breathless . . . dyspnoea. *Nursing Times, 91*(27): 46–47.

Hickey J.V. (2013) *The Clinical Practice of Neurological and Neurosurgical Nursing* (7th edition). Lippincott Williams & Wilkins, Philadelphia, PA.

Hill-Smith I. and Johnson G. (2021) *Little Book of Red Flags*. National Minor Illness Centre, Bedfordshire.

Kambarami R.A., Rusakaniko S. and Mahomva L.A. (1996) Ability of caregivers to recognise signs of pneumonia in coughing children aged below five years. *Central African Journal of Medicine, 42*(10): 291–294.

Letko M.D. (1996) Understanding the APGAR score. *Journal of Obstetric, Gynecologic and Neonatal Nursing, 25*(4): 299–303.

Owen A. (1998) Respiratory assessment revisited. *Nursing, 28*(4): 48–49.

Strohl K.P. (1996) The biology of sleep apnea. *Science and Medicine*, September/October: 32–41.

# 6 Fluid and electrolyte balance

- Introduction
- Water in the body
- Water gain versus water lost
- Fluid balance in children
- Problems of water imbalance
- Electrolyte balance
- Key points
- References

## Introduction

The water molecule (**$H_2O$**; Figure 6.1) has two hydrogen atoms covalently bonded to an oxygen atom. This creates a **dipole** (i.e. 'two poles'), in this case a molecule with a *positive* pole at one end (the hydrogen end), and a *negative* pole at the other end (the oxygen end; Figure 6.1).

This arrangement allows water to have some interesting and biologically valuable properties e.g. it is an excellent solvent for many other molecules and it has a high **heat capacity**. This means that it absorbs and loses large amounts of heat with little change in temperature, important as part of stabilising body temperature (see Chapter 1).

## Water in the body

The adult human body contains 50% to 65% water (males) and 45% to 60% water (females), depending on body size. In very young infants, the average is about 75% to 78%, gradually declining to 65% by the age of 1 year. This water is recycled and renewed multiple times a day. A typical 70 kg person has about 42 litres of water (about 60% of the body weight), and this breaks down to 28 litres of intracellular water (inside the cells) plus 14 litres of extracellular water (outside the cells), i.e. 11 litres as tissue fluid and 3 litres as blood plasma.

DOI: 10.4324/9781003389118-6

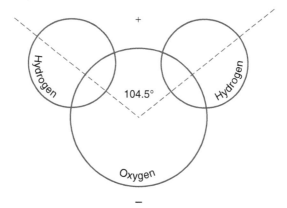

*Figure 6.1* The water molecule ($H_2O$). Two hydrogen atoms are bonded to one oxygen atom at an angle of 104.5° to make one water molecule. The hydrogen end is positively (+) charged, and the oxygen is negatively (−) charged, so the whole molecule becomes a dipole (i.e. two poles).

Water is critical in the body because:

1   Cellular metabolism depends on water. Many chemical reactions involve water, and other reactions that do not use water directly work through the medium of water, i.e. they would not happen if the components were dry
2   Water is vital for movement of substances around the body, notable by the blood and the lymphatic systems, which are both important water-based transport systems. This is because water is an excellent **solvent**, and many compounds are dissolved in water in the human body. At a cellular level, water is instrumental in the movement of dissolved substances across membranes
3   Water is also vital for elimination purposes, not just through urine but also through the other water-based excretory systems: faeces and sweat. Many waste substances for excretion are dissolved in water (e.g. urea)
4   Water helps to keep cells in their correct shape through internal pressures, and water shortage in the cells causes shrinkage with a corresponding reduction in cellular function.

The body requires between 1 and 7 litres of water intake per day to avoid dehydration. The exact amount is dependent on levels of activity, the body and ambient temperatures, the atmospheric humidity and other factors, but averages about 2–2.5 litres per day for most people.

Water occupies three body compartments (Figure 6.2):

1   **Intracellular** i.e. inside the cells, the largest fluid compartment, with an average of about 30 litres of water
2   **Extracellular** i.e. outside or between the cells, also called **tissue fluid**, with an average of about 12 litres of water
3   **Blood**, both inside the blood cells and as the main constituent of plasma, with an average of about 3 litres of water.

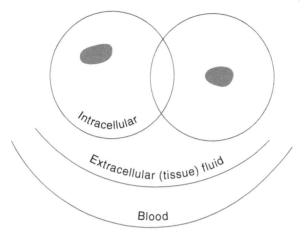

*Figure 6.2* The three body water compartments. Water occupies the intracellular (inside the cells), extracellular (outside the cells, also called tissue fluid) and blood compartments.

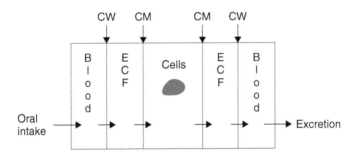

*Figure 6.3* Water passes from input (oral) to output (excretion) through the three body compartments: blood, extracellular fluid (ECF) and cells. CW: capillary wall; CM: cell membrane.

The overall total for all 3 compartments is about 45 litres. However, water is never static in these compartments but moves across **semipermeable membranes** (**SPMs**) from one compartment to another and is also replaced all the time by new water. The movement and replacement sequence for water is as follows: new water entering the digestive system from drinking is absorbed into the blood, then passes into extracellular fluid, then intracellular fluid, back to extracellular fluid, then blood again, either directly or via the lymphatic system and is finally excreted (Figure 6.3).

Water moves down its own concentration gradient, i.e. it flows from areas of high concentration to areas of low concentration, a process called **osmosis** (Figure 6.4).

In addition, water will also move down pressure gradients. This process allows the formation of tissue fluid, derived from the *net outflow* of fluid from plasma at the highest pressure (arterial) end of the capillary. Meanwhile, fluid is returning to the plasma, caused by the *net inflow* of fluid at the lowest-pressure (venous) end of the capillary (Figure 6.5).

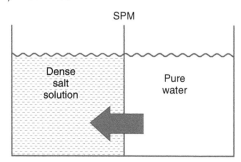

Figure 6.4 Osmosis. In this example, pure water can be considered as a high concentration when compared with the water in the same volume of a dense salt solution. Water will pass through a semipermeable membrane (SPM, water flow shown by large arrow) until the concentration of water is equal on both sides (i.e. water is moving down its own concentration gradient). This would *increase* the volume on the salt side and *decrease* the volume on the pure water side. This process, called osmosis, is in action in the body and is one means by which water moves from one compartment to another.

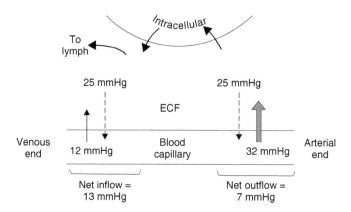

Figure 6.5 The formation and return of tissue fluid. Blood pressure in the capillary forces water out of plasma into the extracellular fluid (ECF). The pressure at the arterial end (32 mmHg) is higher than the pressure at the venous end (12 mmHg) as blood pressure falls throughout the capillary bed. The plasma proteins pull water back into the capillary with an attractive force (measured as a pressure of 25 mmHg) across the capillary bed. Therefore, at the arterial end, there is a net *outflow* from the capillary (i.e. 32 − 25 = 7 mmHg), which constantly creates new tissue fluid from blood plasma, and at the venous end there is a net *inflow* into the capillary (i.e. 25 − 12 = 13 mmHg), which constantly returns water back to the blood plasma. The cells interchange water with the ECF, and some extra water escapes the ECF to become lymphatic fluid.

## Water gain versus water lost

### The fluid balance chart

Humans gain and lose water constantly throughout the day. Some of these gains and losses are known to us, and to some extent they are under our control. However, other gains and losses are invisible, known as **insensible** gains or losses, and they function without any conscious control by us.

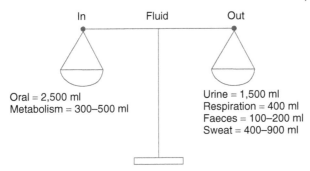

*Figure 6.6* Fluid balance. To balance on both sides, input (oral and metabolism) must equal output (urine, faeces, respiration and sweat).

Humans gain water mainly through drinking (oral intake, about 2,500 ml per day) at regular intervals throughout the day (Figure 6.6). This may be as plain water or flavoured as in tea, coffee or soft drinks. Even alcoholic drinks contain a large proportion of water, notably beer. Drinking water is not only driven by thirst, but we take in fluids for pleasure and comfort. Thirst is the *bottom line* as a driving force for drinking fluids, i.e. we should never wait for thirst to occur before taking fluids by mouth.

Apart from oral intake of fluids, we also gain much smaller quantities (about 300–500 ml per day) from tissue metabolism. In Chapter 1, Figure 1.4 shows the formation of metabolic water from energy production. At the end of the electron transport chain, two hydrogen protons ($2H^+$) join with oxygen (half $O_2$, i.e. O) to produce water ($H_2O$). This quantity of water is too small to sustain life, so oral intake daily becomes essential.

Humans lose much of our daily fluids through urine output, i.e. about 1,500 ml per day (Figure 6.6 and Chapter 8), but an important loss is also through the skin by evaporation of sweat (400–900 ml per day; see Chapters 1 and 10). This skin loss is part of our **insensible loss** since it cannot be directly measured and has to be estimated. Other forms of insensible loss are water vapour exhaled through the lungs (about 400 ml per day) and water lost in faeces (about 100–200 ml per day). These insensible losses must be part of the estimation.

Fluid balance records the amount of intake versus output to see if there is net gain or loss of fluid over a 24-hour period. Everything the patient drinks and passes as urine for 24 hours is measured (in millilitres, ml) and recorded on a fluid balance chart (see Figure 6.7).

The insensible losses and gains are estimated and recorded, and a net total is achieved. The object is to try to maintain a *neutral* fluid balance over 24 hours, i.e. no excess of intake, *positive* balance or excess of output, *negative* balance. Excess water intake or output over one or two periods of 24 hours is not normally a problem in health as the body makes adjustments (usually to urine output) to correct any deficits (see Chapter 8).

Producing a lower urine output will conserve water if intake is low. Similarly, a higher urine output will correct the balance if oral intake is high, e.g. the person drinking lots of beer who then needs to go to the toilet frequently! The physiology of these changes can be found in Chapter 8.

If fluid balance recordings show a persistent excessive loss or gain of fluid over several days or weeks, this will indicate that there is a problem which needs investigation and

**Fluid Balance Chart**

Date _____

| Oral/IV/enteral intake | | | | | Output | | | | |
|---|---|---|---|---|---|---|---|---|---|
| Time | Description | Oral | IV/enteral | Total | Time | Urine | Stool | Other | Total |
| | | | | | | | | | |
| | | | | | | | | | |
| | | | | | | | | | |
| | | | | | | | | | |
| | | | | | | | | | |
| | | | | | | | | | |
| | | | | | | | | | |
| | | | | | | | | | |
| | | | | | | | | | |
| | | | | | | | | | |
| | | | | | | | | | |
| | | | | | | | | | |
| | | | | | | | | | |
| | | | | | | | | | |
| | | | | | | | | | |
| | | | | | | | | | |
| | | | | | | | | | |
| | | | | | | | | | |
| | | | | | | | | | |
| | | | | | | | | | |
| | | | | | | | | | |
| | | | | | | | | | |
| | | | | | | | | | |
| | | | | | | | | | |
| | | | | | | | | | |
| | | | | | | | | | |
| | | | | | | | | | |
| | | | | | | | | | |
| | | | | | | | | | |
| | | Total | | | Total | | | | |

Oral/IV/enteral intake
24 hour total _____

Output 24 hour
total _____

*Figure 6.7* The 24-hour fluid balance chart. The patient's input and output are measured and entered on the chart along with the time. Totals for the 24 hours are calculated, taking into account the insensible losses. IV: intravenous.

attention. Special considerations must be made in relation to fluid balance under certain circumstances, as follows:

- Patients on **intravenous** (**IV**) infusions and **blood transfusions** must have the volumes of administered fluid measured and included in the fluid balance record. Giving fluids by intravenous route is an effective way of rehydrating patients who cannot drink enough, but it raises the risk of rapid fluid overload if renal output is poor. Intravenous overload must be avoided as it puts unnecessary strain on the heart and kidneys.
- Patients who are designated as **nil by mouth** (**NBM**) i.e. eating or drinking nothing for longer than a few hours require careful fluid monitoring to identify any risk of dehydration. Patients who cannot eat or drink long term will need alternative fluid replacement, either by IV route or by feeding tube. This includes coma patients and those in critical care. Short term NBM, e.g. during the perioperative period, i.e. just before and just after surgery is not normally a problem for otherwise healthy individuals.
- Patients who are vomiting have little or no appetite for food and drink. A single bout of vomiting is not a major problem for fluid balance, but if this persists for more than a few hours then fluid balance may need to be monitored and an alternative to oral fluid input considered. Because of their smaller size, children may be particularly prone to rapid dehydration due to persistent vomiting.

**Central venous pressure** (**CVP**) is a measure of the pressure of the *venous blood* returning to the heart, i.e. the blood pressure in the major *veins* close to the right atrium. Normal CVP is 3–10 mmHg (or 5–12 cmH$_2$O). CVP will be altered (higher or lower) when blood volume changes occur, and severe under-hydration or overhydration will affect blood volumes, as will significant blood loss. CVP changes may well occur earlier than blood pressure changes, and as such they will act as an early warning of problems with cardiovascular pressures. Therefore, CVP measurements may be important when rehydrating patients rapidly. CVP is covered in more detail in Chapter 3 (see page 56).

### Fluid balance in children

The first years of life are the time for the fastest changes occurring in water physiology, but these changes slow down gradually throughout childhood until adult levels are reached. The foetus has the highest total body water content per kg of body weight (i.e. as much as 90% of total body weight is water). The extracellular fluid (ECF) compartment (see page 122) accounts for 65% of this water. This slowly adjusts by the time of birth when water accounts for 75% of body weight. As they get older, there are further changes (e.g. water makes up 65% of body weight by 6 months old and 60% by the end of the first year). Young children also have an ability to concentrate urine lower than an adult's, which again changes to near adult values by the age of 2 years, and they have less losses through sweating than adults (mainly in boys). Contrary to this, children have a higher insensible water loss (see page 125) than adults, and again this reduces as they get older. This all amounts to a faster water turnover in very young children than at any other age, especially within the first few weeks of life.

## Problems of water imbalance

*Oedema*

**Oedema** is excessive fluid in the tissues causing the tissues to swell. This excess of water is mostly in the extracellular (tissue fluid) compartment, with very little extra fluid in the intracellular compartment, as the cell membranes would rupture if they took on too much water. Some extra fluid can be housed in the blood compartment, but this is limited because excess water in circulation boosts blood volume and thus raises blood pressure, and the excess would normally be removed by the kidneys. High blood pressure (**hypertension**) can be treated using drugs that promote water loss from the blood compartment through the kidneys (drugs called **diuretics**; see Chapters 3 and 8).

Oedema results either from the intake of water persistently exceeding the output, i.e. a *positive* fluid balance, over several days or weeks or due to the body's failure to handle water properly, i.e. heart or kidney failure. A poor diagnostic outcome in acute renal failure has been linked to positive fluid balance (Payen *et al.* 2008). In normal health, it is difficult to achieve a persistent positive balance because the kidneys remove the excess water and therefore improve the output, thus restoring the balance, i.e. the more water drunk, the more urine passed (see Chapter 8). There are also *local* causes of oedema, i.e. specific causes of oedema occurring in a particular part of the body, e.g. **ascites**, which is oedema in the peritoneal space resulting in abdominal swelling. Oedema is therefore a pathological state, i.e. a symptom of some underlying pathology. The problem of tissue oedema can be narrowed down to five causes:

1  *Obstructed venous return* of blood, as seen in **heart failure**. *Right* heart failure causes a backlog of blood waiting to get into the right side of the heart, and this backlog can increase venous pressure sufficiently that the veins cannot accept any more blood from the capillaries, which then engorge and leak fluid into the tissues (called **systemic oedema**). *Left* heart failure causes a backlog of blood from the lungs waiting to enter the left ventricle, and this increases the venous blood pressure coming from the lungs, which then causes fluid to leak out of the capillaries into the lungs. Fluid then collects in the alveoli (called **pulmonary oedema**). At a more local level, congestion of venous return can occur if there are any tight restrictions to a limb preventing venous return, e.g. an inflated blood pressure cuff left on for too long
2  *Excess sodium* in circulation and the tissues. The kidneys remove excess sodium from the body by excreting it in the urine (see Chapter 8). Kidney problems can cause a failure to remove sodium, which then accumulates in the blood (called **hypernatraemia**) and in the tissues. One property of sodium is that it attracts water. If sodium is retained in the body, so will be water, causing an oedematous state. Excessive sodium intake will also contribute to oedema, especially again if the kidneys are unable to excrete it all. The hormone **aldosterone** (from the adrenal cortex) conserves sodium in the body (see Chapter 8), and excess of this hormone may also contribute to a hypernatraemia and thus oedema
3  *Inadequate plasma protein* concentration. One of the vital functions of proteins in plasma is to attract fluid back to the blood from the extracellular compartment (see plasma proteins, Chapter 4, page 67). This attracting force draws water back at a pressure of 25 mmHg along the capillary length (Figure 6.5). Capillaries have semipermeable walls to allow this water to pass through. In the event of low plasma proteins, this

attracting force is reduced, i.e. the 25 mmHg pressure drops, and water is then added to the tissues faster than it is withdrawn, and thus it accumulates in the tissues. Low plasma proteins can occur in starvation – especially very low dietary protein intake – and in liver disease since the liver produces **albumen**, the most abundant of the plasma proteins (see Chapter 4, page 67).

4 *Obstructed lymphatic drainage* of the tissues. Normally, the lymphatic system drains away any excess fluid from the extracellular tissue space, thus preventing any fluid build-up (Figure 6.5). Anything that obstructs this drainage will cause oedema. Examples of this are new growths or inflammation of the lymphatic glands (or nodes) and any external pressures on the lymphatic vessels.

5 *Increased capillary wall permeability*. This occurs as a process of **inflammation**. The normally permeable capillary wall becomes even more permeable (i.e. 'leaky') as a result of the inflammatory process. This causes more water to escape into the tissues. Proteins in the plasma are normally too big to pass through the capillary wall, but in inflammation capillaries can become leaky enough to allow proteins to escape the plasma into the tissue fluid. The protein-rich environment surrounding the capillaries attracts even more water out of the capillaries and causes local swelling (**localised oedema**) of the tissues. Swelling is one of the cardinal signs of inflammation, along with redness, pain and heat (see Chapter 10).

*Pulmonary* oedema is a very serious problem that is recognised by acute **dyspnoea** (breathlessness), severe **cyanosis** (due to **shunting**; see Chapter 5, page 109) and cough. Fluid collects in the air sacs (alveoli), reducing the surface area available for oxygen and carbon dioxide exchange (see Chapter 5, page 99). The surprise is the fact that symptoms of pulmonary oedema occur so quickly after left heart failure has occurred. This is because the distance between the left heart and the lungs is very short, and any backlog of blood flow reaches the lungs rapidly. **Loop diuretics** (see Chapter 8) are drugs used to treat pulmonary oedema caused by left ventricular failure. They work by promoting fluid loss from the kidneys, which in turn withdraws fluid from the lungs.

*Systemic* fluid overload can be identified by the following observations: weight gain, raised CVP and raised blood pressure, fast pulse and breathing rates, raised urine output if the kidneys are functioning normally or lower urine output if the heart is in failure and oedematous swelling of tissues (Mooney 2007). The swelling of the tissues is mostly in the limbs (i.e. tissues farthest from the heart), especially the legs and ankles as fluid drains downwards to the lowest points due to gravity. This gravity-driven oedema is known as **dependent** oedema. Dependent oedema also occurs in the back and sacral areas in patients lying on their backs while confined to bed and may contribute towards pressure sore formation. Systemic oedema can also be recognised by applying gentle pressure from a finger to create a shallow dent. Normally the dent should rebound back to normal levels when the finger is removed. If this dent remains the problem is systemic oedema. Reduction of this oedema in the legs (the commonest site) can be assisted by seating the patient with legs elevated, thus employing gravity to gradually drain the tissue fluid back into circulation. Also, it can be prevented by the application of bandages or pressure stockings, which provide enough external pressure to stop fluid leakage into the tissues.

**Cerebral oedema** is swelling of the brain, due to inflammation of the brain or its coverings, or sometimes due to head injury, i.e. **concussion**, which is 'brain shaking' (see Chapter 11). Because the brain is encased in the skull, the problem with swelling is the risk of increasing intracranial pressure (**raised intracranial pressure**, **RICP**) which will put the brain under pressure (see Chapter 11, page 239).

### Dehydration

Insufficient fluid in any or all of the three tissue compartments is called **dehydration**. This is due to the following three conditions:

1  A *persistent negative fluid balance*, where output exceeds input for more than a few days. The exact time it takes to establish dehydration depends on how poor the fluid intake is or how large the fluid loss is. A total lack of all fluid intake will start to cause minor dehydration within hours. Thirst is the normal body response to early dehydration (i.e. before tissue harm is caused) in an attempt to correct the fluid balance by increasing oral intake. The causes of negative fluid loss include persistent vomiting, diarrhoea, both diabetes mellitus and diabetes insipidus (see Chapter 8), polyurea (a large urine output) (see Chapter 8), excessive use of diuretic drugs (see Chapter 8) and fever (see Chapter 1)
2  *Extensive blood loss* causing **hypovolaemia** (low blood volume), usually rapidly (i.e. before the volume loss can be corrected). Blood volume losses can be from internal or external haemorrhage or plasma loss from extensive burns (see Chapter 10)
3  *Maldistribution of fluid* (i.e. fluid is unevenly distributed around the body), with accumulation in some areas while other areas suffer dehydration (Kreimeier 2000).

Severe dehydration causes weight loss, reduced pulse pressure (see Chapter 3, page 47), rapid shallow breathing, fast weak pulse, low volumes of highly concentrated urine, dry wrinkled skin, poor production of thick saliva from a dry mouth (see page 307), thirst and shrunken tissues (Mooney 2007). Folds of skin formed by gentle external digital pressure remain as folds when the finger pressure is removed, instead of returning to the original flat position rapidly as expected in full hydration. This is known as testing for skin **turgor**. Tissues around the eyes shrink and the eyes appear sunken in their sockets in severe depletion of fluids. The mouth in particular becomes very dry, with little or no saliva. This causes the mouth to become very dirty and at risk of oral infections. This is partly because oral fluid intake is an important cleansing mechanism for the mouth, and absence predisposes the mouth to poor hygiene. The dehydrated dirty mouth becomes very hard to clean properly. An oral infection leads to throat, chest, middle ear and even brain infections if left untreated. Management of dehydration is, of course, rehydration, preferably by mouth. However, some patients require an alternative route for fluid replacement, which is normally the intravenous (IV) route. These patients include:

• those who are severely dehydrated and need urgent rehydration, and oral intake is not adequate enough to rehydrate the patient quickly
• those unable to drink and swallow properly (e.g. unconscious, nil by mouth and post-operative patients).

## Electrolyte balance

Water balance in the body is linked to the balance of electrolytes within the three body compartments (cells, tissue fluid and blood; Figure 6.8).

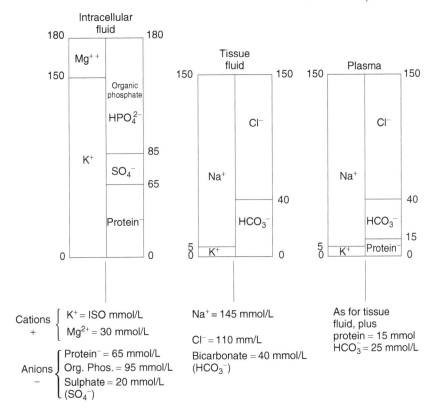

*Figure 6.8* The relative concentrations and values of the major electrolytes are shown in the three body compartments.

**Electrolytes** are ionised elements in solution. They are usually minerals derived from the diet, such as sodium, potassium and calcium. In Chapter 7, Table 7.4 lists the major minerals in the diet. Minerals are commonly consumed in compound form, i.e. two or more minerals elements bound together chemically, e.g. NaCl, sodium chloride. In this form, they are usually electrically neutral (i.e. they have no charge). In the body, these compounds are often dissolved in water (e.g. in blood and tissue fluid), where they normally disassociate (i.e. break up) into their component elements (e.g. NaCl $\rightarrow$ Na$^+$ + Cl$^-$). In this process, each of the separate elements takes on a charge. For example, in the dissociation of sodium chloride, sodium (Na) loses an electron and becomes a positively charged ion (Na$^+$). Positively charged ions are known as **cations**. Chlorine (Cl) gains an electron and becomes a negatively charged ion (now called chloride, Cl$^-$). Negatively charged ions are known as **anions**. These are now electrolytes, dissolved in solution. The electrolyte contents and amounts that are found in body fluids are shown in Figure 6.8. From these figures, it becomes obvious that the bulk of the potassium is inside the cells (intracellular), while the bulk of the sodium is outside the cells (extracellular), e.g. tissue fluid and blood plasma.

The majority of the electrolytes in the body are minerals, such as sodium (Na$^+$), potassium (K$^+$), chloride (Cl$^-$), magnesium (Mg$^{2+}$) and calcium (Ca$^{2+}$). Magnesium (Mg$^{2+}$) and calcium ($Ca^{2+}$) have a double positive charge because they each lose two electrons when their compounds disassociate, rather than a single electron in the case of sodium and potassium. In addition to minerals, blood plasma has proteins that carry negative charges, and are thus considered to be anions, while intracellular fluid has **organic phosphates** (**$HPO_4{}^{2-}$**), which are also negatively charged. Blood and tissue fluid have **bicarbonate** (**$HCO_3{}^-$**), which is an electrolyte important in buffering acids, by binding **hydrogen ions**, **$H^+$**, to prevent excessive acidity (see Chapter 8).

Some important electrolyte functions include:

- Sodium ($Na^+$) is essential for nerve conduction and water balance (see no. 2 on the causes of oedema list, page 128).
- Potassium ($K^+$) is also essential for nerve conduction and is important in muscle contraction (including the heart muscle) and regulation of blood pressure.
- Chloride ($Cl^-$) works in chemical combination with sodium (as **sodium chloride**, **NaCl**) and with potassium (as **potassium chloride**, **KCl**). As sodium chloride, it is essential for maintenance of fluid balance in blood and extracellular fluids.
- Calcium ($Ca^{2+}$) is essential for nerve conduction, muscle contraction, blood clotting and as part of the mineralisation of bones and teeth.
- Magnesium ($Mg^{2+}$) is essential for more than 300 metabolic reactions, including energy production and muscle relaxation between contractions.

**Electrolyte balance** is the term used when stabilising electrolyte levels within normal limits in the body. Ill health, including serious disturbances of fluid balance, disturbance of cardiac and neurological function and adverse changes in acid-base (pH) balance, is caused by disturbance of electrolyte levels in the blood and tissue fluids, either excess or deficiency of one or more electrolytes (Table 7.4, page 144).

Electrolyte imbalance can be caused by:

- Body fluid loss as a result of prolonged vomiting, diarrhoea, excessive sweating or high fever.
- Poor diet, including inadequate mineral, vitamin and fluid intake.
- Poor absorption of these nutrients.
- Endocrine (hormone) disorders, e.g. any disorder that disturbs **aldosterone** function.
- Renal disease, because the kidney normally regulates electrolyte levels by excreting the excess or conserving electrolytes if they are low, and this function may be lost in kidney disorders (see Chapter 8).
- Some drugs (e.g. diuretics, those that promote electrolyte loss) and hydrocortisone.
- Prolonged or excessive intravenous infusion of sodium chloride causing **hypernatraemia** (excess sodium in the blood) or **hyperchloraemia** (excess chloride in the blood; see Chapter 4). Medical staff must be careful about balancing electrolyte input for those patients on long term intravenous infusions. Hyperchloraemia may cause an acidosis (excessive acid conditions in the blood and tissue fluids), but this may have some beneficial effect by causing extra down load of oxygen from the blood into the cells (see *Bohr effect*, Chapter 5; Handy and Soni 2008).

Table 6.1 shows the terms used to describe the various abnormal levels of the major electrolytes and the symptoms that they produce.

*Table 6.1* Four major electrolytes present in body fluids, the terms used to denote excess and insufficiency and the symptoms

| Electrolyte | Excess | Symptoms of excess | Insufficient | Symptoms of insufficiency |
|---|---|---|---|---|
| Sodium ($Na^+$) | Hypernatraemia | Weakness, irritability, oedema, fits, coma | Hyponatraemia | Headache, confusion, fits, muscle cramps, tiredness, nausea, vomiting, restlessness |
| Potassium ($K^+$) | Hyperkalaemia | Nausea, fatigue, muscle weakness, bradycardia, cardiac arrest | Hypokalaemia | Muscle weakness, aches and cramps, palpitations, cardiac arrhythmias |
| Chloride ($Cl^-$) | Hyperchloraemia | Vomiting, dehydration, diarrhoea, Kussmaul beathing (see Chapter 4), weakness, thirst, possibly acidosis | Hypochloraemia | Vomiting, dehydration, diarrhoea |
| Magnesium ($Mg^{2+}$) | Hypermagnesaemia | Loss of deep tendon reflexes, flaccid paralysis, apnoea, urinary retention, bradycardia, hypotension | Hypomagnesaemia | Hypokalaemia, hypocalcaemia, tetany, fits, cardiac arrhythmias |

**Key points**

- The body contains 50% to 65% water (males) and 45% to 60% water (females).
- A 70 kg person has about 45 litres of water, about 70% of the body weight.
- Water occupies three body compartments; intracellular, extracellular (tissue fluid) and the blood.
- Water moves down its own concentration gradient, from high concentration to low concentration, a process called osmosis.
- Humans gain water through drinking about 2,500 ml per day, with some additional gain from metabolism.
- Humans lose fluids through urine output (about 1,500 ml per day) but with additional losses through the skin (400–900 ml per day), through respiration (about 400 ml per day) and in faeces (about 100–200 ml per day).
- Fluid balance records the amount of intake and output to see if there is net gain or loss of fluid over a 24-hour period.
- Central venous pressure (CVP) is a measure of the pressure of the venous blood returning to the heart.
- Oedema is excessive fluid in the tissues causing the tissues to swell.

- There are five causes of oedema: poor venous return, low plasma proteins, excess sodium in the tissues, obstructed lymphatic drainage and increased capillary wall permeability.
- Dehydration is insufficient water in the tissues.
- Dehydration is caused either by persistent low oral fluid intake, severe blood loss or uneven water distribution in the tissues.
- Dehydration causes tissues to shrink and the mouth to become dry.
- Dry mouths can get infected, leading to throat, chest, middle ear and even brain infections.
- A dehydrated patient needs regular mouth hygiene to promote oral moisture and to prevent infection.
- Rehydration is required urgently, preferably by mouth but supplemented by intravenous intake if oral fluids are insufficient or the patient cannot swallow.
- Water balance is linked to electrolyte balance in the three compartments: the cells, tissue fluid and blood.
- Electrolytes are ionised (charged) particles in solution.

### References

Handy J.M. and Soni N. (2008) Physiological effects of hyperchloraemia and acidosis. *British Journal of Anaesthesia, 101*(2): 141–150.

Kreimeier U. (2000) Pathophysiology of fluid imbalance. *Critical Care, 4*(Suppl. 2): S3–S7.

Mooney G.P. (2007) *Fluid Balance*. www.nursingtimes.net/199391.article

Payen D., Cornélie de Pont A., Sakr Y., Spies C., Reinhart K. and Vincent J.L. (2008) A positive fluid balance is associated with a worse outcome in patients with acute renal failure. *Critical Care, 12*: R74.

# 7  Nutrition

## Introduction

Observing the nutritional status of patients involves a number of specific assessments that together will give insight into their dietary needs. Nutritional assessment often starts with the *diet*, i.e. including the *dietary history*. Information on nutritional status can be obtained from the patient and relatives, including whether or not they have been eating a **balanced diet**. This means a diet containing all the necessary daily portions of protein, carbohydrate, fats, fluids and fibre. Vitamin and mineral intake is harder to judge, and if deficiency is suspected this would require investigation. The patient is weighed, and any previous weight gain or loss is identified.

Every cell needs **energy** to function, and therefore cells must produce it. This requires energy-giving foods in the daily diet (Chapter 1).

The energy value of specific foods is measured in **kilojoules (KJ)** or **kilocalories (kcal)**, where 1 kcal = 4.184 kJ. **Energy balance** refers to the person's energy intake compared with their energy use. If the balance is *neutral*, then their energy intake matches their energy use. Overall, they neither gain nor lose energy. In *positive* balance, the energy

DOI: 10.4324/9781003389118-7

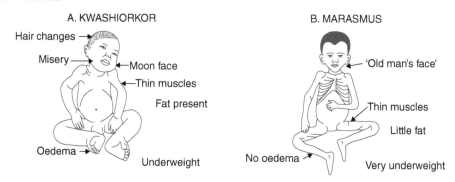

*Figure 7.1* (A) Kwashiorkor (protein deficiency). (B) Marasmus (energy deficiency) in children.

intake exceeds the amount used and surplus energy must be stored in the body, often as fat. This is not a problem in the short term, but persistent and long-term positive balance leads to obesity. In *negative* balance, the intake is less than the energy used. Again, in the short term this is not a problem and the shortfall can be made up. However, in the long term, chronic negative balance leads to severe weight loss and can result in death. The body uses glucose (a simple carbohydrate) as the *first-line energy source*, but if this is not available, e.g. due to a poor diet of low energy foods, the body turns to fats as a *secondary* source of energy. Ultimately and as a last resort, protein from skeletal muscle can be used as an energy source. This only happens in critical situations, e.g. in severe ill health when the patient is deteriorating towards the end of life. **Marasmus** (Figure 7.1B) is a disorder of prolonged negative energy balance, where there is a lack of energy (low calorie) intake, seen mostly in very young children. It causes depletion of glucose and fat stores in the body, and this leads to muscle wasting. There is severe weight loss and failure of growth. This is a long-term chronic disorder because it takes time to convert first fat then muscle to energy. Equally, it takes time to replenish the energy stores; therefore, treatment improves the condition gradually.

## Proteins

Proteins are the body's source of **nitrogen** (see *protein*, Chapter 1, page 7). Since the body is largely made from protein, a component of every body tissue including blood, it makes sense that we need a regular daily intake of protein to satisfy demands made by cells during metabolism, cell replacement, tissue growth and repair. Proteins are made from **amino acids**, which contain the **amino group** ($NH_2$), a **carboxyl group** (**COOH**) and a **radical group** that differs from one amino acid type to another (Figure 7.2).

Proteins, as part of our diet, are reduced by digestive enzymes to 23 different types of amino acids (Table 7.1), and these are absorbed into the blood and taken, initially, to the liver.

The liver uses a large number of amino acids to produce blood proteins (largely **albumin**) (see Chapter 4) and also stores many more amino acids (known as the liver's **amino acid pool**). The liver has some ability to convert one amino acid type to another type as the body requires. Human proteins are assembled inside the body's cells by the process called **protein synthesis**, using the **deoxyribonucleic acid** (**DNA**) code provided by the

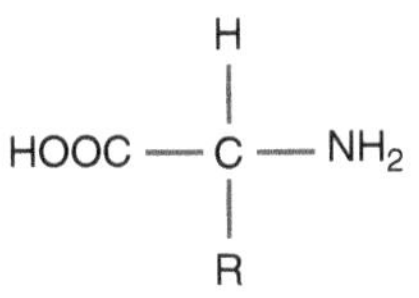

$$HOOC - \underset{\underset{R}{|}}{\overset{\overset{H}{|}}{C}} - NH_2$$

*Figure 7.2* The amino acid molecule with an amino group (NH$_2$), a carboxyl group (COOH) and a variable radical (R).

*Table 7.1* Essential and non-essential amino acids. Essential means they must be present in the diet because the liver cannot synthesise them. Non-essential amino acids can be synthesised by the liver if they are lacking in the diet

| *ESSENTIAL* | *NON-ESSENTIAL* | |
|---|---|---|
| ISOLEUCINE | ALANINE | SELENOCYSTEINE |
| LEUCINE | ASPARAGINE | SERINE |
| LYSINE | ASPARTIC ACID | TYROSINE |
| METHIONINE | CYSTEINE | ARGININE |
| PHENYLALANINE | GLUTAMIC ACID | HISTIDINE |
| THREONINE | GLUTAMINE | ORNITHINE |
| TRYPTOPHAN | GLYCINE | TAURINE |
| VALINE | PROLINE | |

genetics of the cell. Each individual **gene** codes for one type of protein, which will be any of the wide range of possible proteins:

- **hormones**, which regulate tissue function
- **antibodies**, which fight infections
- **enzymes**, which drive cellular metabolism
- **plasma proteins**, which have multiple functions in the blood (see Chapter 4)
- **structural proteins**, which build and support our body, and many other protein types.

A shortage of protein in the diet results in a severe lack of amino acids and therefore an inability for the cells to sustain protein synthesis. This causes disturbed metabolism, poor hormonal function, high risk of infections, potential body structural weaknesses and multiple other problems. On a chronic (i.e. long-term) basis, this causes a condition known as **kwashiorkor** (Figures 7.1A and 7.3). In this disorder, the deficiency is mainly protein, but vitamin deficiency may also be present. A significant stress level is also involved in the cause of this disorder. The symptoms include moon-shaped face, oedema due to low blood proteins (see Chapters 4 and 6), retarded growth and mental development, muscle wasting with retained fat, poor immunity (which increases the risk of infections), delayed wound healing, anaemia, hair loss, mild weight loss and liver degeneration.

A mild form of kwashiorkor could be happening in some patients in hospital. Contributing to this is the fact that hospital patients may be having insufficient dietary intake, especially protein, due to nausea and vomiting, prolonged periods of nil by mouth or anorexia (loss of appetite). Added to this is the presence of stress, mostly from pain, surgery,

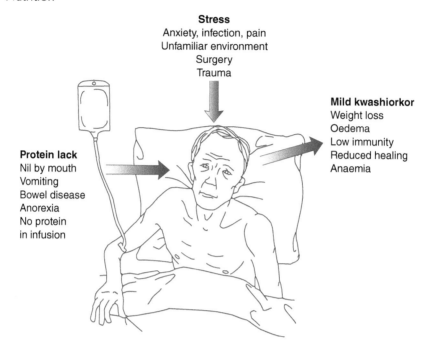

**Stress**
Anxiety, infection, pain
Unfamiliar environment
Surgery
Trauma

**Mild kwashiorkor**
Weight loss
Oedema
Low immunity
Reduced healing
Anaemia

**Protein lack**
Nil by mouth
Vomiting
Bowel disease
Anorexia
No protein
in infusion

*Figure 7.3* Mild kwashiorkor in hospital patients due to protein lack and stress.

abrupt change of environment on admission, infection and injury. Protein deficiency in hospitalised patients will delay healing – especially wounds and fractures – and allow for increased risk of infections. Assessment of the nutritional status of the hospitalised patient should specifically consider the possibility that they may be lacking protein.

### Fats

Fats are our *second-line energy source* (see Chapter 1, page 4) and are made from carbon, hydrogen and oxygen. Fats are **triglycerides** (Figures 1.7 and 7.4) i.e. molecules composed of a glycerol backbone to which is attached three fatty acids. Fatty acids are long chains of carbon atoms ending in a **carboxyl group** (**COOH**), which can liberate hydrogen and hence is acidic. The addition of hydrogen to the long carbon chains varies between *saturated* and *unsaturated* fats. **Saturated** fatty acids have the general formula $CH_3(CH_2)_nCOOH$, indicating that a carbon atom with three attached hydrogen atoms ($CH_3$) occupies one end of the molecule and is followed by a chain of $n$ carbons each with two hydrogens ($CH_2$; where the number $n$ varies between different fatty acids), followed by the carboxyl group (COOH). Fats that are based on saturated fatty acids tend to be solid at room temperature (e.g. lard).

In **unsaturated** fats (Figure 7.5), one or more pairs of carbon atoms in the fatty acid chain are linked by a *double* rather than a *single* bond, i.e. a single bonded $CH_2CH_2$ group in saturated fats differs from unsaturated fats by a double bonded $HC = CH$, with two fewer hydrogens (Figure 7.5). Thus, 'saturated' means that all the carbons are saturated with hydrogen, while 'unsaturated' means that some carbons are missing hydrogen. In a **monounsaturated** fatty acid, only one carbon = carbon double bond exists. In a **polyunsaturated** fatty acid, double bonds occur at more than one place in the carbon chain. Polyunsaturated fats tend to be liquid at room temperature (i.e. oils, such as cooking oil).

In an unsaturated fatty acid, the **omega** ($\omega$) count indicates the position of the first double bond in the chain, counted from the end furthest from the carboxyl group (the omega end), which is the most stable during physiological reactions (Figure 7.5 and Table 7.2). In a triglyceride molecule, the omega end is farthest from the glycerol backbone (Figure 7.4).

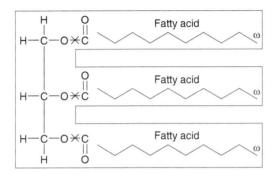

*Figure 7.4* The triglyceride molecule consists of three fatty acids attached to a glycerol backbone. The free ends of the fatty acids are the omega ($\omega$) ends.

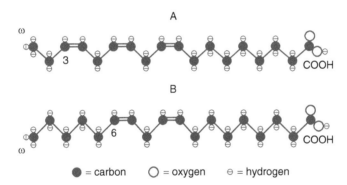

● = carbon    ○ = oxygen    ⊖ = hydrogen

*Figure 7.5* Unsaturated fatty acids showing omega ($\omega$) 3 and 6. Omega 3 has the first double bond at the third carbon counted from the omega end, and omega 6 has the first double bond at the sixth carbon counted from the omega end.

*Table 7.2* Eicosapentaenoic acid (EPA) and linoleic acid, showing omega numbers

| Fatty acid | Molecule | Omega |
|---|---|---|
| Eicosapentaenoic acid (EPA) | | Omega 3 |
| Linoleic acid | | Omega 6 |

Fats are essential in the diet because from them are derived the steroid hormones, e.g. cortisol, the oestrogens, the testosterones and others, structural fats (e.g. cell membranes and adipose tissue) and cytokines (cell-signalling molecules) and because they allow the intake of fat-soluble vitamins, i.e. vitamins A, D, E and K. Generally, the healthier option is to reduce the intake of saturated fats and make up the difference with unsaturated fats. This is because saturated fats have been linked to obesity and to coronary arterial disease, which causes potentially fatal heart disorders.

## Carbohydrates

Similar to fats, carbohydrates are made from carbon, hydrogen and oxygen. The difference is that the hydrogen and oxygen have the same ratio as water, i.e. two hydrogen for every oxygen, 2H:O. Carbohydrates therefore could be viewed as *hydrated carbon*, hence the name. They exist at three levels of complexity:

1 **Monosaccharides** are simple sugars made from three to seven carbons bonded to hydrogen and oxygen. They may exist in straight line or ring structures. **Glucose** is the best-known monosaccharide in human physiology as it is the *first-line energy source* used in cellular metabolism (see Chapter 1, Figure 1.2A).
2 **Oligosaccharides** are more complex molecules made from various numbers of monosaccharide subunits bonded together. The simplest oligosaccharides are the **disaccharides**, sugars that are built from two monosaccharides (di = two) (e.g. **maltose**, made from two glucose molecules, and **sucrose**, made from one glucose and one **fructose**). Sucrose (disaccharide) is table sugar, maltose (disaccharide) is a constituent of malt (Figure 7.6) and fructose (monosaccharide) is fruit sugar. More complex

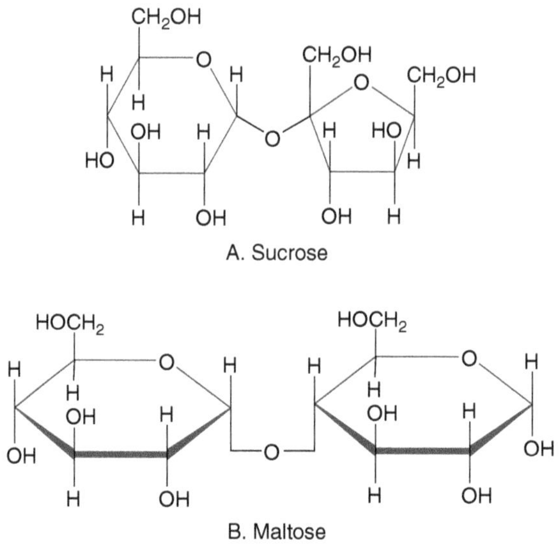

*Figure 7.6* Disaccharides. (A) Sucrose. (B) Maltose. Sucrose is made from a combination of a single glucose (shown here on the left of the sucrose molecule) and a fructose molecule (on the right). Maltose is made from a combination of two glucose molecules.

oligosaccharides consist of three or more monosaccharide molecules, and these are found commonly in plants. They occur regularly in the human diet. Some of these can be digested in humans; others cannot. The undigested molecules become dietary fibre (see fibre, page 143).

3  **Polysaccharides** (also known as **glycans**) are the most complex and the most common carbohydrate structures found in nature. They are built from multiple monosaccharide subunits, of which glucose is the most common. Polysaccharides are important in humans as energy storage as well as structural and protective components. **Starch** is a well-known form of polysaccharide that comes in two forms: **amylose** and **amylopectin**. Plants store starch, and therefore it is eaten regularly in the human diet. Digestive enzymes break down starch, starting in the mouth with the enzyme **salivary amylase**,[1] a component of saliva. **Glycogen** is the main energy storage in humans. It is a polysaccharide made from large numbers of **glucose** molecules linked together. It is found in the liver and skeletal muscles, the two structures that need high energy levels, and it can be broken down by enzymes to release glucose, which is used to provide cellular energy and to stabilise blood sugar levels. **Cellulose** is one of nature's most common structural polysaccharides, being a major component of plants. Because it is found in plant cell walls, it becomes another component of our diet. Cellulose cannot be digested in humans by our enzymic action, and it therefore becomes a major part of our fibre intake (see fibre, page 143). Normal bacteria in the digestive system of some animals (i.e. the ruminants such as cattle) can digest cellulose-releasing glucose that the animal can then absorb. Many human structural polysaccharides are bonded to protein or lipid (fat) molecules.

## Vitamins

The word **vitamin** comes from the two words 'vital amine'. Two aspects make them a cohesive group of nutrients:

1  Vitamins are organic nutrients required in small quantities, unlike proteins and carbohydrates, which are required in much larger daily amounts
2  Vitamins are necessary in the diet since the body cannot synthesise them for itself.

Vitamins have a name but are given a letter of the alphabet for convenience (e.g. ascorbic acid is vitamin C), but several of these vitamins include a number of closely related compounds, of which one is usually the active form and the others can be converted to this active form (e.g. vitamins A and D). Some vitamins are water-soluble (e.g. the vitamins of the B group and C), and others are fat-soluble (e.g. vitamins A, D, E and K). These fat-soluble vitamins are stored in the liver and are therefore not necessarily needed every day. Taking high-dose supplements of them may even cause harmful effects. Table 7.3 shows details of the main vitamins in the human diet, including the important vitamin deficiency disorders.

## Minerals

Minerals are *inorganic*[2] chemical elements required in the diet in varying quantities, some in quite small daily amounts called **trace elements**. They are essential because the body cannot produce these for itself. Some minerals, e.g. sodium and potassium, become

*Table 7.3* The major vitamins, food sources, need and deficiency

| Vitamin | Full name | Food source | (1) Vitamin needed for / (2) Effects from lack of vitamin |
|---|---|---|---|
| **A** | **Retinol** | Liver, fish liver oils, butter, cream, cheese, whole milk, egg yolk. | (1) Growth, vision, healthy tissues, immunity. <br> (2) Night blindness, dry and itching skin, reduced taste, bone growth failure. |
| **B$_1$** | **Thiamin** | Yeast, cereals, legumes. | (1) Heart and circulation, growth, nervous system, energy. <br> (2) **Beriberi** (fatigue, low appetite, weight loss, muscle wasting, diarrhoea, heart failure, oedema, paralysis), plus parasthesia, **depression**. |
| **B$_2$** | **Riboflavin** | Cereals, yeast, milk, eggs, green vegetable leaves, lean meat. | (1) Healthy skin, tissue healing, immunity, red blood cells. <br> (2) **Cheilosis** (oral cracks and fissures, scaling of lips), sore tongue (**glossitis**), sensitivity to light (**photophobia**), **dermatitis**. |
| **B$_3$** | **Niacin or niacinamide** | Yeast, liver, kidney, meat, cereals, green vegetables, bran. | (1) Energy, skin, nervous system, cell metabolism. <br> (2) Weakness, skin rash, memory loss irritability, insomnia, **pellagra** (dermatitis, glossitis, diarrhoea, mental disturbance, e.g. depression, confusion, hallucinations, delirium, leading to death). |
| **B$_5$** | **Pantothenic acid** | All plant and animal foods, especially eggs, kidney, liver, salmon, yeast. | (1) Energy production, immunity, hormones. <br> (2) Weakness, depression, low infection resistance |
| **B$_6$** | **Pyridoxine** | Pork, organ meats, fish, corn, legumes, seeds, grains, wheat, leafy vegetables, green beans, bananas. | (1) Protein metabolism, haemoglobin, nervous system. <br> (2) Fatigue, nervous dysfunction, anaemia, irritability, skin lesions. |
| **B$_9$** | **Folic acid** | Green leafy vegetables, liver, beef, fish, lentils, asparagus, broccoli. | (1) RBC maturation, growth, healthy tissues. <br> (2) Anaemia, neural tube defects during very early pregnancy. |
| **B$_{12}$** | **Cyanocobalamin** | Only from animal foods, liver, meat, milk, eggs, oysters. | (1) RBC (haemoglobin), growth, nervous system. <br> (2) **Pernicious anaemia**: fatigue, glossitis, nerve degeneration. |
| **B$_{15}$** | **Pangamic acid** | Sesame seeds, pumpkin seeds, whole brown rice, liver, organ meats. | (1) Unknown function. <br> (2) No deficiency symptoms known. |
| **B-factor** | **Choline** | Yeast, milk, eggs, wheat germ, soya, organ meats. | (1) Nerve transmission, liver, cell membranes. <br> (2) Growth problems, reduced liver and nerve function. |

| Vitamin | Full name | Food source | (1) Vitamin needed for / (2) Effects from lack of vitamin |
|---|---|---|---|
| **B-factor** | **Inositol** | Milk, yeast, meat, fruit, nuts. | (1) Nerve transmission, fat metabolism <br> (2) Eye problems, constipation, hair loss. |
| C | **Ascorbic acid** | Citrus fruits, strawberries, tomatoes, cabbage, potatoes, parsley, broccoli, sweet peppers. | (1) Collagen maturity, wound healing, maintains healthy gums, skin, immunity, blood. <br> (2) Bruising, slow wound healing, anaemia, gingivitis, **scurvy** (fatigue and bleeding, later gum disorder). |
| D | **Calciferol** | Milk, fish oil, liver, butter, egg yolk, ultraviolet light (UVL) in sunlight acting on skin. | (1) Absorption of calcium from the diet, good bones and teeth. <br> (2) **Rickets** (children): soft bent and fragile bones, deformity. **Osteomalacia** (adults): soft and painful bones, fractures. |
| E | **Tocopherol** | Vegetable oil, whole grains, wheat germ, egg yolk. | (1) Antioxidant, maintenance of circulation and cell protection. <br> (2) Poor muscle performance and circulation, RBC haemolysis. |
| F | **Unsaturated fatty acids** | All sources of unsaturated fatty acids. | (1) Skin, blood and glandular products. <br> (2) **Acne**, allergies, dry skin, brittle hair, **eczema**, brittle nails. |
| H | **Biotin** | Liver, meat, eggs, nuts, milk, most vegetables, tomatoes, grapefruit, watermelon, strawberries. | (1) Skin, blood circulation, metabolism. <br> (2) **Depression**, anorexia, non-specific skin rashes. |
| K | **Phylloquinone** | Lettuce, spinach, cauliflower, cabbage, egg yolk, soya bean oil, liver. | (1) Blood clotting mechanism. <br> (2) Bleeding and diarrhoea. |
| P | **Bioflavonoids** | Fruit, especially citrus. | (1) Healthy blood vessel walls. <br> (2) Bleeding and bruising, colds, **eczema**. |

**electrolytes** in the blood and tissue fluids, and these are discussed under electrolyte balance (see Chapter 6, page 130).

Table 7.4 gives details of the main minerals required by the body, including the important disorders and symptoms linked to deficiency of these minerals.

### Fibre

Dietary fibre, or **roughage**, is a mix of large molecules in the diet that remain largely unchanged throughout the digestive system, and therefore they are not absorbed and so provide no direct nutritional value. By remaining in the digestive system, they become a major component of faeces (see Chapter 9). The term *fibre* includes some **oligosaccharides** and many of the

*Table 7.4* The major minerals

| Mineral (chemical symbol) | Mineral function | (1) Food source (2) Effects from lack of mineral |
|---|---|---|
| **Calcium (Ca)** | Bones, teeth, muscle and nerve function, blood clotting mechanism. | (1) Milk and other milk products.<br>(2) Weak bones and teeth, weak muscles, bleeding, poor nerve function. Severe loss of blood calcium levels causes **tetany** (a state of continuous muscle contraction). |
| **Chloride (Cl)** | Important electrolyte (as Cl⁻), usually in compound with sodium or potassium, helps to maintain tissue fluid balance, nerve impulses. | (1) In compound with sodium in salt (NaCl), also vegetables, tomatoes, lettuce, celery and olives.<br>(2) Deficiency is rare, can cause alkalosis, muscle weakness, irritability, anorexia, dehydration, lethargy. |
| **Chromium (Cr)** | Glucose metabolism, amino acid transportation, blood lipid and glucose levels. | (1) Full cream milk, seafood (e.g. oysters), wholegrain, cheese, fresh fruit, nuts, vegetables, brewer's yeast and variable amounts in water.<br>(2) Glucose imbalance, impaired growth, obesity, tiredness, increased cancer risk, heart disease and diabetes. |
| **Copper (Cu)** | Haemoglobin in blood, collagen, heart function, energy production, iron absorption. | (1) Grains, nuts, liver, oysters and legumes.<br>(2) Anaemia, muscle weakness, abnormal collagen synthesis, neurological defects. |
| **Iodine (I)** | Thyroid hormones. | (1) Seafood.<br>(2) Low thyroid hormone levels, goitre, cretinism, **myxoedema**. |
| **Iron (Fe)** | Haemoglobin in blood, immunity, brain function. | (1) Liver, shellfish, oysters, lean meat, poultry, kidney, fish, beans and vegetables.<br>(2) **Anaemia**, attention and learning difficulties, increased risk of infections. |
| **Magnesium (Mg)** | Nerve and muscle function, bone formation. | (1) Leafy green vegetables, nuts, wholegrain, peas, beans, dairy products, fish, cereals, legumes, meats.<br>(2) Weakness, dizziness, abdominal distension, convulsions. |
| **Manganese (Mn)** | Involved in calcium and phosphorus metabolism and bone formation. | (1) Legumes, nuts, wholegrain cereal, tea, green leafy vegetables.<br>(2) No specific deficiency syndrome identified. |
| **Phosphorus (P)** | Bones and teeth, energy production, DNA formation, metabolism. | (1) Meat, poultry, fish, eggs, peanuts.<br>(2) Serious problems with the nerve supply to muscles; skeletal, blood and kidney problems. |

| Mineral (chemical symbol) | Mineral function | (1) Food source<br>(2) Effects from lack of mineral |
|---|---|---|
| **Potassium (K)** | Intracellular electrolyte, factor in nerve conduction. | (1) Bananas, oranges, grapefruit juice, melons, nectarines, prunes, pears, avocados, cucumbers, potatoes, peas, beans, tomatoes, nuts, legumes, seeds, milk products, meats of all kinds.<br>(2) Fatigue, depression, weakness, heart irregularities, dry skin, low blood pressure, oedema, muscle cramps. |
| **Selenium (Se)** | Antioxidant, heart muscle, fat metabolism, tissue elasticity. | (1) Cereals, Brazil nuts, wholegrains, seafood, meat, poultry, fish, dairy products.<br>(2) Increased risk of cancer, myalgia (muscle pain) and muscle tenderness, heart disease (e.g. **Keshan disease** in China), premature ageing. |
| **Sodium (Na)** | Extracellular electrolyte, factor in fluid balance, blood pressure, muscle contraction, nerve conduction. | (1) Found widely in the diet, especially table salt, animal foods, processed foods.<br>(2) Deficiency very rare. |
| **Zinc (Zn)** | Gene expression in tissue growth/repair, cell reproduction, child growth, sperm and testosterone. | (1) Meat, poultry, fish, oysters, eggs, legumes, nuts, milk, yoghurt, wholegrain cereals.<br>(2) Rare. **Acrodermatitis enteropathica** (rash over face, anus and distal parts), growth retardation in children, anorexia with diarrhoea, poor wound healing, depression, reduced reproductive ability. |

**polysaccharides**, e.g. **cellulose**, **hemicellulose** and **pectin** and also **lignin**, the tough component of wood – but also found in plant stalks – and **gums** that are also mostly derived from plant foods. Bacteria, normally present in the digestive tract, known as the **intestinal flora**, are *commensals* of the colon and caecum. Commensals are harmless, even useful, organisms active in specific body sites. They are able to break down some of the fibre. These bacteria synthesise some nutrients, notably **niacin** (**nicotinic acid**), **thiamine** (**vitamin B$_1$**) and **vitamin K**, which we can then absorb and use. Fibre is covered in more detail in Chapter 9.

## Nutrition in the young and the elderly

### Nutrition in the young

The child from birth up to about 6 months old should be fed with breast milk preferably or given formula (bottle) food if breastfeeding is not an option. Children of this age cannot cope well with fibre in their diet, and fibre increases the risk of malabsorption of nutrients.

Therefore, fibre in the diet should be avoided. Generally, children aged from 6 months can be weaned on to more solid foods, although the actual age may vary between different children. Young children should avoid certain foods (Table 7.5).

Adequate nutrients to sustain growth is essential throughout childhood, especially during growth spurts when an increased rate of cell division and energy use puts greater demands on the diet.

In schoolchildren aged 5 years to teenage, growth rates slow down a little until the teenage growth spurt starts somewhere between 11 and 13 years old. Energy requirements reflect these changes in growth rate. For example:

- a boy aged 1 year requires about 234.3 kJ/kg/day (56 kcal/kg/day)
- a boy aged 10 years requires about 159 kJ/kg/day (38 kcal/kg/day).

These figures are given in kilojoules per kilogram per day (kJ/kg/day) and kilocalories per kilogram per day (kcal/kg/day). They reflect growth requirements, and variations in activity levels would add to these figures. Iron deficiency appears to be the most common dietary problem in adolescence, aggravated in girls by the onset of menstruation. Iron from animal sources is better absorbed than iron from plant sources, a point to consider in vegetarian diets. The addition of vitamin C and extra protein helps in iron absorption. During the adolescent growth spurt, the skeleton requires a great deal of calcium. This is because the skeleton stores 99% of the body's calcium, and 45% of the adult bone mass is added during the teenage years. The biggest gains in bone mass occur between 10 and 14 years in girls and between 12 and 15 years in boys. About 30% of the dietary calcium is absorbed, and retention of calcium in the body is about 200 mg/day in girls and about 300 mg/day in boys. In children and in adults, unrefined carbohydrates, e.g. bread and

*Table 7.5* Foods young children should avoid

| Food that should be avoided | Reason |
| --- | --- |
| **High fibre** | High fibre in a child's diet increases the risk of malabsorption of nutrients and may possibly lead to constipation or obstruction. Small children's bowel cannot cope with much fibre, and very young babies should have very low fibre content. |
| **Honey** | Honey may have spores of dangerous organisms. |
| **Refined carbohydrates** | Refined sugars (table sugar, sweets, etc.) release energy rapidly, which then triggers insulin release, and the blood sugar then falls quickly. This destabilises blood sugar levels. Unrefined carbohydrates (e.g. potatoes, bread, pasta and rice) release energy gradually, which does not trigger a large insulin release, and the blood sugar is better controlled. |
| **Peanut butter** | Any thick, sticky and oily food such as peanut butter may be hard for children to eat and swallow. |
| **Cow's milk** | Under 12 months of age, cow's milk is inappropriate and children should be preferably breastfed or given a baby formula food. The reason is that cow's milk contains proteins that small babies cannot digest and has mineral levels too high for immature kidneys to cope with. |
| | Over 12 months, children need the fat and calories found in whole milk for growth, so low-fat milk is inappropriate. |

potatoes, are better than refined sugars (as in table sugar and sweets) because unrefined carbohydrates release glucose slowly and thus sustain energy over longer periods than do the refined sugars, which release glucose rapidly for short periods only.

### Nutrition in the elderly

In the elderly, the advancing years provide three reasons why energy food consumption should be reduced:

1 A reduction in physical activity results in the need for less energy-rich food
2 The lean (protein) body mass declines, mainly protein in skeletal muscle, and this results in reduced muscle activity and therefore less energy requirements
3 The gradual reduction in the basal metabolic rate (BMR) also leads to lower energy requirement.

Table 7.6 shows an example of the energy input reduction expected with advancing years.
  A high-energy food diet continued into older age could result in chronic positive energy intake, and this leads to weight increase, even obesity. Protein requirements in adults of all ages remains about the same, i.e. about 57 g/day for men and 41 g/day for women. Fat gradually increases as stored adipose tissue with age, e.g. around the abdomen in men, and on the buttocks and thighs in women. Adipose deposited around internal organs in either sex may increase the risk of cardiac problems. Vitamin and mineral requirements remain about the same in all adults, the two exceptions being in women, where *less* iron but *more* calcium is required after menopause:

• **Iron**: pre-menopause (especially during menstruation) = 14 mg/day, post-menopause = 7 mg/day, since no further menstrual blood loss after menopause means less iron loss.
• **Calcium**: pre-menopausal requirement = 700 mg/day, post-menopausal requirement = 800–1,000 mg/day, to help prevent thinning of the bone mass (**osteoporosis**), which otherwise may lead to fractures.

Reduced levels of digestive enzymes, lower gastric acidity and fewer bowel movements all occur with age but not normally enough to cause any degree of malnutrition provided the diet is adequate. Absorption of all the major nutrients from the bowel is good well into old age. If malnutrition is occurring in an older patient, it may be caused by poor diet. This could be due to a diet of high carbohydrate and low protein because carbohydrate foods are cheaper to buy than protein. Some observations may reveal other factors involved, such as dental losses, poor salivation – which can be due to dehydration (see Chapter 6) – and

*Table 7.6* Energy requirements at different ages

| Male | | Female | |
|---|---|---|---|
| Age (years) | Kilocalories per day | Age (years) | Kilocalories per day |
| 19–24 | 3,000 | 19–24 | 2,100 |
| 50–74 | 2,300 | 50–74 | 1,800 |
| 75+ | 2,000 | 75+ | 1,500 |

mouth infections due to poor oral hygiene (see Chapter 6). General ill health may also be a cause, especially when patients are unable to get out for shopping or they lack the fitness or motivation to cook. Constipation, which is often common in the elderly, may be an important but relatively easily treated cause of appetite loss (see Chapter 9).

## Disorders of nutrition

### *Weight loss*

Weight loss may be due to dehydration in the first instance if the patient does not drink enough. Additional weight loss can initially involve body fat losses, followed later by protein reduction in the form of **muscle wasting**. This occurs when muscle breakdown, also known as muscle **atrophy**, exceeds muscle-building (**muscle synthesis**) and is accompanied by a corresponding loss of muscle strength and power. It is often due to inadequate muscle activity, as is the case when being confined to bed for weeks. There are also some muscle-wasting diseases, including those that cause a loss of the motor nerve control of muscles (neurological disorders). It may simply be due to a low-protein diet as occurs in starvation, digestive disorders or absorption abnormalities. The patient is obviously thin, with the outline of bones being seen under the skin. They are generally weak and tired and are likely to find difficulty with movement, such as walking. This causes the patient to have a high risk of injury due to falls.

Not all weight loss is due to poor dietary intake. Sometimes pathological changes in the body metabolism result in reduced body mass from muscle wasting, severe weight loss, weakness and fatigue, anorexia, immobility and anaemia. The term **cachexia** refers to this moribund state of metabolic malfunction, and it is usually found in terminally ill patients or those who fail to absorb nutrients. Cachexia puts the patient's life at great risk, and it cannot easily be reversed, even by giving nutrition, either by mouth or another route. It most often therefore becomes a terminal state, and it is usually seen in diseases such as incurable cancer or **acquired immune deficiency syndrome** (**AIDS**). This is not the same as **starvation**. Cachexia patients tend to respond poorly – or not at all – to the administration of nutrition, whilst giving nutrition in pure starvation will reverse the problem and restore health in most cases. In starvation, the immediate problem faced by the body is to get energy nutrients to the cells and tissues before they malfunction and die. Glucose and glycogen stores are quite quickly used up (i.e. within 24 hours), and the body starts to use other stored energy sources, notably fatty acids and glycerol from triglycerides stored in adipose tissue (see page 139). Both ketone production (see *ketoacidosis*, Chapter 8) and fatty acid levels in the blood become increased (i.e. a **hyperlipidaemia**) as stored fats are mobilised by enzymes to provide energy. If all the fat has been used the body must then turn to using amino acids from proteins for energy. This involves using up the stored amino acids in the liver (the **amino acid pool**), then releasing amino acids from both skeletal and smooth muscle. There is considerable overlap between these two processes. Muscle breakdown, a **catabolic** process (see page 79), causes muscle wastage and organ dysfunction.

**Anorexia** and **bulimia** are two eating disorders that often result in nutritional problems. Anorexia is a failure to consume adequate nutrients, seen most often in young women. They starve themselves, and therefore lack many of the vital nutrients, especially energy and protein. Chronic stress is involved although this may not always be identified or admitted by the patient. Bulimia is an eating disorder where the patient has food binges during which they eat all they can. This is followed by a period of guilt feelings during which they make efforts to recover the food by inducing vomiting or by using laxatives. There are often periods of normal eating between bouts of binge eating. The biology of food intake regulation is very complex and not entirely understood; consequently, not much is known about the pathophysiology of these eating disorders, especially bulimia (Blows 2011, 2022). The two best-known control mechanisms, both involving the hypothalamus, are shown in Figure 7.7.

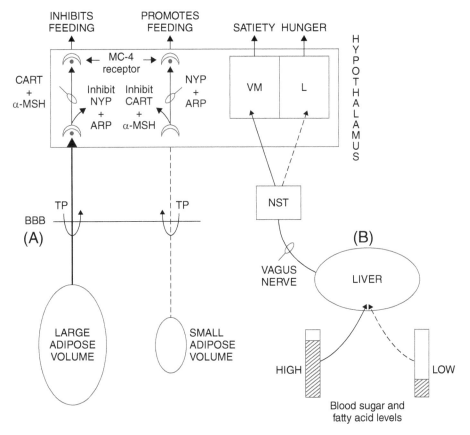

*Figure 7.7* Two of the major pathways for regulating food intake. (A) Large adipose mass produces bigger volumes (thick arrow) of a hormone called **leptin** than small adipose volumes (broken arrow) in the body. Leptin must be transported across the blood – brain barrier (BBB) by a transport protein (TP) before entering the hypothalamus. Leptin binds to the leptin receptor in the hypothalamus. If a substantial quantity of leptin is available for binding, this will cause the production of two hormones – cocaine- and amphetamine-regulated transcript (CART) and alpha-melanocyte-stimulating hormone (α-MSH) – which bind to the MC-4 receptor, and this inhibits feeding. At the same time, two other substances – neuropeptide Y (NPY) and agouti-related protein (ARP) – are inhibited. If there is very little leptin to bind, this will cause the production of ARP and NPY, which bind to the MC-4 receptor, and these promote feeding. At the same time, CART and α-MSH are inhibited. This is a long-term regulator of feeding behaviour, acting over a period of months or years. (B) The liver monitors the blood fatty acid and glucose levels and sends this information via the vagus nerve to the nucleus of the solitary tract (NST) within the brainstem. If the blood levels are high (as after a meal), the NST sends this information to the ventromedial nucleus (VM) of the hypothalamus (solid line), and this nucleus causes satiety (a feeling of fullness). If the blood levels are low (as before a meal), the NST sends this information to the lateral nucleus (L) of the hypothalamus (broken line), and this nucleus causes hunger. Hormones, such as **orexin** act in the lateral nucleus to cause hunger and thus feeding. This is a short-term regulator of feeding behaviour acting over a period of minutes or hours.

*Weight gain: obesity*

Obesity is on the increase, particularly in the Western world. Anyone having a **body mass index** (**BMI**) greater than 30 (see page 152) is considered to be clinically obese. It is the result of chronic consumption of excess calorific food coupled with inadequate energy expenditure, i.e. a state of long-term positive energy balance (see page 135). The mechanism of food intake regulation, and the eating-satiety cycle, have been poorly understood (Figure 7.7). There is also limited understanding of the genetic causes (i.e. the gene mutations, Table 7.7) that upset the feeding-satiety cycle and thus promote eating (Blows 2022).

The problems and complications associated with obesity are:

1  *Increased risk of mortality* due to the serious medical conditions linked to being overweight. These are **diabetes** (see Chapter 8), **hypertension, myocardial infarction, angina pectoris** and **congested cardiac failure** (**CCF**). Obesity puts a lot of strain on the heart, and it carries a 20% increase in sudden death when compared with those of normal weight
2  Increased *metabolic disorders* such as diabetes and gout
3  *Musculoskeletal problems* such as joint disorders (**osteoarthritis**) and flat feet
4  *Respiratory problems* as the ribs may be impeded, thus making breathing more difficult
5  *Accidents* are more common due to balance and movement coordination difficulties
6  *Poor surgical risk*, which means obese patients carry a greater risk of dying under anaesthesia and may suffer more complications following surgery.

*Nutritional deficiencies*

Normal diets will supply all the nutrients required by the body for its daily needs. Apart from areas of the world where food is scarce, dietary deficiencies of all kinds can occur in hospital patients. These are patients who are nil by mouth (NBM) for long periods or on dextrose or saline intravenous infusions which lack nutrients such as amino acids. Vomiting (see page 188) and pain will reduce the appetite, and digestive disorders may make feeding or digestion difficult. Some hospital patients, especially the frail, may suffer a mild degree of kwashiorkor (see page 136; i.e. a lack of protein accompanied by stress). Inadequate food

*Table 7.7* Gene mutations possibly involved in weight gain. This table should be viewed in conjunction with Figure 7.7

| Gene | Possible role for gene mutation in obesity |
| --- | --- |
| Leptin gene (*Ob* gene) | May produce a leptin type that does not activate the leptin receptor very well |
| Leptin receptor gene (*Db* gene) | May produce a receptor that does not respond to leptin very well |
| Leptin transporter gene | May produce a transporter protein that does not transport leptin across the blood-brain barrier |
| MC-4 receptor gene | May produce MC-4 receptors that do not function properly |
| Orexin gene | May cause orexin to stimulate increased amounts of food intake |
| UCP2 gene | May cause malfunction of energy production and thus contribute to obesity |

intake and the stress of admission, pain, investigations and surgery all contribute to this condition. It is important to recognise that vitamin and mineral deficiencies (Tables 7.3 and 7.4), dehydration (see Chapter 6) and a lack of fibre can also occur in hospitals.

## Observations of the nutritional state

More than 50 published screening tools are now available for nurses to assess the patient's nutritional status (Bell 2007; Perry 2009). While at home or in hospital, the simplest observations are often the best. For example:

1 Ensure that the patient is physically able to eat (e.g. they can hold and use cutlery adequately, can they can chew properly or do they need assistance?)
2 Ensure that the patient eats adequately and drinks enough to sustain fluid balance, including, if required, a measurement of the calorific and protein intake per 24 hours
3 Observe the patient's mouth daily to assess the state of cleanliness and to identify any dental pain, oral infections or cracking at the corners of the mouth or lips that may cause pain on eating and may therefore reduce the appetite or ability to eat. Poor mouth hygiene not only contributes to poor nutrition, but it can also lead to throat, chest, ear and even brain infections. Mouth dryness – and therefore risk of oral infection – increases if the patient is nil by mouth for any significant period of time (Wilson 2011)
4 Check that false teeth are clean, well fitting and that the patient uses them
5 Check hair, nails and skin (see Chapter 10) for abnormalities (e.g. hair loss or cracked nails), which may be linked to poor nutrition
6 Daily weighing recorded on a weight chart will permit weight loss to be detected.

### Body weight

Weighing the patient is the standard measurement of assessing their general nutritional status, i.e. it is a guide indicating if the patient has been in positive, neutral or negative energy balance over the last few weeks or months (see page 135 and Table 7.6). *Weight loss* programmes to combat overweight or obesity usually require appropriate adjustments to the diet, i.e. typically involving lower fat and carbohydrate intake. This is coupled with an increase in physical activity within the patient's ability. These measures should be aimed at putting the patient into a slight negative energy balance so the body must mobilise stored energy to make up the shortfall, and weight is therefore lost. *Weight gain* programmes, as in anorexia, involve increasing energy-rich foods in the diet (i.e. a positive energy balance) so the body can replace the energy stores such as adipose tissue. Promoting weight gain in anorexia, however, is not an easy task since the patient's negative approach to eating creates a psychological barrier that is difficult to circumvent. It becomes a major challenge for both the healthcare professional and the patient's family.

### Basal metabolic rate (BMR) and body mass index (BMI)

BMR measures the rate of energy expenditure required to maintain cellular metabolism *at rest* after fasting for 12 hours. This means that the BMR will increase with activity, as cells need and create extra energy as activity increases, especially muscle cells (e.g. BMR increases fourfold during a brisk walk). Calculating the BMR is complicated and involves special clinical conditions that are not always available; therefore, this observation is not undertaken regularly. The results also vary from one patient to another and are therefore specific to the individual involved.

The BMI is more widely adopted as it is easy to calculate at home as well as in the clinical setting. It estimates body fat by comparison of body weight with height. The BMI is calculated by the formula:

BMI = body weight in kilograms (kg) ÷ (height in metres)$^2$

After measuring the person's body weight in kilograms, and their height in metres, it is just a matter of multiplying the height by the height (i.e. height$^2$), then dividing this result into the weight. As an example, a man weighing 78 kg is 1.8 metres tall:

height$^2$ = 1.8 × 1.8 = 3.24 (warning: *do not* convert the metres to centimetres!)
BMI = 78 ÷ 3.24 = 24 (there are no units)

It can also be done easily on BMI calculators that do the arithmetic for you. They can be downloaded from the Internet or obtained from healthcare product suppliers.

The results are usually interpreted in this manner:

- BMI below 18.5 = underweight
- BMI 18.5–24.9 = normal weight
- BMI 25–30 = overweight
- BMI more than 30 = obese.

### Bioelectrical impedance analysis (BIA)

**Bioelectrical impedance analysis** (**BIA**) uses a piece of equipment that passes a safe, low-voltage electrical current through the body. This current is not enough to be felt by the subject. Because electrical currents flow faster through water-rich areas of the body (e.g. muscle), fat tissue (which has low water content) will impede the flow. These variations in flow rates are measured by the machine, which, together with information on the subject's height, weight, age and gender, allows the instrument to calculate the percentage of body fat (Haroun *et al.* 2010).

### Total parental nutrition (TPN)

**Total parental nutrition** (**TPN**) is a treatment regime that is used to replace oral food intake in those patients who are unable to take any food or fluid by mouth. The nutrition and fluids are administered by intravenous cannula directly into a main venous blood vessel, usually a central vein. Smaller veins are not recommended as they may get blocked as a result of the fluid administered. The nutrition provided must be in the same form that would be absorbed from the digestive tract, i.e. glucose, fatty acids, amino acids, vitamins and minerals. It gives the staff the opportunity to measure and record nutritional and fluid intake very accurately and thus to work out the nutritional and fluid balances. Very careful mouth observations and oral management must be made to prevent dryness and infection since a major part of normal mouth cleanliness from drinking fluids will be missing.

## Key points

*Energy*

- Energy balance is the energy intake compared with the energy used.
- Neutral energy balance means the intake equals the energy used.
- Positive balance (i.e. greater energy input than used) can lead to being overweight.
- Negative balance (i.e. less energy input than used) can lead to weight loss.

*Proteins*

- Amino acids are the components of proteins; they contain an amino group ($NH_2$), a carboxyl group (COOH) and a radical that differs between the various amino acids.
- Proteins in the body function as structures (e.g. muscle), hormones, antibodies, plasma proteins, enzymes and other important elements.
- Proteins are not used for energy except as a last resort.
- Some hospital patients may develop a mild form of kwashiorkor, which should be considered when assessing patients in hospital.

*Fats*

- Fats (notably fatty acids) are our secondary energy source.
- It is the healthier option to reduce the intake of saturated fats.

*Carbohydrates*

- Carbohydrates (notably glucose) are our primary energy source.

*Vitamins*

- Vitamins are organic nutrients required in small quantities in the diet.
- Vitamins A, D, E and K are fat-soluble, and their presence requires some fat in the diet. Other vitamins are water-soluble.

*Minerals*

- Minerals are inorganic chemical elements required in the diet.
- Electrolytes are charged particles in solution.

*Fibre*

- Fibre remains unchanged in the digestive system; it is not absorbed and provides no direct nutritional value.
- Fibre is very important for elimination and healthy bowel function.

*Nutrition in the young and the elderly*

- Adequate nutrition is essential to sustain growth throughout childhood.
- Energy food consumption should be reduced as people get older, particularly fats and sugars.
- Women after menopause require less iron but more calcium.

*Disorders of nutrition*

- Cachexia is a moribund state of critical malnutrition caused by a metabolic malfunction.
- Starvation is a lack of foods that, if it continues, results in weight loss, muscle wasting and possibly death.
- Anorexia is starvation due to an eating disorder, more often seen in young women.
- Bulimia is an eating disorder where eating binges are followed by periods of guilt during which the patients try to retrieve the food by vomiting and the use of laxatives.
- Obesity causes multiple long-term complications to health and shortens the lifespan.

*Observations of the nutritional state*

- Simple observations of nutritional status include the dietary history, observing the patient eat and ensuring they are able to eat adequately.
- Other observations include body weight, the body mass index (BMI) and bioelectrical impedance analysis (BIA) to measure fat percentage.

## Notes

1 Don't get amylose and amylase muddled. Any chemical word ending in 'ose' is usually a sugar, and the word ending in 'ase' is the enzyme acting on that sugar.
2 Inorganic means not derived from a living source, i.e. originally derived from a geological source.

## References

Bell J. (2007) Nutritional screening during hospital admission: 1. *Nursing Times*, *103*(37): 30–31.

Blows W.T. (2011) The physiology of food intake regulation and eating disorders. *Journal of Gastrointestinal Nursing*, 9(6): 40–45.

Blows W.T. (2022) *The Biological Basis of Mental Health Nursing* (4th edition). Routledge, Abingdon and New York.

Haroun D., Taylor S.J., Viner R.M., Hayward R.S., Darch T.S., Eaton S., Cole T.J. and Wells J.C. (2010) Validation of bioelectrical impedance analysis in adolescents across different ethnic groups. *Obesity*, *18*(6): 1252–1259.

Perry L. (2009) Using nutritional screening tools to identify malnourished patients. *Nursing Times*. www.nursingtimes.net/clinical-archive/nutrition/using-nutritional-screening-tools-to-identify-malnourished-patients-06-01-2009/ (Accessed 19th February 2023).

Wilson A. (2011) How to provide effective oral care. *Nursing Times*, *107*(6): 14–21.

# 8 Elimination (I)

## Urinary observations

- Introduction
- Urine formation
- The urinary system in youth
- Urinary observations and tests
- Urinalysis
- Other urine tests
- When to test urine
- Drugs active on the urinary system
- Key points
- Notes
- References

## Introduction

The eliminatory systems, the bowel and kidneys, are the principal excretory pathways for many surplus and toxic substances produced by the tissues. Their functions maintain the body's tissues and blood at permanently optimum levels. The systems also excrete products from disease, i.e. the urine offers insights into many pathologies. Accurate observations of urine can reveal much about the individual at that time, both the factors affecting the system and the underlying metabolism.

### The renal system

The renal system consists of two kidneys attached to the posterior abdominal wall, one each side of the lumbar vertebrae (Figure 8.1). Each kidney consists of around one million nephrons which filter water and other substances (**filtrate**) from the blood. This will be acted on by the nephron until it becomes urine. Urine drains from the kidneys down a **ureter** on each side, to the bladder where it is temporarily stored **bladder**. The final passageway to the outside world is via the single **urethra** (Figure 8.1).

DOI: 10.4324/9781003389118-8

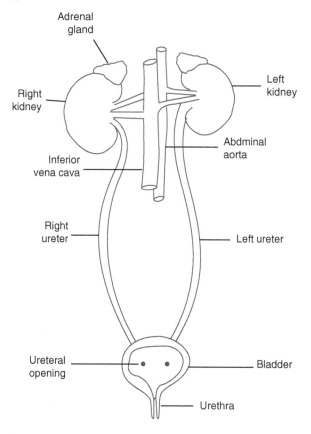

*Figure 8.1* The renal system consists of a left and right kidney with ureters, the urinary bladder within the bony pelvis below and a single urethra.

The kidney, when seen in cross section, shows an outer **cortex** and an inner **medulla** (Figure 8.2). The cortex is the site where nephrons are housed, and the medulla is made of renal collecting ducts. These ducts empty into the **renal pelvis** from where urine drains down the ureters to the bladder (Figure 8.2).

### Urine formation

Urine is formed by **nephron** (Figure 8.3), of which there are about one million in each kidney. Urine production takes place in three distinct steps.

*Step 1* is **filtration under pressure** within the **glomerulus,** which is surrounded by the **glomerular (Bowman's) capsule** (Figure 8.4). Blood plasma passing through the glomerular arterioles is subject to **hydrostatic pressure**, i.e. blood pressure as it occurs in the glomerular arterioles, causing filtration by forcing water and other substances through the **glomerular membrane**. The resulting filtrate is collected in the capsule at a rate known as the **glomerular filtration rate** (**GFR**), which is about 120 ml per minute, measured

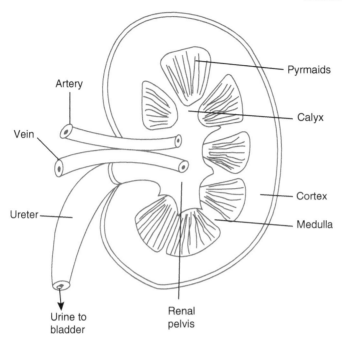

*Figure 8.2* The kidney in cross section. The cortex is mostly nephrons and the medulla is mostly straight collecting ducts set in pyramids. These pyramids drain urine into the calyces and the renal pelvis. Urine then passes to the ureters and onto the bladder.

as a total of all 2 million nephrons. Water and other small molecules may pass through the membrane but large molecules, such as most proteins and blood cells, cannot pass through the normal membrane and remain in the blood.

*Step 2* is the reabsorption of required substances, including much of the water, back into the circulation from the **proximal convoluted tubule** (Figure 8.5). Water returns to the blood at a rate of about 105 ml per minute, measured as a total of all 2 million nephrons. Other substances returned include some sodium and all of the glucose.

The remaining filtrate passes into the **loop of Henle**, which has the effect of causing an osmotic gradient across the renal cortex that becomes important to water reabsorption from the straight collecting ducts (Figure 8.6).

Filtrate then passes into the **distal convoluted tubule**, where further reabsorption of substances takes place, some of which is under hormonal control. The reabsorption of water is controlled by **antidiuretic hormone** (**ADH**) and that of sodium by **aldosterone** (Figure 8.5). ADH is also active along the straight collecting ducts controlling water reabsorption in response to the osmotic gradient.

*Step 3* involves the addition of certain substances, notably hydrogen ions ($H^+$) (see page 173), ammonia ($NH_3$) (see page 76) and potassium ions ($K^+$) into the filtrate from the blood by means of **tubular secretion**, which takes place in the **straight collecting ducts**. The resultant filtrate is now urine, which then passes first to the renal pelvis and then into the bladder.

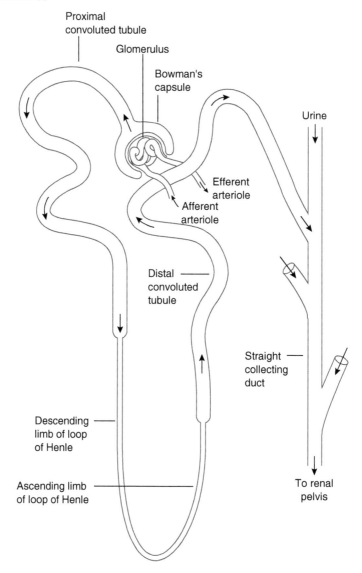

*Figure 8.3* The renal nephron. The glomerulus, inside the Bowman's capsule, is formed from a tuft of arterioles. The blood enters via the afferent arteriole and leaves via the efferent arteriole. Filtrate flows along the proximal convoluted tubule to the loop of Henle. The distal convoluted tubule conveys filtrate to the straight collecting duct, where, as urine, it flows to the renal pelvis and to the bladder.

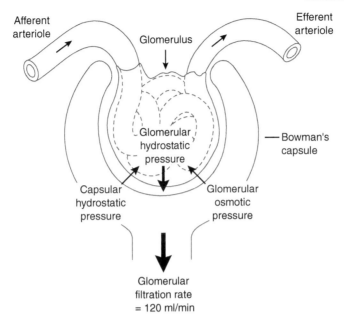

Figure 8.4 The glomerulus and Bowman's capsule. Water is pushed out of the blood and into the Bowman's capsule by the glomerular hydrostatic pressure (GHP). Two other forces are returning water to the blood. The capsular hydrostatic pressure is produced by the fluid within the capsule, and the glomerular osmotic pressure is the force exerted by the proteins within the blood to attract water back. The GHP is greater than the sum of the other two, creating a glomerular filtration rate of approximately 120 ml/min, measured as a sum total for all 2 million nephrons.

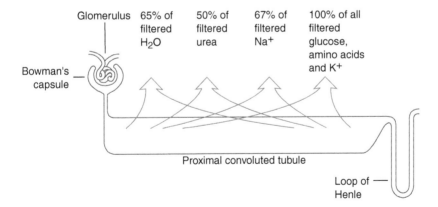

Figure 8.5 The proximal convoluted tubule, between the Bowman's capsule and the loop of Henle, reabsorbs water, urea, sodium and other substances. The percentage shown is that of the amount filtered by the glomerulus.

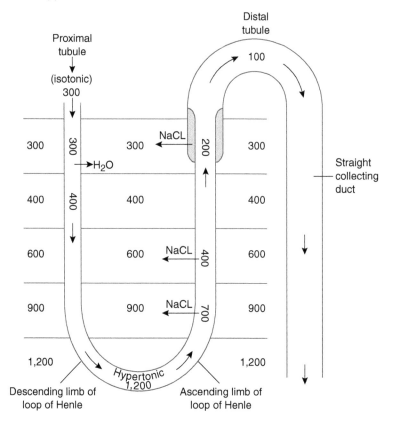

All figures in mosmol/l
(milliosmoles per litre)

*Figure 8.6* The loop of Henle passes through a sodium concentration gradient outside the loop caused by blood capillaries called the vasa recta, which follow the loop closely (not shown). The concentration gradient is shown from 300 to 1,200 mosmol/l. Water can pass out of the descending limb but not the ascending limb, and sodium is unable to pass out of the descending limb but is actively transported out of the ascending limb. The filtrate passing down the descending limb is isotonic to begin with but becomes more concentrated in sodium (i.e. hypertonic) as water is lost. As the filtrate returns up the ascending limb, sodium is lost and the filtrate becomes less concentrated. The resultant dilution of the filtrate in the distal convoluted tubule (100 mosmol/l) allows the kidney to excrete urine more diluted than body fluids (hypotonic) when necessary. The gradient along the straight collecting duct allows the kidney to reclaim water (under antidiuretic hormone control) and therefore excrete urine more concentrated than body fluids (hypertonic) when necessary (Figures 8.7–8.9).

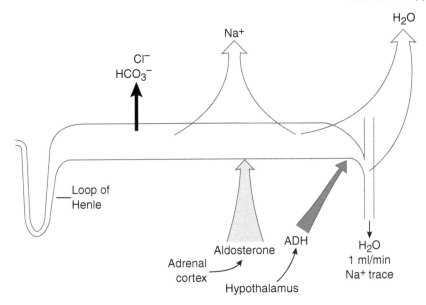

*Figure 8.7* The distal convoluted tubule. After the loop of Henle, the distal tubule absorbs chlorine (Cl⁻) and bicarbonate ($HCO_3^-$). Sodium (Na⁺) is reabsorbed under aldosterone control from the adrenal cortex, and water is reabsorbed under antidiuretic hormone (ADH) control from the hypothalamus. The amount of water returned to the blood allows an average of 1 ml per minute as urine production.

### The urinary system in youth

After birth, the kidneys are anatomically complete but remain underdeveloped and imma-ture and only reach maturity of function by 2 years of age. Normally, the conscious con-trol of urination arises somewhere about 2 or 3 years of age, and by 12 years micturition reaches adult standards. In the teenage years, the risk of urinary tract infections is higher for girls than for boys. Young women aged over 15 years old are at the highest risk, with 1 in 5 becoming affected. This is largely due to the short urethra in girls which allows quick and easy access for bacteria to reach the bladder. The urethral opening is not far from the anus, the major source of the bowel commensal ***Escherichia coli*** (***E. coli***), which causes 70–80% of infections. ***Staphylococcus saprophyticus*** is the second most common cause of urinary tract infections in young women.

### Urinary observations and tests

Urinary observations are made on the volume, colour, smell, deposits and specific gravity of the urine, and there are chemical tests, in the form of reagent pads on a strip, testing for glu-cose, pH, protein, blood, bilirubin, urobilinogen, ketones, nitrite, leucocytes and vitamin C. Collecting urinary specimens and the use of reagent testing strips are described by Simerville *et al*. (2005). The reagent test strips are calibrated to perform accurately within precise limits, and they will give false results if used wrongly. These limits include the need to use the strips before the expiry dates, store them in a dry environment and to read the results at the speci-fied time limit (usually 60 seconds). Testing freshly voided urine is important since constituents change with time when left standing, especially when exposed to the air.

*Urinary volume*

The two kidneys produce urine at the average rate of about 1 ml per minute (close to 1,500 ml per day, with a normal range from 1,000–2,000 ml) given an average daily oral intake of 2,000 ml of fluids. Variations in oral intake will change this output volume by adjusting the levels of ADH in the blood (Figures 8.8 and 8.9). ADH is produced by the hypothalamus of the brain and moves to the posterior pituitary gland. It is released into the circulation and acts on the straight collecting ducts. The role of ADH is to facilitate the return of water from the urinary filtrate back to the blood, thus controlling the concentration of urine, and it is therefore a major influence on fluid balance in the body (see Chapter 6). It works by binding to $V_2$ (ADH) receptors on the surface of cells lining the straight

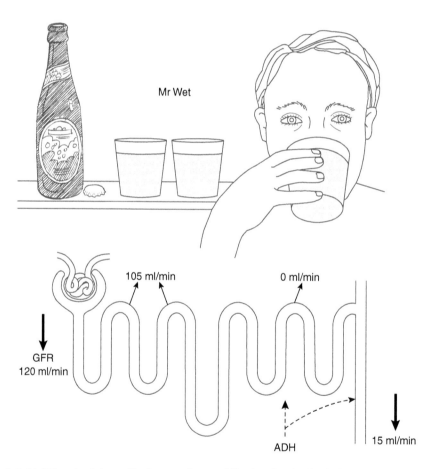

*Figure 8.8* Mr Wet physiology. If a large volume of fluid is drunk, the kidney can compensate by excreting more urine. The figures are totals for the 2 million nephrons (1 million per kidney). The glomerular filtration rate (GFR) is approximately 120 ml/min, and the first tubule reabsorption rate is approximately 105 ml/min. The variations begin in the distal tubule because of very low levels of antidiuretic hormone (ADH). Signals to the brain have caused a shutdown of ADH production and release, resulting in little or none of the water in the distal tubule being returned to the blood. This gives a urine output of 15 ml/min (i.e. 120 minus 105), the renal maximum.

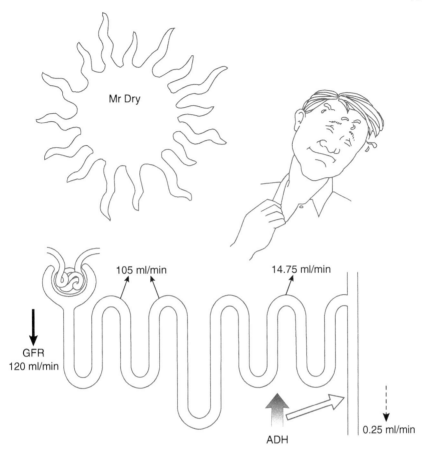

*Figure 8.9* Mr Dry physiology. If the oral intake of fluids is very low, the kidney can compensate to prevent unnecessary water loss. The figures shown are totals for the 2 million nephrons across both kidneys. The glomerular filtration rate (GFR) is approximately 120 ml/min; the reabsorption rate from the first tubule is about 105 ml/min. The difference begins in the second tubule when large amounts of antidiuretic hormone (ADH) are active, returning up to 14.75 ml/min water to the blood and creating a urine output of only 0.25 ml/min, the renal minimum.

collecting duct. After the GFR of 120 ml per minute and the reabsorption of water from the proximal convoluted tubule, the remaining filtrate has a water volume of about 15 ml per minute. Average ADH levels, as found in those who are drinking normal amounts daily, return about 14 ml per minute to the blood, leaving an average of 1 ml per minute as urine. The extremes of ADH activity are seen in those persons with very different oral intakes of fluid (Figures 8.8 and 8.9).

Mr Wet is drinking large quantities of fluid quick succession (Figure 8.8). His high oral intake of fluid sends stimuli to the hypothalamus to reduce ADH production and release, and it therefore lowers the amount that is active on the kidneys. A minimum of ADH release can be achieved if the oral intake is high enough. Less water is returned from the collecting duct as a result, i.e. little or no post-loop reabsorption occurs, and the urine output increases to a maximum of 15 ml per minute, the **renal maximum**, causing a large urine output called a **polyuria**, or **diuresis**. Outputs higher than this suggest that the kidneys have lost control of fluid balance, a feature of **chronic renal failure**. Failure here means *failure to control fluid balance*. High outputs should return to normal as fluid balance is restored, but outputs remaining consistently high, or exceeding 15 ml per minute (900 ml per hour), particularly if the input is not high, should seek medical advice. As Mr Wet's drink contains alcohol, this will have a further dehydrating effect by suppressing ADH production. Dehydration is said to be one of the causes of the hangover.

Meanwhile, Mr Dry (Figure 8.9) has no oral fluids, and he may be losing a great deal of water through his skin by sweating. His very low oral intake of fluid causes stimuli to pass to the hypothalamus, creating an increase in the production and release of ADH, therefore boosting his ADH activity on the kidneys.

Up to 14.75 ml per minute of the post-loop 15 ml per minute filtrate can be returned to the blood, leaving a urine output of about 0.25 ml per minute, the **renal minimum** (causing a very low output called an **oliguria**). No output (**anuria**) is not possible in normal renal physiology as this would cause retention of wastes, especially urea, a feature of **acute renal failure**. The word failure in acute renal failure means *failure to produce urine*, otherwise known as *renal shutdown*. Observations of urine output volume are made in those patients most at risk of imbalance, i.e. those who are nil by mouth or are not drinking well, those on intravenous infusion, those with excessive fluid losses from sweating, over breathing, bleeding or drains and those with renal disease or children with diarrhoea and vomiting (see Chapter 6). Outputs falling below 1 ml per minute (60 ml per hour) should be monitored closely and medical advice sought if the output reaches 30 ml or less per hour.

### Diabetes

One important cause of polyuria, hyperglycaemia, glycosuria and ketonuria is **diabetes**. The word *diabetes* means a disease characterised by a large urine output (**polyuria**). Since more than one disorder causes polyuria, at least two distinct diabetic diseases, *diabetes insipidus* and *diabetes mellitus*, are known. In addition, diabetes mellitus is subdivided into *type 1* and *type 2*.[1]

**Diabetes insipidus** is a polyuria caused by a lack of ADH due to a failure of the hypothalamus or the pituitary gland. Inadequate ADH means that water in the distal convoluted tubule cannot be returned to the blood and is then lost in the urine. The urine tests negative for glucose (thus *insipidus*, i.e. insipid = not sweet)[2] because glucose metabolism is not involved.

**Diabetes mellitus** (melli = honey) is divided into *type 1* and *type 2* (see note 1, page 179). *Diabetes mellitus type 1* is a disorder of carbohydrate metabolism caused by a lack of insulin from degenerating beta (β) cells[3] in the pancreas (Figure 8.10). The blood has a raised glucose level (**hyperglycaemia**) and the urine also contains glucose (**glycosuria**).

Insulin production normally responds to the current blood glucose levels, i.e. an increase in blood glucose causes more insulin to be released. Insulin lowers blood glucose levels by promoting the uptake of glucose into cells. It does this by binding to **insulin receptors** on the cell surface, and this activates **glucose transport molecules** (called **GLUTs**), which then transport the glucose into the cell as an energy source (see *glucose*, Figures 1.2A and 1.3 and *carbohydrates*, Chapter 7). A lack of insulin results in the inactivity of GLUTs and the glucose remains in the blood, causing hyperglycaemia (raised blood glucose level), i.e. 5.5 mmol/L or 100 mg/dL or higher (Chapter 4;

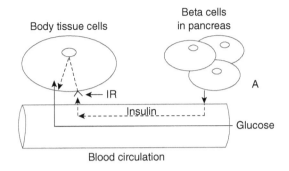

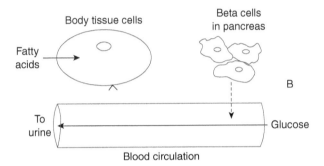

*Figure 8.10* The effect of insulin on glucose. (A) Normally, insulin released from the beta cells enters the blood and promotes glucose uptake into the body cells by binding to insulin receptors (IRs) on the cells. (B) In type I diabetes, the beta cells are producing inadequate insulin, and glucose remains in circulation and is excreted in the urine. The cells then must use fatty acids for energy.

Table 8.1). Excess glucose is excreted in the urine. Glucose is normally filtered via the glomerulus and absorbed back into the blood from the proximal convoluted tubule. This return of glucose to circulation is total, leaving no glucose in the filtrate or urine (Figure 8.5). The process of absorption involves glucose transport molecules within the cells that line the tubule, and these molecules move glucose from the filtrate back into the blood. A set amount of transport molecules means that glucose movement is finite, but this is adequate for the average volume of glucose found in the filtrate under normal conditions. It is possible for glomerular filtration to exceed this **renal threshold** for glucose, and the surplus glucose remaining in the filtrate passes through the remaining nephron and into the urine (**glycosuria**). This will happen mostly when there is excess glucose occurring in the blood (hyperglycaemia), as in diabetes mellitus. Glycosuria can also occur during pregnancy (Chapter 16) – but it is usually of no significance – or in individuals with naturally fewer transport molecules but who do not have diabetes.

High glucose-laden filtrate within the nephron tubule exerts an osmotic force that retains the water present in the filtrate and attracts more water out of the blood, all of which escapes as urine. The resultant large urine loss causes a state of dehydration that results in thirst (**polydipsia**) to replace this water. In diabetes the polyuria causes thirst and an increase in oral intake (Figure 8.11). So, the patient suffers the two main symptoms of the disorder: constant thirst and frequent urination.

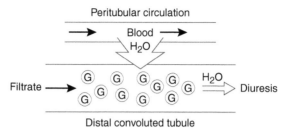

Peritubular circulation

*Figure 8.11* Mechanism of the large urine loss (diuresis) in uncontrolled diabetes. Glucose is not normally present in the distal convoluted tubule, so if glucose molecules (G) do get through to this part of the nephron, they cause a return of water ($H_2O$) from the peritubular blood circulation to the filtrate. This osmotic increase in filtrate water causes the large urine loss that is seen in uncontrolled diabetes.

At the same time, because glucose is no longer available as an energy source, cells must find an alternative, i.e. stored fat (**adipose**), which, if used for energy, releases **ketones**. Adipose is then broken down by enzymes in a process called **lipolysis**, and this releases more of the fatty acids. Ketones are the end product of excess adipose breakdown in the body. Adipose stores fats in the form of **triglyceride**, which has three fatty acids attached to a glycerol molecule (Figure 1.7, page 6). Fatty acids can be used as an additional (secondary) energy supply by entering the tricarboxylic acid (Krebs) cycle (Figure 1.3, page 4), and in the presence of oxygen they are used to create energy in the form of **adenosine triphosphate** (**ATP**) (see Chapter 1). A large release of fatty acids into circulation from lipolysis results in the liver converting the excess into any of the three **ketones**; **acetone, acetoacetic acid** and **beta-hydroxybutyric acid**. Acetone, being the largest amount produced, is excreted via both the kidneys (**ketonuria**) and the lungs, giving a sweet pear drop smell to the urine and the breath, as noted in diabetes mellitus. Urine is therefore tested for ketones as a measure of fat metabolism. At normal levels of ketone production, the urine should have no ketones present. Excess ketones in circulation (and therefore also in the urine) in diabetes is **diabetic ketoacidosis** (**DKA**). The acidosis is a lowering of blood pH to below 7.35 and is caused by the acidic nature of the ketones in the absence of adequate insulin. The symptoms include thirst and dehydration, abdominal pain, nausea and vomiting, flushed and dry skin, sweet pear drop smell to the breath and confusion. **Ketosis** is a slightly raised ketone level but not enough to cause acidosis.

The condition of low blood glucose (hypoglycaemia), i.e. below 70 mg/dL or 3.9 mmol/L can also cause a state of collapse with sweating, tremors, pallor, headache, palpitations, hunger and fatigue (Table 8.1).

In *diabetes mellitus type 2*, the insulin production varies and does not always respond to the blood glucose levels. The beta cells appear to have become less sensitive to the blood glucose level, and insulin release is more haphazard, often rising above normal in the early stages (see Chapter 4). There is a varying amount of *insulin resistance*, which means that when insulin binds to the receptors, it does not always activate GLUTS, and therefore blood glucose levels fluctuate. Insulin resistance in type 2 is strongly linked to obesity, i.e. weight loss improves insulin receptor sensitivity and reduces symptoms, and it occurs mostly in the older age group. Patients do not generally require insulin therapy since their blood glucose can be controlled by a combination of diet, weight loss and oral medication. If not well controlled, type 2 diabetes may gradually degenerate towards type 1, and insulin therapy may then become necessary.

*Table 8.1* Red flag warnings of deteriorating diabetic condition

℈ **Red Flag = serious situation which needs urgent medical attention.**

| Flag warning | Details |
| --- | --- |
| ℈ **Red Flag** | **Diabetic hyperglycaemia (blood glucose level too high):** collapse, rapid breathing, vomiting, thirst, dehydration, abdominal pain, flushed and dry skin, pear drop smell to breath, confusion and ultimately coma. **Diabetic hypoglycaemia (blood glucose level too low):** collapse, pallor, sweating, palpitations, tremor, hunger, headache, fatigue and ultimately coma. |

(After Hill-Smith and Johnson 2021, with permission)

**Maturity onset diabetes of the young** (**MODY**) is a related disorder often misdiagnosed as diabetes mellitus type 1 or 2. The disorder affects mostly those under 25 years old, causing a non-insulin-dependent mild diabetes with a fasting hyperglycaemia. There is a distinct genetic history (autosomal dominant inheritance) involving genes linked to beta-cell activity. There are 10 genetic mutations, of which the most common (94%) are:

- MODY 3: HNF-1-alpha gene (52% of cases)
- MODY 2: GCK gene (32% of cases)
- MODY 1: HNF-4-alpha (10% of cases).

(HNF = hepatocyte nuclear factor; GCK = glucokinase)

Because the genes have a high degree of penetrance,[4] it is likely that any child inheriting the gene mutation will develop the disease early in life. The symptoms are similar to type 1 diabetes mellitus, but are mild and some symptoms are absent. The C-peptide test (see Chapter 4) is useful to distinguish between MODY and diabetes mellitus type 1 because C-peptide falls (along with the insulin) in type 1 but remains normal in MODY (Morris and Morris 2017).

Some causes of diabetes involve **autoantibodies**, i.e. antibodies that attack and destroy normal body tissues. They are part of the immune system that goes wrong, creating an **autoimmune disease**. In diabetes these are usually anti-beta-cell antibodies that attack and degrade the beta cells in the pancreas. **Latent autoimmune disease in adults** (**LADA**) is a disorder similar to type 1 diabetes but lacking some of the features. It occurs mostly in the over-35-years age group. The autoantibodies that attack the beta cells in LADA are:

- anti-**glutamic acid decarboxylase** (anti-GAD) antibody
- anti-**islet cell cytoplasm** (anti-ICA) antibody
- anti-**tyrosine phosphatase-like protein IA2** (anti-IA2) antibody.

LADA can be seen as a slow variation of type 1 diabetes, with the need for insulin being delayed anything from months to several years after diagnosis. Other autoimmune disorders may be present alongside LADA (e.g. pernicious anaemia, thyroid autoimmune disease and coeliac disease), and the presence of these disorders further suggests the autoantibody nature of LADA (Morris 2017).

Diabetic patients may, in the future, be assigned to one of five distinct clusters of the disease. This would allow more individualised treatment tailor-made for their specific disorder. The clusters are:

1   Severe autoimmune diabetes with early age onset and producing no insulin
2   Severe insulin-deficient diabetes, similar to cluster 1 but with no immune involvement
3   Severe insulin-resistant diabetes in overweight patients who are making insulin but the cells are not responding to it
4   obese patients with mild diabetes whose metabolism is closer to normal than those in cluster 3
5   mild, age-related diabetes, developing symptoms in old age.

A close link between the digestive tract and diabetes has been identified (Rubino 2017). Surgery on the digestive system to reduce weight has become an effective treatment for type 2 diabetes. The operation re-routes and shortens the passage of food and bile through the digestive system. The mechanism by which the surgery reduces diabetes is not fully understood, but it may be due to the effect on the neural circuits, the gut microbes, the function of bile acids, the hormones that control bowel function or the mechanism of glucose transport across the bowel wall. This surgery is now gaining ground in the treatment of type 2 diabetes.

### Colour, smell and deposits

The normal colour of urine is a clear pale yellow with no clouding or deposits. Urine density affects the colour: the more dilute the urine is with water, the weaker the colour. Concentrated urine becomes darker, depending on how much solutes are present (see *specific gravity*, page 169). This is normal, but the colour can also change when unusual substances are present (Table 8.2 and Plate 1).

**Bilirubin** will colour the urine strong yellow, and when seen in bulk in concentrated urine it can appear to be black (Plate 1). Bilirubin is the end product of the breakdown of haemoglobin from erythrocytes (red blood cells) in circulation (see *bilirubin in the urine*, page 172).

Whole blood will change the colour according to the amount present and how long it has been mixed with urine. Small amounts of blood added to the urine during formation (i.e. well mixed with the filtrate within the nephron) may give a grey smoky appearance, whereas larger amounts of blood added lower down the renal tract, especially in the bladder, will appear as red urine (**haematuria**; Plate 1). Red urine may also be a feature of excessive beetroot consumption in the diet, and some drugs may affect the colour (e.g. **anthraquinones** in laxatives such as **senna** may turn urine yellow, brown or orange). Simerville *et al.* (2005) give a comprehensive list of urine colours and the causes, including some drugs (Table 8.2).

Both **urea** and **ammonia** are nitrogenous (i.e. contains nitrogen) wastes of protein metabolism, normally produced by the liver from excess protein. Ammonia is more toxic than urea and gives a more powerful smell. The ammonia smell associated with some urine specimens is due to infective organisms in the urinary tract (a **urinary tract infection**, or **UTI**) that split the urea molecules present in urine into ammonia. Urine can smell of **acetone** (see page 166) if left to stand for some hours. It is the result of collecting organisms from the environment and a good reason for testing only fresh samples. **Ketones** (such as acetone) are waste products of fat (lipid) metabolism. Acetone is the main ketone produced, and this adds a smell of pear drops or nail polish remover to the urine. This is usually present in association with glycosuria in diabetes mellitus.

*Table 8.2* Urine colour

| Urine colour | Possible causes |
| --- | --- |
| Dark yellow | Concentrated (inadequate fluid intake, i.e. dehydration), jaundice (bilirubin) from hepatic disease |
| Neon yellow | Excessive vitamin B group intake |
| Orange | Excess carotene (carrots); vitamin C, blackberries, beetroot or rhubarb in the diet; some drugs (antibiotics, laxatives, some chemotherapy agents) |
| Brown | Jaundice (bilirubin), excess fava beans in diet, copper poisoning, melanoma, laxatives |
| Red/pink | Blood (haematuria) due to trauma, renal calculi (stones), urinary tract infection (UTI), neoplasms, excess beetroot, blackberries, rhubarb in diet; red food dye in sweets and medication |
| Black | Severe jaundice (bilirubin) from hepatic disease |
| Very pale | Very dilute urine from excessive fluid intake |
| Green | Urinary tract infection (UTI), bilirubin, excess vitamin B intake, artificial food colouring |
| Blue | Pseudomonas urinary tract infection (UTI); excess calcium in urine, dyes in some drugs, artificial food colouring |
| Cloudy | Urinary tract infection (UTI), excess calcium in urine, renal calculi (stones) debris |

Deposits are another indication of a potential problem with urine. Cloudy urine in UTIs is caused by the presence of inflammatory cells (leucocytes), bacteria (both live and dead), pus, mucus and cellular debris. Alternatively, excessive calcium excretion can give a cloudy effect and leave a chalky deposit on standing (Plate 1). This may be due to excessive calcium in the diet or to any of the decalcifying bone diseases, such as **osteoporosis**. Here, too much calcium leaves the bone and passes to the kidneys via the blood and is excreted in the urine. In this case patients are said to be *urinating their skeleton*. Excessive calcium lost in urine also increases that person's risk of forming renal stones (see page 175) (Arshad and Shar-Baloch 2007). Phosphates and **urates** (salts of **uric acid**) can produce cloudy effects in urine. Uric acid is the excretory product from the breakdown of nucleic acids such as **deoxyribonucleic acid (DNA)** and **ribonucleic acid (RNA)**. **Casts** can also leave a visible deposit when urine is left to stand. Casts are made from a matrix of a mucoprotein produced by the distal tubular epithelium that fills and takes the shape of the tubule lumen. Cells get incorporated into this matrix, which can then be washed out by the urine. When excreted, these casts indicate a potentially high protein content and a low urinary pH. When cloudy urine is observed, a sample should be collected for laboratory analysis to determine the exact component.

*Specific gravity*

The **density** of urine identifies how much **solute** there is present. Solutes are chemical substances that are dissolved in water, such as sodium chloride (found in trace quantities in urine). Specific gravity is the measure of urine density compared with the density of pure water (Plate 2). By using water as a baseline density, the specific gravity of urine states just how much denser than water a urine sample is. Since the fluid component of urine is water, the specific gravity measures the dissolved solutes in that water. The baseline density of water is 1,000 (or 1.000, labelled 0 on some hydrometers), and a particular urine sample will measure greater than this (e.g. 1,010, or 1.010) if the hydrometer reads 10. The normal range of specific gravity for urine is 1,002 (or 1.002) for dilute urine to

1,035 (or 1.035) for concentrated urine (see page 162). The **hydrometer** (or **urinometer**) floats in the urine sample and measurement is made from where the urine surface crosses the stem scale (Plate 2). How high (in dense urine) or how low (in dilute urine) the urinometer floats is an indication of how much the urine is pushing back against the weight of the instrument, and this is the effect of the solute content. Think of the difference between a body floating in the swimming pool (low solute density) and floating in the Dead Sea (high solute density). Now, the use of a hydrometer has been replaced by a specific gravity test pad on the urinalysis stick (see *urinalysis*).

The specific gravity is affected by both the water concentration and the solute concentration in the urine sample. The water concentration varies as described (see page 162 and Chapter 6). Solutes vary in concentration depending on several factors because many different solutes are involved. **Sodium (Na⁺)** is naturally excreted from the kidneys in amounts according to blood levels of sodium and its controlling hormone, **aldosterone**. A high oral intake of sodium chloride (NaCl) increases the blood level, which promotes removal of more sodium by glomerular filtration. The majority of the filtered sodium will return to the blood from the proximal convoluted tubule; most of the remainder will be reabsorbed from the distal convoluted tubule under aldosterone control. Aldosterone comes from the adrenal cortex and is released according to blood sodium levels: higher levels reduce aldosterone release; lower levels increase its release. Aldosterone acts to facilitate sodium reabsorption back into the blood. In high blood sodium levels (**hypernatraemia**), less aldosterone allows more sodium to escape in the urine and reduce the blood level. In low blood sodium levels (**hyponatraemia**), the higher aldosterone release allows more sodium to return to the blood and thereby increase the blood level. Aldosterone release is also facilitated by the **renin-angiotensin-aldosterone cycle**, whereby the kidney emergency hormone renin is produced under low blood pressure or low blood sodium conditions. Renin activates the blood protein angiotensin (a vasoconstrictive agent that raises blood pressure), which in turn also stimulates aldosterone release to conserve sodium. Sodium is filtered and reabsorbed under aldosterone control (Table 8.3) which also has an exchange mechanism with potassium (Figure 8.12).

**Calcium (Ca²⁺)**, phosphates and other solutes are eliminated in the filtrate and contribute to the specific gravity.

## Urinalysis

Eight different chemical tests measure the amounts of solutes in urine that may indicate disease. These are impregnated into pads and mounted on strips in a convenient manner for urine testing (Plate 3). Glucose and ketones in urine were discussed under diabetes (see page 164).

*Table 8.3* Water and sodium in urine

| Substance | Glomerular filtered | Proximal tubule | Hormone | Distal tubule | Amount in urine |
|---|---|---|---|---|---|
| Water | Yes | Most is reabsorbed | ADH | Average 15 ml/min | Average 1 ml/min |
| Sodium | Yes | Most is reabsorbed | Aldosterone | Most is reabsorbed | Trace |

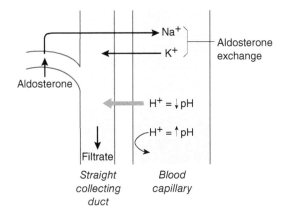

*Figure 8.12* Mechanism of sodium and hydrogen loss. The return of sodium (Na⁺) to the blood by aldosterone in the distal convoluted tubule is accompanied by the return of potassium (K⁺) to the filtrate (aldosterone exchange). Thus, aldosterone influences the potassium balance. In addition, hydrogen ions (H⁺) can be returned to the filtrate from the straight collecting duct or retained in the blood, according to the need to maintain the blood pH balance at pH 7.4. Under low pH conditions (e.g. acidosis), hydrogen ions are excreted, and under high pH conditions (alkalosis) hydrogen ions are retained in circulation.

### Protein in urine

**Protein** does not normally appear in the urine (Plate 3). Blood proteins include **albumin**, **globulin**, **fibrinogen** and **prothrombin** (the last two are also clotting factors; see Chapter 4). Protein molecules are too large (7–9 nm) to pass through the glomerular membrane pores (about 3 nm across). Albumin could pass through the pores but is mostly repelled back into the circulation by the strong negative charges associated with the glycoproteins of the glomerular membrane. What few proteins do appear in the filtrate can be reclaimed by the urinary cells, a process called **pinocytosis**. Protein in the urine (**proteinuria**, or more specifically **albuminuria**) can be caused by damage to the glomerular membrane, resulting in a larger pore size – as seen in glomerular infections (**glomerulonephritis**) – and damage by nephrotoxic agents. Systemic hypertension raises the intraglomerular blood pressure and forces more protein into the filtrate. The presence of blood in urine also means protein is there as well and therefore urine with blood added will show a positive protein result. **Nephrotic syndrome** is a condition recognised by a persistent protein loss in the urine (3.5 g or more of protein lost per day) and can result in a reduced blood protein level with the consequence of possible tissue oedema (see Chapter 6).

### Blood in the urine

**Blood** in the urine (**haematuria**; Plate 3) may be expected in some circumstances, e.g. blood contamination of urine during menstruation or immediately after bladder, renal or prostate surgery, but otherwise urine should be free of blood. If present, it may be a manifestation of a pathology that requires investigation. Blood in the urine can occur as a result of trauma to any part of the renal system (Pfitzenmaier *et al.* 2008) or can be caused by the effects of renal stones damaging the urinary tract wall (see page 175) (Arshad and Shar-Baloch 2007). Blood can also occur as a result of infections or new growths within the bladder, kidney or prostate gland. The test pad for blood on clinical sticks is sensitive to haemoglobin, ensuring a positive result even when red blood cells have been broken down. Haematuria from surgery or trauma often appears as bright red urine (*frank* blood) at first, diminishing in intensity over several days until the urine appears normal and blood can only be detected by testing. An uncomplicated recovery aided by a good fluid input during the post-operative period results in a blood-free urinalysis.

### Bilirubin in the urine

Bilirubin and urobilinogen are products of haemoglobin breakdown when it is released from old destroyed red blood cells (Figure 8.13).

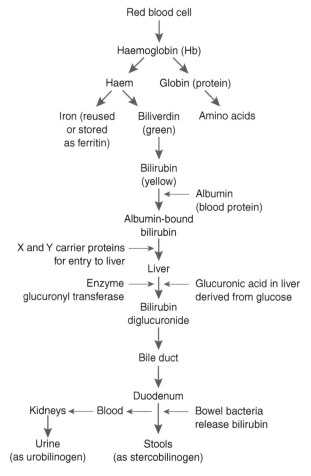

Figure 8.13 The natural history of bilirubin. Red cell breakdown causes the release of haemoglobin, which breaks down into a *haem* group and the protein globin. Globin can be further reduced to amino acids; the haem group, which contains iron, releases the iron which can be stored or reused. The remainder is biliverdin, which is green, and this is converted to yellow bilirubin. Albumin, a blood protein, binds bilirubin, and other proteins called X and Y help to transport the bilirubin to the liver. Here, the enzyme glucuronyl transferase causes the bilirubin to combine with the glucuronic acid to form bilirubin diglucuronide, which becomes one component of bile. Bile arrives in the duodenum, where further conversion of bilirubin creates *stercobilinogen*, a component of stools. Some bilirubin is reabsorbed into the blood and filtered in the urine as *urobilinogen*.

**Erythrocytes** (red blood cells) degrade and release haemoglobin after about 120 days in circulation. The metabolism of the haemoglobin is shown in Figure 8.13. Normal uro-bilinogen levels in urine are small (0.09–4.23 µmol per 24 hours), but levels will increase in **jaundice**. This condition occurs if the liver is no longer able to accept or handle biliru-bin adequately (i.e. **hepatic jaundice** as in **liver failure**, **cirrhosis** or **hepatitis**) or if the bile drainage is obstructed (i.e. **post-hepatic jaundice**, caused by an impacted **biliary stone** or **pancreatic cancer**). **Pre-hepatic jaundice** can also occur when the breakdown of red cells, or **haemolysis**, is happening too quickly, as in **haemolytic anaemia**, and bilirubin is produced faster than the liver can accept. In any of these conditions, the surplus is removed by the kidney and lost in the urine but not before the excess bilirubin colours yellow the skin and **sclera** (the white of the eyes). Bilirubin, being not normally found in urine, will appear to make urine very dark (Plate 1) along with the raised urobilinogen.

*Acid-base measurement of urine (pH)*

**pH**[5] is a scale of acidity or alkalinity (or base)[6] of a substance. The pH scale (Figure 8.14) is a measure of the **hydrogen ion** (**H⁺**) concentration (sometimes written [pH] as square brackets mean 'concentration').

Strong concentrations give an acid solution (low pH 1–6, pH 1 being the strongest acid) and a weak concentration gives an alkaline solution (high pH 8–14, pH 14 being the strongest alkaline). pH 7 is neutral and is the value found in most water samples tested, especially distilled water. In urine, the hydrogen ion concentration normally varies from pH 5 to pH 8 according to the diet and tissue metabolism, but usually stabilises around pH 6 (Plate 3). Hydrogen ions are the end waste product of energy (ATP) production by the cells, from glucose or fatty acids (see Chapter 1) and also from ketone production (see page 168) and from acids taken in the diet. Because hydrogen ions cause acidity they are potentially hazardous. They have to be transported in the blood to the kidneys and need to be excreted. Blood pH is critical at pH 7.35–7.45 (see Chapter 4), and it must be stabilised within this range. Hydrogen ions entering the blood must be *buffered* then removed by the kidneys for excretion. **Buffers** are a means of 'tying up' hydrogen ions into compounds so that they are unable to contribute to the hydrogen ion concentration. This allows them to be carried safely in the blood without affecting the blood pH. Examples are bicarbonate, proteins, haemoglobin and

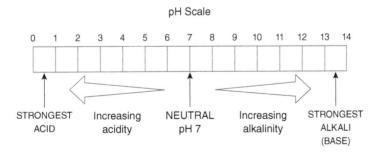

*Figure 8.14* The pH scale. The lower part of the scale (shown here on the left) is acidic, with the lowest numbers being the strongest acid (pH 1). The higher part of the scale (shown on the right) is alkaline, with the highest numbers being the strongest alkaline (pH 14). Neutral is pH 7 on the scale (centre).

phosphate buffers. Of these, haemoglobin (Hb) is very important for buffering hydrogen ions in the blood (Hb + $H^+$ → HHb), followed by blood proteins, which have a nitrogenous component ($NH_2$) which is able to take up surplus $H^+$ ($NH_2$ + $H^+$ → $NH_3^+$). Bicarbonates ($HCO_3^-$) are filtered from the blood in the glomerulus and serve to buffer urine in the proximal tubule ($HCO_3^-$ + $H^+$ → $H_2CO_3$ → $H_2O$ + $CO_2$), where $CO_2$ is absorbed back into the tubular cells and then into the blood. It is finally excreted from the blood via the lungs. The water ($H_2O$) remains in the filtrate and is excreted in the urine. Phosphates ($HPO_4^{2-}$) are major buffers in the renal filtrate of the distal tubular cells ($HPO_4^{2-}$ + $H^+$ + $Na^+$ → $NaH_2PO_4$). Phosphates prevent urine from becoming too acidic or alkaline, which would otherwise damage the tract lining and cause great discomfort, especially when passing urine (**micturition**). Increased urinary pH (above pH 8, i.e. alkaline urine) occurs in **alkalosis** (high blood pH, as may occur in a vegetarian diet). It occurs naturally soon after a meal. Low urinary pH (below pH 5, i.e. acidic urine) appears in **acidosis**, i.e. low blood pH as in diabetic ketoacidosis or aspirin overdose or after the consumption of prunes or cranberries or as a result of starvation. Disturbance of blood pH (and thus urinary pH) can happen in various therapies that influence the fluid balance of the body (see Chapter 6). Since $H^+$ and $K^+$ share the same excretory mechanism in the distal tubule and collecting duct cells, the excretion of large quantities of $K^+$ (as may be the case with excessive intravenous potassium chloride [KC1] treatment or diuretic therapy) may cause retention of $H^+$.

### Nitrites in urine

Nitrites can be tested for as an indicator of the presence of a **urinary tract infection** (**UTI**). Nitrites are the result of the breakdown of nitrates in the urinary system. Nitrates[7] are a component of our diet and are excreted normally in the urine. The presence of nitrites, however, indicates that there is a bacterial infection by a type of organism that is capable of producing an enzyme, **nitrate reductase**, necessary for converting nitrate to nitrite. Ninety per cent of UTIs are caused by organisms of this type (e.g. gram-negative bacteria such as *Escherichia coli*), and therefore the nitrite test stick is of increasing clinical importance as a quick, accurate means of detecting UTIs. The remaining 10% of urinary infections include staphylococci, *Pseudomonas* species and enterococci. These are organisms that do not produce the enzyme, and therefore the test is not sensitive to them. Chemical stick reagent tests can often replace the more expensive laboratory tests and give quicker results. The problems have centred around the accuracy of the chemical test strip. If they are used routinely for the identification of UTIs before laboratory cultures are taken, the risk is that they may miss some clinically significant infections. Stick analysis of urine for infection is now accurate enough to be used to identify only those urines that need laboratory culture and analysis (Doley and Nelligan 2003).

### Leucocytes in urine

**Leucocytes** (white blood cells; see Chapter 4) of the granulocyte type (especially **neutrophils**) produce another enzyme, **leucocyte esterase**, that can be detected in urine. This test will identify the presence of intact and lysed (broken down) granulocytes in the urine either with or without infection. The presence of leucocytes indicates an inflammation, either with organisms (infection) or without (sterile).

## Other urine tests

**Midstream urine** (**MSU**) is the procedure for collecting a clinically clean sample of urine for laboratory culture. Ideally, the sample collected is as clean as possible. However, even though urine is produced sterile, it does pick up contaminants (mostly bacterial organisms) from the urethra. Therefore, at the start of urination, the first flush of urine will gather most of these contaminants and wash these out of the urethra. This first part of the urine stream is then discarded. A sterile container is then used to collect the next stream of urine (the midstream sample), which will now flow down a cleaner urethra and therefore will have far fewer contaminants. Any remaining urine in the bladder after that can then be discarded as usual. This midstream specimen is then sent to the laboratory, and any organisms grown from it are most likely to be from a urinary infection requiring treatment and not just a urethral contaminant (Gilbert 2006).

**Creatinine clearance** is a test to assess the amount of creatinine that is lost through the kidneys. The test requires urine collected over a 24-hour period. The result is compared with the creatinine present in the blood (see *Test: Creatinine*, Chapter 4). In Chapter 4, creatinine was described as a breakdown product of **creatine**, a molecule in muscle essential for energy recycling. The amount of creatine present is dependent on the person's size, age, sex and muscle bulk. Measuring creatinine clearance not only estimates creatinine levels (an indication of the rate of muscle cell breakdown and renewal; see *muscle wasting*, page 148), but it also is a measure of renal function. This is because creatinine removal from the blood depends on the glomerular filtration rate (GFR; the average adult GFR is about 120 ml per minute; see page 159). A poor GFR gives a low creatinine clearance value.

**Renal** (or **urinary**) **stones** (called **calculi**) that form in the urinary tract, anywhere from the renal pelvis down to the bladder. They have several different compositions and therefore different causes (Table 8.4).

Renal calculi can cause extreme pain when passing down the urinary tract, especially down the narrow ureters and urethra. Stones passing down the ureters often cause very severe pain in the loins known as **renal colic**. They may also cause trauma to the lining of the tract, which then bleeds creating a haematuria. They may obstruct urine flow, and this can dam back to the kidney, causing a **hydronephrosis**, i.e. excessive urine accumulation within the kidney, with resulting loss of renal function.

**Pregnancy tests** can detect the presence of **human chorionic gonadotropin** (**hCG**) in urine. Human chorionic gonadotropin is produced by the developing placenta, which

*Table 8.4* Types of renal stones

| Type of renal stone | Notes (percentages are approximate) |
| --- | --- |
| Calcium oxalate (CAOX) | The most common of the stones (67%). Dietary oxalate is found in many fruits and vegetables. |
| Calcium phosphate | 8% of stones. They form in alkaline (pH higher than 7) urine. |
| Uric acid | 8% of stones. Made from uric acid, they form in acidic urine (pH below 6). They occur with diets rich in proteins and purines. |
| Cystine | 2% of stones. Caused by a rare genetic disorder (cystinuria) that allows the amino acid cystine to leak into urine and form crystals. |
| Struvite | 15% of stones. Made from magnesium ammonium phosphate. Caused by renal tract infections. Often large stones, sometimes called 'staghorn calculi'. More common in women. |

can only happen after implantation of the fertilised ovum into the uterine lining (i.e. after 10 days following fertilisation). Before this, the fertilised ovum is still in the fallopian tube and the test is liable to create a false negative result.

### When to test urine

Urinalysis has become a standard routine test carried out on admission to hospital and in the doctor's surgery. The tests are quick, cheap and non-invasive, with instant results, and they can provide a wealth of information by virtue of there being multiple tests on one stick. For reagent strip analysis, all that is required is a very small quantity of fresh urine, one stick and a few minutes of time. If the results are recorded as *nothing abnormal detected* (NAD), then it is known that the renal system appears to be functioning normally, the chance of trauma is less and there is probably no diabetes, ketoacidosis, bleeding or jaundice. For these reasons, methods for putting other urine tests on a reagent strip are being considered. The nitrite and leucocyte tests are two of the results of these initiatives. Laboratory analysis will still be necessary to identify the organism and the antibiotic required for treatment. By making it possible to do a test in the clinical area, the test itself becomes far less labour-intensive, more cost-effective and reduces the time factor to minutes, an important point for patient comfort and recovery.

**Ascorbic acid** (**vitamin C**) has become a common food supplement that is excreted in the urine and can interfere with urine tests results. Ascorbic acid test pads are now added to some urine test sticks to test for vitamin C levels in urine. High levels of ascorbic acid in the urine can cause false negative results for several of the other tests, notably the glucose, blood, nitrite and bilirubin test pads. By testing for ascorbic acid in the urine at the same time as the other tests, it becomes possible to say if the other tests results are reliable, provided the ascorbic acid level remains below 20mg/dL.

As a standard screening device, reagent strip urinalysis can be carried out as routine almost anywhere, e.g. test strip urinalysis done in the accident department can quickly rule out injury to the kidneys (Worrall 2009). In the community, it can be used in the doctor's surgery or in the patient's own home.

New and potential urine tests which would require laboratory tests include identifying disorders not directly affecting the urinary system:

* Testing for a distinctive metabolite pattern in urine produced by the bacteria *staphylococcus pneumonia*. This is an important organism for causing community-acquired pneumonia (CAP), a serious lung disease. Early detection of this organism can result in rapid treatment and the saving of many lives (Watt *et al.* 2010).
* The possibility of testing for the protein biomarker called leucine-rich alpha-2-glyco-protein (LRG), which, if present, indicates the presence of appendicitis in young children's urine (Kentsis *et al.* 2010).
* The levels of 4-(methylnitrosamino)-1-(3-pyridyl)-1-butanol (NNAL) can be measured in urine. NNAL is a metabolite of 4-(methylnitrosamino)-1-(3-pyridyl)-1-butanone (NNK), a component of tobacco smoke. Both NNK and NNAL are potent pulmonary carcinogens and the presence of raised NNAL in urine can suggest a higher risk of lung cancer (Hecht *et al.* 2001).
* A '**PCA3 assay**' test identifies genetic evidence of prostate cancer in urine. The test identifies a small piece of **ribonucleic acid** (**RNA**) from an overactive gene that is 95% specific to prostate cancer. Therefore, it can significantly reduce the need for painful prostatic biopsies. However, more recently, questions have arisen concerning the accuracy of this test, but combining it with tests looking for two other genes that are

linked to high-risk cancer increases the reliability. These two genes (**TMPRSS2** with **ERG**) are abnormally fused in prostate cancer (called '**TMPRSS2:ERG fusion**'). If this fusion is found in the urine, it is highly specific for prostate cancer. In another development, a urine test called '*urine exosome gene expression assay*' also improves the reliability of the PCA3 test by combining it with tests for *ERG* and another gene called *SPDEF*. This test requires a 'first-catch' urine sample, i.e. the first flush of urine to leave the urethra.

* **Motor neuron disease** (**MND**) is a neurodegenerative disorder affecting several motor systems (see Chapter 14), causing progressive limb weakness and leading to paralysis, muscle wasting, gradual loss of speech and swallowing. Sufferers may live for two to five years depending on the different types of the disease (see Chapter 14, page 302), and there is no known cure. There is a confirmed genetic basis to some forms of the disease (see page 301) and relatives of the sufferer may carry the gene involved. A new urine test has been developed to identify the presence of a protein in the urine of sufferers with one type of MND called **amyotrophic lateral sclerosis** (**ALS**; see page 302). The protein is called '**p75NTRECD**', often abbreviated to '75ECD' or even 'p7'. Protein is not normally found in urine, so any protein found there suggests an abnormality is present. 75ECD is not only present in the urine of MND sufferers, but it increases as the disease get worse, making it a useful measure of the disorder's progress. It can also be used to screen other members of the sufferer's family to see if they are at risk before symptoms begin. If the protein was found, early administration of an anti-glutamate medication may help to protect neurons and slow the onset of symptoms (Shepheard *et al.* 2017).

### Drugs active on the urinary system

**Diuretic** drugs are those that induce a diuresis (a large urine output) for medical purposes, i.e. to treat **oedema**, **hypertension** or **cardiac failure** that is causing oedema (see Chapter 6). Several groups of drugs achieve a large urine output, and the patient should be warned that he/she will be passing a lot of urine. Where relevant, diuretics could make incontinence of urine worse.

* The **thiazides** (e.g. **Bendroflumethiazide**, Chapter 3, Table 3.8) prevent the reabsorption of sodium from the distal parts of the tubule. The sodium remains in the filtrate and is lost in the urine. Water follows sodium, so a sodium loss creates a diuresis.
* **Loop diuretics** (e.g. **furosemide** [**frusemide**]) and **bumetanide**, Table 8.5) work by preventing reabsorption of sodium at the loop of Henle. They are the most potent diuretics, producing the largest urine output but with the greatest potential for causing unwanted reactions. They may promote the loss of potassium as well, and this can be a complication. The **potassium-sparing** diuretics (e.g. **amiloride** and **spironolactone**) conserve potassium while causing mild diuresis as a result of sodium loss.
* Some drugs (e.g. **spironolactone**; Table 8.6) are aldosterone **antagonists**, i.e. they reduce the activity of aldosterone and this promotes further sodium and water loss. They are referred to as *potassium-sparing diuretics* because they significantly reduce the loss of potassium in the urine, a problem that may occur with other diuretics. They can be used to reduce the circulatory volume and therefore reduce the work load on the heart and to relieve oedema in specific sites (e.g. **ascites** = oedema of the abdomen).

*Table 8.5* Loop diuretic drugs

| Drug | Possible side effects | Use and other notes |
|---|---|---|
| Bumetanide | Dehydration, skin rash, hypotension. | Oedema. |
| Co-amilofruse | Acute urinary retention, nausea, headache, bowel disturbance. | Oedema. |
| Furosemide (Frusemide) | Fever, skin and mucosal reactions, malaise. | Oedema and hypertension. With or without triamterene (Table 8.5). |
| Torasemide | Gastric disturbance, asthenia (loss of energy), urinary retention. | Oedema and hypertension. |

*Table 8.6* Aldosterone antagonists

| Drug | Possible side effects | Use and other notes |
|---|---|---|
| Co-flumactone | Gut disturbance, tiredness, confusion, headache. | Congestive heart failure. A combination of hydroflumethiazide and spironolactone. |
| Eplerenone | Arrhythmias, cough, nausea, diarrhoea, dizziness, insomnia. | Specific situations related to heart failure. |
| Spironolactone | Hair loss, confusion, cramp, skin reaction, dizziness, malaise. | Oedema, heart failure, ascites, hypertension. With or without furosemide. |

**Key points**

- The functional unit of the kidney is the nephron. About 1 million nephrons exist in each of the two kidneys.
- Urine forms in three steps: filtration from the glomerulus, reabsorption from the convoluted tubules and secretion from the straight collecting ducts.
- Urine is formed at an average rate of 1 ml per minute.
- For accurate results, urine must be tested when fresh using the correct technique.
- Normal urine is a pale straw colour, clear with no deposits.
- On testing, normal urine should show negative results for glucose, blood, protein, ketones and bilirubin.
- Urinary pH ranges from 5 to 8, with an average about 6.
- The specific gravity measures the density of dissolved solutes in urine compared with water, normally about 1,010 (water = 1,000).
- Nitrite and leucocyte tests for infection or inflammatory cells in urine.
- Diabetes is an important cause of polyuria (causing thirst) and glycosuria (due to hyperglycaemia).
- Some diseases cause polyuria (diuresis), including diabetes insipidus, diabetes mellitus (types 1 and 2), maturity onset diabetes of the young (MODY) and latent autoimmune disease in adults (LADA).
- Diuretic drugs induce a large urine output as a treatment for hypertension, oedema or cardiac failure.

## Notes

1 Proposed additional types of diabetes mellitus (e.g. type 3, type 4 etc.) are not officially recognised as they lack an internationally accepted solid research base confirming their existence. Some are linked to autoimmune conditions and others to insulin receptor resistance.
2 Sweet refers to the old days when the only way to test for sugar in the urine was to taste it. Fortunately, this practice has stopped thanks to the introduction of chemical reagent tests.
3 Beta (β) cells, along with alpha (α) and delta (δ) cells, form the islets of Langerhans in the pancreas. Beta cells produce insulin.
4 Penetrance is the degree (or amount) the gene product affects the body. With low penetrance the gene has little effect, but in high penetrance the gene has a big effect on the body.
5 This must always be small p and capital H, not any other combination, as explained in Chapter 4, note 5.
6 Base is any substance that reacts with acids and neutralises them, and an alkali is a base dissolved in solution.
7 Don't get nitrates muddled with nitrites.

## References

Arshad I. and Shar-Baloch K. (2007) Renal stones. *The Annals of the Royal College of Surgeons of England*, *89*(3): 326. https://doi.org/10.1308/rcsann.2007.89.3.326a

Doley A. and Nelligan M. (2003) Is a negative dipstick urinalysis good enough to exclude urinary tract infection in paediatric emergency department patients? *Emergency Medicine Fremantle WA*, *15*(1): 77–80.

Gilbert R. (2006) Taking a midstream specimen of urine. *Nursing Times*, *102*(18): 22.

Hecht S.S., Ye M., Carmella S.G., Fredrickson A., Adgate J.L., Greaves I.A., Church T.R., Ryan A.D., Mongin S.J. and Sexton K. (2001) Metabolites of a tobacco-specific lung carcinogen in the urine of elementary school-aged children. *Cancer Epidemiology Biomarkers Prevention*, *10*(11): 1109–1116 (a publication of the American Association for Cancer Research co-sponsored by the American Society of Preventive Oncology).

Hill-Smith I. and Johnson G. (2021) *Little book of Red Flags*. National Minor Illness Centre, Bedfordshire.

Kentsis A., Lin Y.Y., Kurek K., Calicchio M., Wang Y.Y., Monigatti F., Campagne F., Lee R., Horwitz B., Steen H. and Bachur R. (2010) Discovery and validation of urine markers of acute pediatric appendicitis using high-accuracy mass spectrometry. *Annals of Emergency Medicine*, *55*(1): 62–70.e4.

Morris D. (2017) Latent autoimmune disease in adults as a cause of diabetes. *Independent Nurse*, 21 August: 13–15.

Morris J. and Morris D. (2017) MODY: One of the most easily missed causes of diabetes. *Independent Nurse*, 17 July: 13–15.

Pfitzenmaier J., Buse S., Haferkamp A., Pahernik S., Djakovic N. and Hohenfellner M. (2008) Kidney trauma. *Der Urologe Ausg A*, *47*(6): 759–767; quiz 768. Available at: www.ncbi.nlm.nih.gov/pubmed/18478197 or http://doi.org/10.1007/s00120-008-1766-6 (Accessed 19th February 2023).

Rubino F. (2017) Operation: Diabetes. *Scientific American*, *317*(1): 53–57.

Shepheard S.R., Wuu J., Cardoso M., Wiklendt L., Dinning P.G., Chataway T., Schultz D., Benatar M. and Rogers M.-L. (2017) Urinary p75ECD: A prognostic, disease progression, and pharmacodynamic biomarker in ALS. *Neurology*, *88*(12): 1137–1143. http://doi.org/10.1212/WNL.0000000000003741

Simerville J.A., Maxted W.C. and Pahira J.J. (2005) Urinalysis: A comprehensive review. *American Family Physician*, *71*(6): 1153–1162.

Watt J.P., Moïsi J.C., Donaldson R.L.A., Reid R., Ferro S., Whitney C.G., Santosham M. and O'Brien K.L. (2010) Use of serology and urine antigen detection to estimate the proportion of adult community-acquired pneumonia attributable to Streptococcus pneumoniae. *Epidemiology and Infection*, *138*(12): 1796–1803. https://doi.org/10.1017/S0950268810000555

Worrall J.C. (2009) Emergency department visual urinalysis versus laboratory urinalysis. *CJEM Canadian Journal of Emergency Medical Care; JCMU Journal Canadien de Soins Medicaux Durgence*, *11*(6): 540–543.

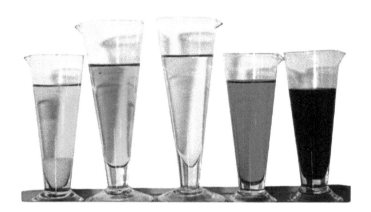

*Plate 1* Different colours of urine and sedimentation. Far left: chalky sedimentation, which may indicate the excretion of too much calcium. Left of centre: concentrated urine, as may be passed on a hot day or because of reduced fluid intake. Centre: dilute urine, as may be passed when fluid intake is high. Right of centre: blood in the urine (frank haematuria). Far right: dark urine seen in jaundice, when the urine is rich in bilirubin.

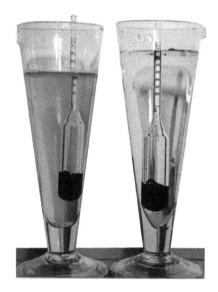

*Plate 2* Different densities of urine and specific gravity. Left: dense (darker) urine, which indicates less water is lost through the kidneys, as occurs when dehydrated. Right: dilute urine, as may be passed when fluid intake is high. Note the hydrometer (urinometer) floats lower on the right than on the left, and deeper urine on the right is needed to stop the hydrometer from touching the bottom. The hydrometer is a measure of the density observed. Left: the dense urine measures between 30 and 40 on the hydrometer scale (where the urine level crosses the scale). Right: the dilute urine measures close to 0 on the scale. Zero on this scale (or 1,000 on other scales) is the specific gravity of pure water, so the urine on the right is not much denser than pure water. Note that the hydrometer appears 'broken' in the left sample due to the different refraction (bending) of light seen through dense urine.

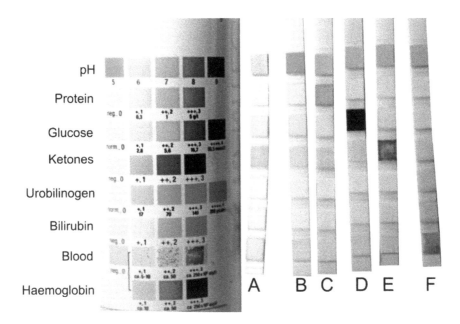

*Plate 3* Urine testing strips. The colour chart (shown left) is for comparing the colour changes seen on the strips after immersion in urine. The tests are, from top to bottom, pH (measuring the acidity or alkalinity of urine), protein, glucose, ketones, urobilinogen, bilirubin, blood and haemoglobin. (A) A stick essentially normal with pH approximately 7 (neutral). (B) A stick with pH 5 (acidic). (C) Protein is present. (D) Large amounts of glucose. (E) Positive for ketones. (F) Positive for blood.

# 9 Elimination (II)

## Digestive observations

### Introduction

The digestive system consists of the mouth, oesophagus, stomach, duodenum, jejunum, ileum, colon (ascending, transverse and descending), caecum, rectum and anus (Figure 9.1). The function of the system, i.e. the digestion and absorption of food nutrients, is controlled through enzymes from various glands and by the nervous system. The enzymes are **catabolic**, i.e. they breakdown the food to the simplest forms for absorption into the blood (Chapter 7). The nervous system causes the smooth muscles in the gut wall to contract in waves (called **peristalsis**) in order to propel the contents forward.

The inside of the gut, i.e. the gut lumen, is technically part of the outside world. That sounds strange, but for anything to get *into* the body it must first be absorbed through the gut wall. Swallowing food does not mean it is entering the body, it is simply entering the gut. So the gut wall is the interface between the outside world (inside the lumen) and the body (the blood and tissues). This is why the gut contents contain millions of bacterial and viral organisms (called the **intestinal flora**), whilst the internal body remains sterile. Also, the solid waste eliminated from the anus has passed *through* the body without actually *entering* the body.

Abnormal elimination, such as diarrhoea and vomiting, indicates that important changes have occurred within the digestive system. It is essential to establish if it is a passing phase or a symptom of something more persistent and potentially serious. The history that led up to the event coupled with the observations made at the time are paramount.

DOI: 10.4324/9781003389118-9

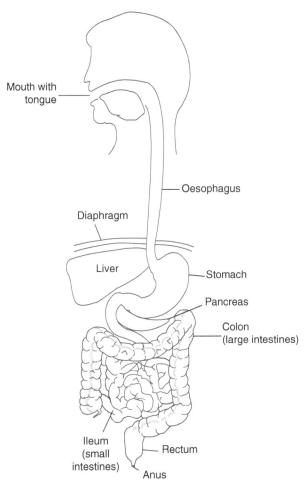

Mouth with tongue

Oesophagus

Diaphragm

Liver

Stomach

Pancreas

Colon
(large intestines)

Ileum
(small
intestines)

Rectum

Anus

*Figure 9.1* The digestive system begins at the mouth. Food passes down the oesophagus to the stomach. The ileum (small intestines) completes digestion, but food remnants are processed through the colon before elimination at the anus. The intestines are drawn lower than normal to expose the liver and pancreas which are subsidiary organs of digestion.

## Faeces

**Faeces** is waste material obtained primarily from ingested food. It normally contains **fibre**, a term for several indigestible components of the diet that provides the bulk of the stool. Fibre is derived mostly from the plant substances in the diet (i.e. fruit and vegetables), but less is found in meats. The varieties of fibre include **cellulose, hemicellulose, pectins, gums** and **lignins** (Chapter 7, page 145). These are mostly large-molecular **polysaccharides** that form the walls of plant cells. These particular polysaccharides are complex carbohydrate molecules that are indigestible by any of the digestive enzymes in the small bowel (**ileum**), but some can be broken down (**catabolised**) to a certain extent by digestive bacteria present in the large bowel (**colon**). These bacteria, the *intestinal flora*, are **commensals**.[1] In fact, human bowel commensals actually produce important vitamins from their activity on bowel contents, e.g. **niacin** (or **nicotinic acid**), **thiamine** (**vitamin B$_1$**) and **vitamin K**, which we can absorb and use (see Chapter 7, Table 7.3, page 142). Fibre has several properties; i.e. it absorbs and holds water, **electrolytes** (see Chapter 6, page 130) and bile salts. Holding water makes it normally soft so that the stool is easy to pass. The action of the colon in absorbing water from the bowel contents prevents the faeces from being too wet. The absorption of electrolytes and bile salts into the fibre itself aids the elimination of these substances. **Refined foods** are those in which the fibre is largely removed or cooked sufficiently to break it down to digestible carbohydrates and provide a greater degree of nutrient efficiency with less waste material. The refining of foods, which is becoming less common in the Western diet, has resulted in an increase in bowel disorders such as colon cancers and **diverticular disease**. The latter is a condition in which the mucous lining of the bowel is pushed through the muscular wall into pouches that can become inflamed. Clearly, fibre has a greater role to play in human digestion than was at first thought, being vital for correct bowel function, and as such it is protective against bowel disease.

### The mechanism of defecation

The rectum is normally empty. Bowel wall movements push faecal matter into the rectum, stretching the rectal wall. This triggers the **defecation reflex** (Figure 9.2), an automatic action involving afferent sensory pathways from stretch receptors in the rectal wall to the spinal cord and efferent motor pathways from the cord to the rectal muscles.

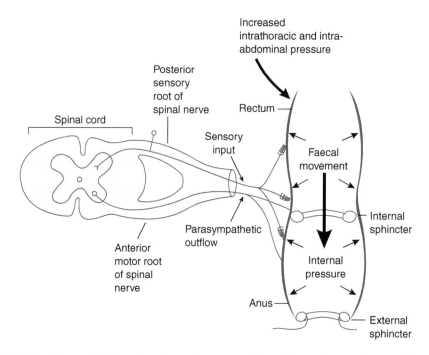

*Figure 9.2* Physiology of defecation. Internal pressure from descending stools into the rectum stretches the rectal wall. Sensory input from stretch receptors triggers a parasympathetic output from the spinal cord, which relaxes the internal sphincter and contracts smooth muscle in the bowel wall. This puts pressure on the external sphincter to open, but being voluntary skeletal muscle, this sphincter opens under conscious control. Increasing intrathoracic and intra-abdominal pressure pushes the bowel contents forward.

Activation of this pathway results in two actions: (1) the contraction of the muscular walls of the sigmoid colon and rectum, pushing the contents further along and (2) the anal sphincters to relax. Relaxation of sphincters causes them to open, and this means opening the escape route for faeces. Whereas the internal anal sphincter is autonomic (smooth muscle), the external requires voluntary control (skeletal muscle), thus allowing the time needed for the sphincter to be opened appropriately. It is this last aspect that is important in childhood, for control of the external sphincter is a skill that has to be learnt. Expulsion of faeces is achieved by contraction of the rectal wall, depression of the diaphragm and contraction of abdominal muscles, the last two causing an increase in the intra-abdominal pressure. Although this is a spinal reflex, achieved by the **parasympathetic nervous system** from the sacral outflow (Figure 9.1), the medulla is involved in coordinating the various muscle activities. It is useful to think of the parasympathetic nervous system as being the neurological control of all three normal emptying mechanisms of the body, i.e. urination, defecation and – in males – ejaculation.

The age by which a child is ready for toilet training is between 18 and 36 months. The average age for girls is 29 months, and for boys it is 31 months. The majority of children will be toilet-trained by 36 months.

## Disorders of faecal elimination

### Diarrhoea

The term '*rrhoea*' arises at the end of several words such as diarrhoea and steatorrhoea (see page 184), and it means 'flow'. **Diarrhoea** is a flow of faeces in fluid form, since the water content is excessive and the fibre bulk is minimal. It often results in multiple bowel evacuations throughout the day and night. Diarrhoea has numerous causes, and some basic observations are needed to establish a possible **aetiology**.[2] These observations are for quantity and number of bowel evacuations that occur per day. This will give an estimate of the fluid loss the patient is experiencing, and fluid balance records (Chapter 6) may be necessary. Identification of any obvious abnormal content (e.g. the presence of blood or mucus) is important, and investigations may be required to establish if any infectious organisms are present.

### Blood and fat in the stools

**Blood** in the stools may be fresh and red, indicating a bleed somewhere within the lower bowel, i.e. the colon or rectum itself. Otherwise, it may be a darker red-brown or even black, called **melaena**. The presence of melaena suggests that the blood has undergone some degree of digestion and has mixed with the stools. In this case, it must come from higher in the digestive system, i.e. a bleed within the stomach or ileum. Digestive bleeds can arise from mucosal ulcerations, polyps or other growths that erode blood vessels, inflammatory bowel disease, ruptures of varicose veins within the oesophagus or rectum or abdominal trauma. Being a liquid itself, blood can provide the necessary water to prevent colonic contents from being converted to solid stool, and blood therefore can become thoroughly integrated with the faecal matter. Of course, heavy digestive bleeds are likely to be accompanied by other symptoms of blood loss, notably pallor, increased and weakened pulse rate, low blood pressure and even shock.

Blood is not always visible in the stool, and in very small quantities it may only be detected by chemical test. This is referred to as **occult blood**[3] and occurs when the bleed into the bowel is very small, sometimes microscopic. It is most likely to have arisen from a bleed higher in the bowel before the stools are fully formed, so the blood gets mixed into the stool. The cause needs to be investigated because it could be from the early stages of a bowel tumour.

Fat present in the stool is called **steatorrhoea**. It is caused by poor fat digestion and a low level of absorption (a fat *malabsorption*), so most of the fat in the diet passes through the digestive tract unchanged. Poor digestion of fat may be due to problems with bile production in the liver or lack of bile drainage through the biliary ducts, since bile is required for fat absorption. It may also be due to failure of the pancreas to produce **lipase**, the enzyme responsible for the breakdown of fat. Lipase may be obstructed from reaching the intestines if the pancreatic duct is obstructed. A high level of fat in the stools has the effect of softening the stool to a pulp and making it lighter in colour. Fat-laden faeces also float on water, making them difficult to flush.

### Mucus in diarrhoea

Mucus is the natural secretion of the mucous membrane and acts as a lubricant in the bowel for the passage of food and faecal content and dissolves some nutrients before it is itself reabsorbed. Mucus in diarrhoea is an indication of excessive inflammatory changes within the mucous membrane that result in overproduction of mucus. **Inflammatory bowel disease** (**IBD**) is a term that encompasses at least two bowel disorders, **ulcerative colitis** and **Crohn's disease** (inflammation of mainly the small bowel but sometimes seen in the colon). Both diseases are characterised by inflammation of the mucous lining of the bowel with blood and mucus present in the diarrhoea.

### Other causes of diarrhoea

Diarrhoea can also be caused by overstimulation of bowel movements by the parasympathetic nervous system, which promotes digestive activity. Normally, bowel contents are propelled along by waves of muscle contraction (called **peristalsis**) at a speed that allows water to be absorbed and therefore faeces to be well formed. If this rate of propulsion is sped up (known as increased bowel **motility**), the contents reach the rectum before all the water is absorbed, and liquid faeces results. This speeding up of peristalsis also causes the other symptom associated with diarrhoea, i.e. very frequent bowel evacuations and abdominal pain that occurs during peristalsis, known as **colic**. A patient suffering from a severe form of IBD e.g. 40 or more diarrhoea bowel evacuations in 24 hours, may often incur sleep loss and restriction of activities. Other symptoms include dehydration and electrolyte imbalance (Chapter 6), with distressing pain and tenderness around the anal sphincter. Infections such as ***Shigella*** – an organism that causes **dysentery** – or food-poisoning organisms such as ***Staphylococcus*** or ***Salmonella*** can have similar effects. Non-infectious causes include the overuse of **purgatives** (or **laxatives**; see page 186), **malabsorption syndromes**, certain foods in the diet that increase bowel propulsion, treatments such as radiation therapy involving the digestive tract and even anxiety ('**nervous diarrhoea**').

Drug-induced diarrhoea is an important cause of the problem, especially in elderly people because this group often requires more medication than younger people, and therefore they suffer more side effects (Ratnaike and Jones 1998). **Antibiotic drugs** can cause diarrhoea as a side effect because their activity against living organisms may also involve killing the natural colonic commensals (see Note 1), i.e. bacteria we need for normal bowel function, known as the *intestinal flora*. This becomes particularly important with oral antibiotics (see Chapter 15).

Diarrhoea normally settles down once the cause has been corrected and the bowel is empty. However, there are occasions when medical intervention is required and it can be relieved with drug therapy. **Loperamide hydrochloride** (Imodium) reduces the bowel motility (i.e. it reduces peristalsis) and therefore calms the bowel propulsive actions. Opium and morphine mixed with kaolin (an adsorbent clay) are sometimes used to help control persistent acute diarrhoea when other treatments fail. Opium (which contains mostly morphine) requires specialist supervision. **Co-phenotrope** is used to help manage faecal consistency as part of stoma management.

*Constipation*

Constipation is the failure to evacuate the bowel adequately, often totally, leading to an increasing collection of faeces in the colon. Possibly as much as 10% of the Western world population suffers from some degree of retained bowel content. Unlike diarrhoea, constipation provides few external clues to its presence, and a history of bowel activity over the previous few days is necessary to identify the problem. There may be some abdominal pain or discomfort. It is important to recognise the patient who is *at risk* of constipation: notably, the patient with reduced mobility, altered levels of consciousness, inadequate fluid or dietary fibre intake, taking medication which has constipation as a side effect, ignoring regular toiletry habits, suffering from a bowel disease or any combination of these. The elderly are most likely to suffer constipation as they may possess more risk factors than the young (Nazarko 2017).

Constipation is *preventable*, not just *curable*, by the identification of the patient's risk status, by the monitoring of bowel movements with intervention if necessary and by the correction of dehydration. In some patients, improvements in their mobility also contributes to the prevention of constipation, as well as the many other complications of immobility (see Chapter 14).

One bowel evacuation each 24 hours is the average, but considerable variation does occur, with some individuals claiming that bowel evacuations of only once or twice per week is normal for them. Others may pass faeces more than once a day. What *is* abnormal is a total absence of any bowel evacuation, and what *may* be abnormal is a significant change in a person's bowel habit, especially if this change is persistent. If once a day is normal for an individual, then three days without evacuation is a potential for constipation, and the reason should be identified if possible. Additional signs to aid the diagnosis of constipation include the presence or absence of **anorexia** (loss of appetite), abdominal pain (especially colic) and distension, nausea and confusion. The presence of confusion is particularly important in elderly people, when the brain becomes especially susceptible to the toxic effects of constipation (i.e. waste products in faeces that are normally excreted are reabsorbed into the blood). Confusion as a result of constipation must be identified as families can think that their elderly relative is becoming demented when all that is required is treatment for constipation. Diet is also important to note, since a lack of oral fluid or fibre in the diet is an important factor leading to constipation. Lack of exercise, especially complete immobility, reduces bowel movement, which, in turn, causes the contents to remain longer in the colon. During this longer stay in the colon, more water is absorbed from the contents, which then get drier and harder to propel and evacuate. Total obstruction of the bowel with hard, solid faeces can follow on from this in some extreme cases, made worse by any condition that narrows the bowel lumen (e.g. new growths). High dosage of some drugs that have a constipating side effect, including **morphine**, as in the management of some terminal disorders, may cause constipation, which then requires additional management. Assessing the risk of constipation requires keen observation of diet and fluid input, mobility, attempts at defecation, abdominal pain and mental alertness, and these are sometimes put together in risk assessment scales, which may be useful in some clinical areas (Duffy and Zernike 1997). Elderly people are always said to be at highest risk because of reduced mobility and a decline in the health status of the bowel with age (Bouras and Tangalos 2009).

Management of constipation may include the use of laxative drugs, enemas or suppositories. Laxative drugs fall into four main groups: (1) Bulk-forming agents, (2) Bowel stimulants, (3) Faecal softeners and lubricants and (4) Osmotic laxatives (Table 9.1).

*Table 9.1* Laxative medications

| Group | Drug | Notes |
|---|---|---|
| 1 | (1) Ispaghula husk (Isogel) <br> (2) Sterculia (with or without frangula) | Bulk-forming agents. These improve the fibre and water content within the bowel (bulk forming) and provide something for the muscle wall to work on. They increase the bowel transit times and soften the stool so it can be passed easier and with more comfort. |
| 2 | (1) Senna (Senokot; with or without ispaghula husk) <br> (2) Bisacodyl <br> (3) Co-danthramer <br> (4) Co-danthrusate <br> (5) Glycerol <br> (6) Sodium acid phosphate with sodium bicarbonate <br> (7) Sodium picosulfate | Bowel stimulants. They act on the bowel wall and its nerve supply, which then increases peristalsis to propel the stools forward. These must not be used regularly on a daily basis since the bowel can become dependent on them to function in the long term and will not function without them. So, they are best used as a one-off treatment. They may also cause bowel cramping pain. |
| 3 | (1) Arachis oil <br> (2) Docusate sodium <br> (3) Liquid paraffin | Faecal softeners. These line the bowel and prevent water absorption so the stools will not dry out. This softens the stools to make them easier to eliminate by lubricating the passage. They should be used only as a short-term, temporary measure since there is evidence that they may prevent the absorption of some important nutrients. |
| 4 | (1) Lactulose <br> (2) Macrogol 3350 (with or without KCl, NaCl and $NaHCO_3$)[4] <br> (3) Magnesium hydroxide <br> (4) Sodium acid phosphate with sodium phosphate | Osmotic laxatives. These attract more water into the bowel to soften and lubricate the stools. |

*Table 9.2* Red and amber flag warnings of deteriorating condition

꘏ **Red Flag = serious situation which needs urgent medical attention.**

꘏ **Amber Flag = Important to get a medical assessment as soon as possible.**

| Flag warning | Details |
|---|---|
| ꘏ **Red Flag** | **Vomiting and/or abdominal swelling with an ongoing history of constipation (possible bowel obstruction).** |
| | **Diarrhoea and/or vomiting associated with dehydration.** |
| | **Melaena stool or blood in the vomit, a symptom of gastrointestinal bleeding.** |
| ꘏ **Amber Flag** | **Possibility of serious bowel disease if there is blood in the stools, unusual alteration of bowel habit, weight loss, abdominal pain and a history of bowel disease.** |
| | **High frequency of diarrhoea, especially associated with blood.** |

(After Hill-Smith and Johnson 2021, with permission)

### Stomas

A **stoma** is an artificial surgical opening into the bowel to allow the excretion of bowel contents into a collection bag worn on the abdominal wall. This is done when normal defecation is not possible due to bowel disease. Stomas are made into the ileum (**ileostomy**) or colon (**colostomy**), depending on the nature of the problem. Stomas are sometimes used in the management of bowel cancers, ulcerative colitis, diverticular disease or after permanent **bowel resection** (removal of part of the bowel). A colostomy opening made into the *proximal* half of the colon, on the right side of abdomen, will initially result in a more liquid stool than an opening into the *distal* half of the colon, on the left side of the abdomen (Figure 9.3).

This is due to the water extraction function of the colon. The proximal half contains liquid stools from the small intestine, whereas the distal half contains stools that have travelled nearly the entire length of the bowel and are therefore much drier. Stoma bags require changing, which the patient can often do themselves after being taught about their stoma. The stoma should be observed for the normal red colour of healthy mucous membrane with no bleeding. Pallor or cyanosis (blue coloration) may indicate reduced blood supply which can cause complications and must be reported. The skin around the stoma is inspected for soreness, inflammation, infection and any broken areas. Some collection devices stick to the skin and this could cause skin problems. The bag contents are observed for the same constituents as faeces, i.e. for diarrhoea, blood, bile or mucus and also colour and quantity. Some drugs may affect the function of stomas or change the colour of the contents. These drugs include laxatives and antacids, both of which are best avoided for most stoma patients unless prescribed and monitored carefully. **Narrow-spectrum antibiotics** are preferable to **broad-spectrum antibiotics** when such drugs are necessary, since narrow spectrum means they will have less effect on the normal bowel commensals with less risk of diarrhoea. Diarrhoea in a stoma patient is very difficult to manage since it requires numerous and frequent bag changes which disrupts normal daily activities and could cause complications of the skin at the stoma site. Skin irritation and breakdown around the stoma should be avoided. Antibiotics can change the faeces to a grey-green colour and irritate the skin. Other colour changes caused by drugs include **iron** (black), **tetracycline** (red), **heparin** (pink or red),

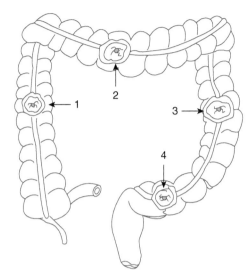

*Figure 9.3* Colonic stoma sites. (1) Within the ascending colon. (2) Within the transverse colon. (3) Within the descending colon. (4) Within the sigmoid colon.

**indometacin** (green) and **aspirin** (pink or red). Aspirin is acidic and may cause mucosal and skin irritation at the stoma site. It also contributes to anticoagulation of blood, i.e. helps to stop blood clotting and promotes bleeding, and is therefore best avoided. Stoma patients will be referred to the care of a stoma specialist nurse who should be consulted on all matters concerning these patients.

### The mechanism of vomiting

Vomiting (or **emesis**) can be regarded generally as a normal physiological response to an abnormal condition affecting either the digestive system or its neurological control. It is protective because it removes from the body any ingested substance that is unwanted and may be potentially dangerous. Stomach and sometimes bowel contents are driven the wrong way up the oesophagus back into the mouth. Accurate observations of the patient and the contents of the vomited matter, plus a history of events leading up to the episode of vomiting, can provide important clues about the nature of the cause.

The brainstem medullary **vomit reflex centres** coordinate what is a relatively complex process involving a range of different stimuli. Also, closely associated with the vomit centres are the **chemoreceptor trigger zones** (**CTZ**; Figure 9.4).

These are a bilateral pair of centres under the floor of the fourth ventricle, within an area called the **area postrema**, and this receives impulses from adverse chemical stimuli in the blood. Chemicals of this type include various drugs (e.g. cytotoxic agents) and other toxins from perhaps food or infectious organisms. Such stimulation of the CTZ causes stimulation of the vomit reflex centres, which then coordinates and controls vomiting.

The vomit centres themselves receive nerve impulses directly from:

1  The **cerebellum**, part of the brain that coordinates muscle activity and balance. The cerebellum obtains sensory information on balance (**vestibular** information) from the semicircular canals in both ears via the vestibular branch of the eighth cranial nerve,

the **vestibulocochlear nerve**. These canals register changes in balance and head movement as nerve impulses that are transmitted first to the **vestibular nuclei** in the medulla, then to the cerebellum (Figure 9.5).

Any disturbing movements or upsets in balance, as in motion sickness, can produce adverse nerve impulses that pass through the vestibular nuclei, the cerebellum and on to the vomit reflex centre, and vomiting occurs. A disease that causes dizziness and vomiting via this route is **Ménière's disease**, a chronic disorder of the inner ear where the amount of the fluid called endolymph becomes excessive. This causes sudden attacks of **vertigo** (dizziness), nausea and vomiting, progressive deafness and **tinnitus** (continuous internal sounds in the ear). The word *vertigo* is usually linked to dizziness caused by heights. The word actually means dizziness linked to a 'whirling round' sensation, i.e. the environment is spinning around. It is not especially related to heights, and people can suffer from vertigo at any height, often at ground level (see also Chapter 15, page 324).

2  The **gag reflex,** a feeling of retching when the back of the tongue or throat is touched with a finger or tongue depressor.
3  Bad sights or odours, fear, brain injury and high pressure within the skull (**raised intercranial pressure**) can all stimulate the vomit reflex centre via the **cerebral cortex**, our conscious part of the brain.
4  Stimuli from the digestive tract itself, especially from the stomach, such as over-distension from eating too much or inflammatory irritation from extra spicy or acidic food. Some drugs or excessive alcohol can cause vomiting. Such stimuli arrive at the vomit centre via the **vagus nerve** (the tenth cranial nerve; Figure 9.6).

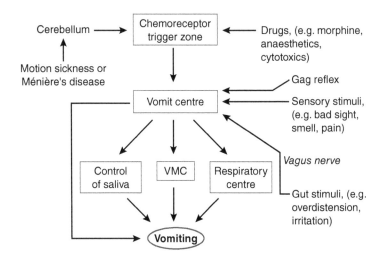

*Figure 9.4* Stimulation of the vomit centre is often via the chemoreceptor trigger zone, which itself is stimulated by motion or drugs. Sometimes the vomit centre is affected directly by bad sensory stimuli (e.g. an unpleasant smell or sight) or by vagal stimuli from the gut. The vomit centre output is via the vasomotor centre (VMC) – which influences the blood pressure during the event – and via the respiratory centre which regulates breathing throughout vomiting. The vomit centre also controls saliva production.

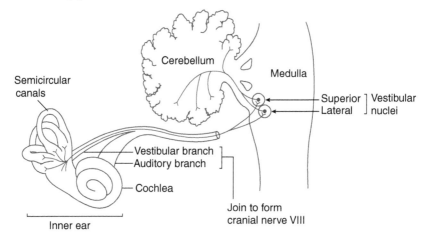

*Figure 9.5* Vestibular stimulation of the cerebellum. Impulses from the semicircular canals of the inner ear pass via the vestibulocochlear nerve (cranial nerve VIII) to the vestibular nuclei of the medulla and then on to the cerebellum.

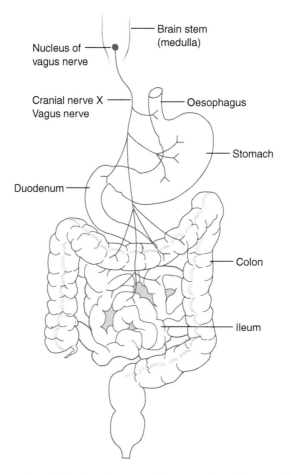

*Figure 9.6* Vagus innervation of the digestive tract. The vagus (cranial nerve X) is the primary visceral sensory nerve. Branches to the stomach increase gastric acidity and the parasympathetic component promotes digestion generally.

The result of initiating activation of the vomit reflex centre is to cause **nausea**, a feeling of sickness without actual vomiting, followed by retching and then finally vomiting. The person will inhale deeply as peristalsis is reversed. **Peristalsis** is the propulsive intermittent waves of smooth muscle contraction that pass along the bowel to push the contents forwards from the stomach towards the colon and rectum. Reversal of the direction of this contraction wave ensures that the digestive contents will be driven towards the mouth during vomiting. Just as with swallowing, the airway must be protected against inhalation during vomiting. Inhalation of vomit would involve not only obstructing the airway, but the gastric acid and digestive enzymes would severely damage the delicate lung tissues and death would occur. To prevent this, the glottis is closed by lowering the epiglottis and raising the hyoid bone and the larynx during the time that the stomach contents are passing through the larynx. The **glottis** is the narrowest part of the airway opening and is found inside the larynx. The **epiglottis** is a flap of cartilage above the glottis that acts as a lid for the glottis by folding downwards at the same time as the **larynx** (voice box) is raised. In this way, the glottis is closed and vomit cannot pass into the lungs. The **soft palate** is raised to close the **nasopharynx**, the passage from the nose to the throat, to prevent vomit entering the nose. If this is not achieved properly vomit may come from the nasal passages as well as the mouth. The top opening into the stomach (called the **cardiac sphincter** because it is close to the heart) is dilated, and the lower opening (the **pyloric sphincter**) is closed. The gastric muscles (smooth type) and abdominal muscles (skeletal type) both contract, forcing the stomach contents upwards towards the mouth. The **diaphragm** (skeletal muscle) also flattens to aid in this process, helping to increase the intra-abdominal pressure. The process leaves the person a little breathless because breathing has been temporarily suspended at a time when energy is being used, the generation of which requires oxygen (see Chapter 1). It is also accompanied and preceded by increases in both salivation and heart rate, the onset of pallor, sweating, pupillary dilation and distress, much of which is caused by **sympathetic nerve** stimulation of the sweat glands, the heart and the pupils.

Nausea, which is simply feeling sick, acts as an early warning that vomiting may happen. It is an unpleasant sensation that may persist alone or quickly result in the act of vomiting. It can occur under all the same pathological conditions that cause vomiting. However, nausea – and sometimes vomiting – can occur in non-pathological conditions, e.g. they are often features of early pregnancy, i.e. **morning sickness**. This is probably due to hormonal changes occurring at that time, especially the introduction of hormones from the placenta, such as **human chorionic gonadotrophic hormone** (**hCG**) – or hormones from the **corpus luteum** – and the gradual decline in these pregnancy-related hormones is associated with the relief of sickness (Coutts 1998). Approximately one-quarter of people coming into hospital for treatment of cancer feel nauseated on arrival, before the therapy has begun. It can happen before second or subsequent treatments where side-effects experienced from the first treatment are anticipated. This is termed **anticipatory nausea and vomiting** (**ANV**) and can sometimes be relieved or prevented in susceptible patients (Aapro *et al.* 2005).

## Observations regarding vomiting

Important observations on vomiting include the volume that is vomited, what the contents are and when vomiting occurs. The quantity is important because the stomach volume is limited and it may not have been full originally. Vomiting should stop once the stomach has been emptied if this was the purpose of the episode. When this happens, it suggests that a cause lies within the stomach itself or its contents. But if vomiting persists beyond this point, it is likely to become unproductive once the stomach is empty, or produce only small volumes of gastrointestinal fluid. **Retching** is an attempt to vomit but with no gastric or duodenal content produced. At this point, it is possible to say that the process of vomiting is not solely to empty the stomach but is caused by factors outside the digestive system continuously stimulating the vomit reflex centre in the brain. This is affecting what is quite possibly a normal stomach (Scorza *et al.* 2007).

It should be established if the vomiting is associated with:

1  Pain, e.g. abdominal pain or migraine (see Chapter 12)
2  The intake of food or specific foods, drugs or alcohol
3  Exposure to motion, as in spinning round, sea or travel sickness
4  Exposure to obnoxious substances or emotionally disturbing experiences, e.g. the sight of blood, someone else vomiting or a foul smell
5  Persistent coughing, since coughing can trigger the vomit reflex. This is mostly seen in children in whom prolonged coughing may stimulate the vomit reflex centre. The cough and vomit centres both occur close together in the **medulla**, part of the brainstem.

How long the vomiting has persisted is vital to confirm because prolonged and persistent vomiting results in fluid and electrolyte losses (Chapter 6), leading to imbalance and various degrees of malnutrition (Chapter 7). This is especially the case for children, especially small children, who will become ill rapidly if the fluid and electrolyte imbalance are not corrected quickly and vomiting is not brought under control. History of the event is taken to identify if it is food (digested or not) or medicines that may be the cause, and observations are made on the vomit to check for blood or bile.

### Food in vomit

Food, when vomited, indicates that the time span between eating and vomiting is relatively short, i.e. within four hours of each other, and generally the shorter the time span, the less digestion has occurred. In this case, either the stomach cannot tolerate the food, or the food itself causes a vomit reaction. The former happens as a result of infection or inflammation of the stomach (**gastritis**) or if the food was accompanied by large quantities of alcohol (a gastric irritant). It may be due to the inability of the stomach to pass food into the bowel because of an obstruction, e.g. **pyloric stenosis**, as sometimes seen in young children. Pyloric stenosis is a restriction of gastric contents passage through a tight or closed pyloric sphincter. Pyloric stenosis can be associated with **projectile vomiting**,[5] when peristalsis attempts to force food through the obstruction but actually ejects it upwards under pressure. Bowel obstructions are also caused by new growths (**neoplasms**) or by compression of the bowel by abdominal muscle contraction, as seen in **strangulated hernias**. Both conditions are often found in the older adult. Some degree of obstruction can occur in distortions of the bowel such as **intussusception** (telescoping of the bowel) or **volvulus** (twisting of the bowel), both of these being conditions found usually in younger children (Figure 9.7).

Where the food itself causes the vomiting, it may occur as a result of infections or toxins in the food (**food poisoning**). A number of different organisms cause food poisoning of varying degrees, some more dangerous than others (e.g. *Clostridium botulinum*, the cause of **botulism**). This is a rare but fatal form of food poisoning often contracted after eating

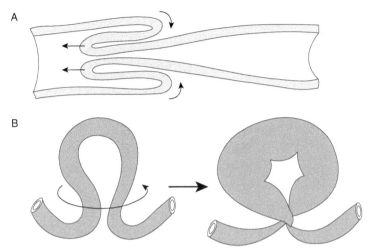

*Figure 9.7* Bowel distortions that occur mostly in children. (A) Intussuception, a telescoping of the bowel. (B) Volvulus, a twisting of a bowel loop causing obstruction of both the bowel and its blood supply.

contaminated canned meat products. Such contamination results from failure of the can-sealing process or ruptured seals on cans during transport. All the seals at the joints in the metal of canned meats should be inspected before purchase and any breaks in these joints reported to shop staff. A less dangerous yet very unpleasant food poisoning is caused by **Staphylococcus aureus**, usually implanted on food by those preparing the food. This gives 24 hours of vomiting and diarrhoea, leaving the person feeling debilitated and very unwell.

*Blood in vomit*

Blood appears in different forms in vomit, depending on where the bleeding is occurring and how much digestion the blood has been subjected to. Fresh bright-red blood in the vomit means it has not been in the stomach for very long – perhaps only minutes – and may indicate a possible gastric bleed, known as a **haematemesis**, from an ulceration or neoplasm. However, swallowed blood, often from an **epistaxis** (nosebleed), can be vomited back since the acidic stomach cannot tolerate large quantities of blood. This is a good reason for holding the head forward when treating nosebleeds, to prevent posterior bleeding which would otherwise be swallowed and cause vomiting. Vomiting blood can continue for some time, i.e. until the patient collapses from shock, and requires urgent intervention. Sudden massive quantities of vomited blood are sometimes seen in ruptured **oesophageal varices**, i.e. varicose veins of the lower oesophagus caused by congestion of hepatic portal venous blood as a result of obstructive liver diseases (Figure 9.8). An important cause of liver obstruction is **cirrhosis**, a gradual loss of liver cells that are replaced by scar tissue which partially obstructs blood passage through the liver and is usually accompanied by **hepatic failure**.

   Blood that has been in the stomach for an hour or more before being vomited has been subject to changes caused by digestion and the hydrochloric acid conditions. In this case, it is described as *coffee grounds*, a reference to its appearance. This type of bleeding indicates low-grade blood loss which the stomach can tolerate for a while, possibly from an ulceration.

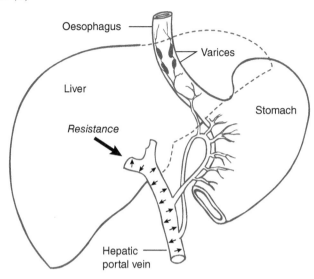

*Figure 9.8* Oesophageal varices caused by portal hypertension. High blood pressure inside the portal vein (shown by small arrows inside the vessel) is due to some resistance to blood flow within the liver, often the result of liver disease. Backflow of blood to the lower end of the oesophagus causes venous dilatations, which can rupture and bleed severely.

### Bile in vomit

Bile and other gastrointestinal fluids do occasionally appear in vomit, especially if persistent vomiting has emptied the stomach and has forced duodenal or even ileal contents up into the mouth. About 500 ml of bile comes from the liver each day into the duodenum, and it gives a strong unpleasant alkaline burning taste in the mouth and throat when vomited. The digestive system as a whole produces 7 litres of fluid secreted into the bowel lumen over 24 hours, which consists of saliva (1.5 litres), gastric juice (2 litres), pancreatic juice (1.5 litres), bile (0.5 litres) and intestinal juice (1.5 litres), which contains digestive enzymes, mucus, cells and other products. Normally, most of this is reabsorbed (6.5 litres from the small intestine and 350 ml from the colon per day), but it can be vomited as a watery fluid, usually seen after heavy or persistent bouts of vomiting.

### Faeces in vomit

Very rarely, it is possible to vomit faeces. This is a very serious complication and it requires urgent medical intervention. It happens only in the event of a severe persistent bowel obstruction, when any form of bowel evacuation has stopped for a significant length of time. The actual time involved may vary from one patient to another. Under these conditions, it becomes necessary to empty the bowel as much as possible while supporting fluid and electrolyte balance (Chapter 6) before urgent surgery to relieve the obstruction.

## Drugs affecting vomiting

Vomiting can be caused or prevented by various drugs. They can induce vomiting by irritating the mucosal lining directly or by stimulating the CTZ once in circulation (see

Chapter 15). **Emetics** are drugs that specifically cause vomiting.[6] However, drugs are no longer used for this purpose and only induce vomiting as a side effect, such as **apomorphine**, which is derived from **morphine** and used in the treatment of Parkinson's disorder. It stimulates receptors on the chemoreceptor trigger zone (Figure 9.4). Some of the other drugs that have emesis as a side effect are **cytotoxic agents** – which are used in cancer therapy – and **opiate analgesics** that act on the brainstem, such as morphine.

Drugs with the opposite effect are the **anti-emetics**, which prevent vomiting in several ways. **Anticholinergics** (e.g. **hyoscine hydrobromide**) block stimuli from the vestibular system and are therefore useful in the treatment of motion sickness.[7] The side effects are sometimes troublesome, notably a dry mouth, blurred vision and drowsiness. Drowsiness is dangerous if driving, and a warning against combining these drugs with driving should be on the pack. The **antihistamines** are also used in motion sickness therapy; they are less effective than hyoscine but produce less side effects. They include **cyclizine** and **promethazine hydrochloride**. These drugs block receptor sites for **histamine** (the $H_1$ receptor), but it is not clear how they prevent sickness. **Cannabinoids**, such as the drug **nabilone**, act on the chemoreceptor trigger zone and are useful in treating sickness during cytotoxic therapy, but they do cause drowsiness, dizziness and a dry mouth. The **dopamine antagonists** work by blocking the dopamine receptors (type $D_2$ **receptors**) in the **area postrema** (see page 188), reducing CTZ stimulation of the vomit reflex centre. They are therefore less useful in treating motion sickness. Included are the non-phenothiazines **metoclopramide hydrochloride** and **domperidone**. Metoclopramide can also act on the stomach, promoting its emptying via the normal pyloric route. The side effects are sedation, **hypotension** (low blood pressure, Chapter 3) and some problems of movement involving the **extrapyramidal tract system** of the brain (see Chapter 14).

Key points

- Diarrhoea and vomiting are indications that changes have occurred in the patterns of physiology within the digestive system.
- Fibre has an important role to play in human digestion, being vital for correct bowel function and protection against bowel disease.
- Blood in the stools may indicate a bleed somewhere within the colon if fresh or a bleed within the stomach or ileum if darker.
- Mucus in diarrhoea is an indication of excessive inflammatory changes within the mucous membrane that result in overproduction of mucus, as in inflammatory bowel disease.
- Diarrhoea can be caused by excessive bowel movements that can occur in bowel infections or food poisoning, the overuse of laxatives, malabsorption syndromes or treatments such as radiation therapy.
- Signs of constipation include anorexia, abdominal pain, distension, nausea and confusion.
- Lack of fluid or fibre in the diet and lack of exercise are important factors leading to constipation.
- A stoma is an artificial opening in the bowel. Stomas open into the ileum (ileostomy) or colon (colostomy).
- In the event of vomiting, checks are important to assess how long it has persisted, whether the vomiting is associated with any pain, food intake, drugs, alcohol, exposure to motion, obnoxious substances or an emotionally disturbing experience or whether there is any persistent coughing.

- Observe and report any food, blood, bile or faeces in vomit.
- Prolonged vomiting results in fluid and electrolyte losses, especially in young children, who will become ill rapidly if the fluid and electrolyte imbalance is not corrected quickly and vomiting is not brought under control.
- Emetics are drugs that cause nausea and vomiting although their use as such is now discouraged. Anti-emetic drugs prevent vomiting.

## Notes

1  Commensals are harmless bacterial organisms which naturally inhabit one part of the body. They are there to produce valuable substances which can be absorbed into the blood. However, if the commensals get into another part of the body, e.g. through a wound, they can become *pathogenic* (e.g. causing infection).
2  Aetiology is the cause of a condition, and involves taking a history of the event, observations and medical investigations.
3  In medicine, occult means not easily seen – or hidden.
4  KCl = Potassium chloride; NaCl = Sodium chloride; $NaHCO_3$ = Sodium bicarbonate.
5  Projectile vomiting means that the stomach contents are forcefully ejected for some distance.
6  Emetics such as ipecacuanha are no longer recommended for use in the management of oral drug overdose.
7  Try checking the ingredients of several brands of travel sickness tablets to see which ones contain hyoscine.

## References

Aapro M.S., Molassiotis A. and Olver I. (2005) Anticipatory nausea and vomiting. *Supportive Care in Cancer (Official Journal of the Multinational Association of Supportive Care in Cancer)*, *13*(2): 117–121.

Bouras E.P. and Tangalos E.G. (2009) Chronic constipation in the elderly. *Gastroenterology Clinics of North America*, *38*(3): 463–480.

Coutts A. (1998) The 'minor' problems of pregnancy: A review. *Professional Care of Mother and Child*, *8*(4): 95–97.

Duffy J. and Zernike W. (1997) Development of a constipation risk assessment scale. *International Journal of Nursing Practice*, *3*(4): 260–263.

Hill-Smith I. and Johnson G. (2021) *Little Book of Red Flags*. National Minor Illness Centre, Bedfordshire.

Nazarko L. (2017) Constipation: A guide to assessment and treatment. *Independent Nurse*, 5 June: 26–29.

Ratnaike R.N. and Jones T.E. (1998) Mechanisms of drug-induced diarrhoea in the elderly. *Drugs-Aging*, *13*(3): 245–253.

Scorza K., Williams A., Phillips J.D. and Shaw J. (2007) Evaluation of nausea and vomiting. *American Family Physician*, *76*(1): 76–84.

# 10 Skin

- Introduction
- Structure and function of skin
- Skin observations
- Skin trauma
- Important skin diseases
- Key points
- Notes
- References

## Introduction

The skin, also known as the **integumentary system**, is the largest organ of the body. It accounts for 16% of the body weight, it is between 1.5 and 2 square meters in area and it mostly averages between 2 and 3 mm thick. In some specific places, such as the soles of the feet, it is often thicker. The skin has its own unique structure and functions.

## Structure and function of skin

There are two major divisions of the skin, the outer **epidermis** and the deeper **dermis**.

### Epidermis

The epidermis has five layers of cells, which are the same cells that started life in the deepest layers and are migrating slowly towards the surface. The five layers, starting with the deepest layer, are (Figure 10.1):

1 **Stratum germinativum**, which is the deepest of the five epidermal layers and rests directly on top of the dermis. The basal cells, next to the dermis, are constantly dividing by **mitosis** (i.e. standard cell division). From here, cells migrate upwards away from the dermis. As they do so, they enter the next layer
2 **Stratum spinosum** ('spiny layer'), where the cells from the stratum germinativum develop a degree of shrinking of the cytoplasm, but many can still continue to divide

DOI: 10.4324/9781003389118-10

3 **Stratum granulosum** ('grainy layer') is where cells migrated from the stratum spinosum show no further cell division. Instead, they produce considerable amounts of a fibrous protein called **keratin** (a process called **keratinisation**). The cell membranes get thicker and the passage of substances through these membranes becomes difficult and declines. Eventually, the nucleus and organelles of the cells disintegrate and the cells die, their cytoplasm filled with keratin. They are called **keratinocytes**. Towards the upper limits of the layer, the cells begin to flatten out and pack closer together as they dehydrate. This is now effectively a layer of dry keratin

4 **Stratum lucidum** is a glassy layer of densely packed keratinised cells derived from the stratum granulosum and only found in thick skin areas (e.g. the sole of the foot)

5 **Stratum corneum** is the outermost layer on the very surface of the skin. These keratinised dead cells, derived either directly from stratum granulosum or via stratum lucidum, form a protective layer for the deeper parts of the skin. Flakes of dead keratin are being shed from the surface all the time, i.e. about 30,000 flakes shed per minute. In the hair, this is referred to as **dandruff**. This outer layer is therefore dead tissue, which means when you look at someone, you are actually looking at a layer of *dead tissue*!

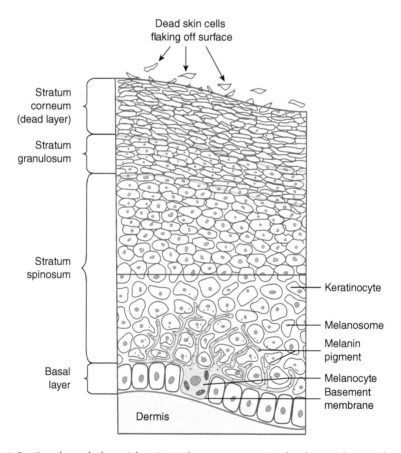

*Figure 10.1* Section through the epidermis. Melanocytes occur in the deepest layers. They produce a pigment called melanin that is packaged in melanosomes. These melanosomes infiltrate into the keratinocytes and help to protect them from sunlight during the early stages of their migration towards the surface. During this migration, the cells flatten and die and fill with keratin.

The epidermis can be thought of as a cell 'escalator', with newly evolved cells in the stratum germinativum moving up through the layers and becoming flat, dead, keratinised cell remnants as they arrive in the stratum corneum. The epidermis is constantly being replaced with new cells from below. It takes anything from 15 to 30 days for cells to move through the epidermis, and they remain as dead cells on the surface for a further two weeks before being shed into the environment.

Other important cells exist at specific layers of the epidermis, particularly **melanocytes** in the stratum germinativum and **Langerhans cells** in the stratum spinosum.

Melanocytes (Figure 10.1) are pigmentation cells producing the dark brown pigment **melanin** from the dietary amino acid **tyrosine**. Melanin is packed inside vesicles called **melanosomes** which are transported into keratinocytes. This protects vital cell structures (e.g. the nucleus) against harmful exposure to ultraviolet (UV) light in sunlight as the keratinocytes migrate towards the surface. Eventually, the melanosomes are destroyed as the keratinocyte nucleus degrades and the cells die. The differences between light and dark skin are that dark-skinned people have larger melanosomes and the melanin levels are higher and persist for longer than in light-skinned people. The concentration of melanocytes in the epidermis is about 1,000 per mm$^2$, but this doubles in more heavily pigmented areas of the body such as the nipples, labia and scrotum.

Langerhans cells are immune cells that fight microorganisms from the environment that have penetrated into the epidermis. The skin surface has its own ecosystem of microorganisms consisting of bacteria, yeasts and viral agents. Each square inch (6.5 cm$^2$) has approximately 50 million bacteria, a figure that rises to 500 million in areas of skin subjected to rich oily secretions. On the surface, they are harmless to the skin because they are incapable of causing harm to the dead keratinised outer layer. But should they penetrate deeper they may cause infection. Langerhans cells are an important part of our protection against these deeper organisms.

Epidermal growth, i.e. the growth of new cells in the stratum germinativum, is promoted by a protein hormone called **epidermal growth factor** (**EGF**). EGF is found in some glands of the body, e.g. submandibular and parotid salivary glands, and in most body secretions, e.g. blood plasma, tears, saliva, urine and breast milk. It has a range of functions throughout the body, notably within the mucosal lining of the digestive system. In the skin it promotes growth and cellular differentiation by increasing cell division and keratin production, and is an important factor in wound healing (see page 205).

*Dermis*

The layer beneath the epidermis is the **dermis**. This is subdivided into two main layers (Figure 10.2).

The *outermost* layer is called the **stratum papillare** made from **areolar** connective tissue. Areolar connective tissue is common in the body, not just the skin, acting as a loose packing material between other structures. It contains random collagen fibres, elastic fibres (called **elastin)** and reticular fibres, with small blood vessels, nerve endings and some open spaces. The junction between the epidermis and the dermis is folded into **dermal papillae**, i.e. extensions of the stratum papillare that push upwards into the basal area of the stratum germinativum (Figure 10.2). Dermal papillae contain blood vessels that mark the closest extension of the blood supply to the skin surface.[1] Dilation and constriction of the blood vessels within the papillae, being so close to the skin surface, affect heat loss (dilation) or heat conservation (constriction), part of the body's temperature control

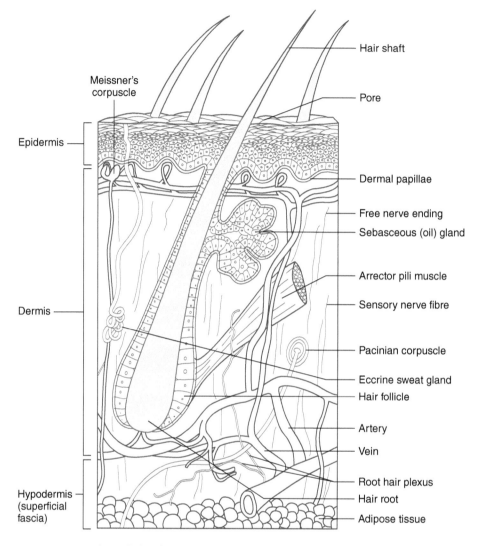

*Figure 10.2* Section through the skin showing the epidermis, dermis and hypodermis. Sweat glands, hair roots and sebaceous glands are shown originating in the dermis. Nerve endings are listed and described in Table 10.1.

mechanism (see Chapter 1). Some dermal papillae contain **Meissner's corpuscles**, sensory nerve endings for the purpose of touch.

The *innermost* of the two layers, the **stratum reticulare**, is made from **collagen** fibres in bundles (for strength) and elastin. Cells embedded within this matrix are **fibroblasts**, i.e. cells for the production of protein fibres, **macrophages** i.e. specialised cells of the immune system and small patches of **adipocytes** (fat cells).

There are some additional embedded structures within the dermis (Figure 10.2). These are:

1 **Sweat glands**, which produce sweat from blood plasma. Sweat is released on to the skin surface and contains water, salts and some urea (see Chapter 8). Sweating

occurs in response to high body temperature, as part of the temperature control mechanism (see Chapter 1) or in response to overactivity of the sympathetic nervous system

2  **Hair follicles** containing hairs, which grow and protect various body areas and provide some, albeit minimal, insulation against heat loss. They are made from a hard keratin outer layer and a soft keratin inner core. There is an average of 5 million hairs, 98% of which are not on the head! Hair shafts, which are part of the follicle, extend from the dermis to the epidermis. They have **sebaceous glands** attached which secrete **sebum**, an oily fluid that lubricates the hair shaft

3  **Nails**, which are made from the same dead keratin protein as epidermal keratino-cytes but are more densely packed for strength. Nails grow slowly from a nail bed and they provide protective and functional appendages at the ends of the fingers and toes

4  Nerve endings, making the skin a vital sensory organ (Table 10.1).

Beneath the dermis is the **subcutaneous** tissue, also called the **hypodermis**, which is, strictly speaking, not part of the integument. It is made from some **areolar** connective tissue with a variable amount of **adipose** (fat) tissue made from **adipocytes**. The dense adipose areas act as an energy store, they provide insulation against heat loss and they have a protective role against skin impacts, i.e. as a shock absorber. Within the outermost section of the hypodermis, immediately below the dermis, there is a network of larger arteries and veins, the **cutaneous plexus**, that supplies blood to the dermis above.

*Table 10.1* Sensory nerve endings in the dermis and their functions

| Nerve ending in dermis | Notes |
|---|---|
| Free dendritic nerve endings | Sensitive to pain, heat, cold and pressure. Found in most body tissues, including the dermis and lower layers of epidermis. |
| Root hair plexus | Sensitive to hair movement. Found around hair roots. |
| Merkel cells with tactile discs | Sensitive to touch and light pressure. Found across the dermis-epidermis border. |
| Meissner's corpuscles | Sensitive to touch, light pressure and low-frequency vibrations. Found in the dermal papillae, especially over sensitive areas such as the nipples, external genitalia, fingertips and eyelids. |
| Krause's end bulb | A modified Meissner's corpuscle. Found in mucous membrane and some skin areas. |
| Pacinian corpuscles | Sensitive to deep pressure, stretching and high-frequency vibrations. Found in the subcutaneous tissues of the skin, especially on the fingers, feet, external genitalia and nipples and also some deeper tissues. |
| Ruffini's corpuscles | Sensitive to deep pressure and stretching. Found in the dermis and subcutaneous tissues and joint capsules. |

*The functions of skin*

The skin functions are as follows:

1  It is a barrier against micro-organisms, a major part of our **non-specific** immune system; non-specific because it does not distinguish between one type of organism or another. Almost all organisms from the environment, i.e. bacteria, viruses and fungi, are incapable of penetrating intact skin. If the skin breaks down, that barrier is lost and infection can enter the body, both locally and systemically. Maintenance of this surface barrier involves the secretion of sebum from sebaceous glands attached to hair follicles
2  The skin is the body's vital touch sense organ. The rich supply of nerve endings in the skin provides a wide range of sensations, including touch, pain, temperature and pressure (Figure 10.2 and Table 10.1). Some areas of skin, e.g. the fingertips, are more sensitive than others as part of their specific sensory functions
3  The skin is an important excretory organ, allowing the controlled loss of salts, water and organic wastes (e.g. **urea**) through sweat glands. Water and salt excretion are involved in fluid balance (see Chapter 6)
4  Skin is part of the temperature regulation mechanism since heat is lost through the skin (see *heat loss mechanism*, Chapter 1). The deeper layers of the skin often have fat present, which provides some insulation against the cold
5  Skin stores some nutrients, e.g. lipids in fat cells
6  It carries out synthesis of vitamin $D_3$ (**cholecalciferol**), which is produced when a naturally occurring substance in the skin, called **7-dehydrocholesterol**, which is derived from cholesterol, is exposed to **ultraviolet B light** (**UVB**). Cholecalciferol is also obtained from the diet. Further processing of cholecalciferol in the liver results in the active form of vitamin D (i.e. **25-hydroxycholecalciferol**; see Chapter 4, Figure 4.4)
7  Skin provides physical protection to underlying structures. The skin has a remarkable shielding effect against injury from the outside that stops damage occurring to delicate structures beneath the skin
8  It is also a water resistance barrier (but *not* waterproof). This water resistance prevents water from washing away important protective skin oils when the surface gets wet. However, prolonged immersion in fresh water, particularly warm fresh water, will cause the skin to become waterlogged as this water resistance function gradually fails and water moves in. This causes the epidermal cells to swell. Alternatively, because the sea is salty, prolonged seawater immersion has the effect of drawing water out of the skin, which then dehydrates the skin.

## Skin observations

Because the skin is the outermost organ of the body it is easy to observe acute and chronic abnormal changes taking place within the skin itself or within body systems. Skin observations involve colour, lesions, rashes, trauma and abnormal temperatures.

*Colour and temperatures*

*Permanent* skin colour varies normally between people of different races, but there are some *temporary* changes in skin colour that indicate deviation from the normal as a result of pathological processes occurring in the body:

- **Cyanosis** is a change of colour to grey at first, then to a blue-purple colour, as a result of a lack of oxygen in the blood (Chapter 5, page 111). Cyanosis varies from mild to severe. There is also a distinction between **peripheral cyanosis**, i.e. cyanosis of the fingers, toes, feet and hands and **central cyanosis**, i.e. the trunk and face. Mild cyanosis occurs in the periphery first, but if the situation gets worse the cyanosis becomes more central. Severe central cyanosis is the worst-case scenario and requires urgent treatment, including additional controlled oxygen delivery (Chapter 5). Causes of cyanosis include respiratory diseases of various kinds, e.g. pneumonia, obstructive airways disease and asthma and heart failure. Local cyanosis, i.e. affecting one part of the body only, will occur if there is any circulatory obstruction to that area, e.g. some form of external compression on a limb. Relief of this compression and restoration of circulation will restore normal skin colour. Cyanosis is sometimes linked to another sign, i.e. finger and toe **clubbing**. This is where the digits expand to form bulb-like swollen ends. The cause is not fully understood, although dilated blood vessels at the ends of the fingers, growth factors and other natural biochemical agents have been suggested (Anoop and George 2011).
- **Jaundice** is a yellow colour to skin usually widespread across the body. It is due to deposits in the skin of a substance called **bilirubin** (Chapter 8, Figure 8.13). Bilirubin results from the breakdown of **haemoglobin** derived from red blood cells (**RBCs**, also called **erythrocytes**; Chapter 8, Figure 8.13). Deposits of excess bilirubin in the skin and other tissues result from abnormally high bilirubin production, more than can be excreted through the kidneys. The cause can be attributed to any of three possible pathological processes (see page 173):

  1 **Pre-hepatic jaundice**, where rapid red cell breakdown takes place in the general circulation, releasing excessive amounts of haemoglobin. This serious condition is called **haemolytic anaemia** and can be part of some blood disorders and also as a consequence of mismatched blood transfusion (see Chapter 4)
  2 **Hepatic jaundice**, where excessive bilirubin builds up as a result of liver disease, as in **liver failure**, liver **cirrhosis** or **hepatitis**
  3 **Post-hepatic jaundice**, where jaundice is caused by failure of bilirubin to drain into the digestive system, and therefore bilirubin is reduced in the faeces. This results from an obstruction of the bile duct, possibly from a biliary stone or tumour. Since there are a significant number of different causes of jaundice, the symptom needs investigations involving blood tests (see Chapter 4) and hepatic function (Lock-In 2006)

- **Redness** of the skin (called **erythema**) is due to increased blood supply to the skin surface. This occurs when the blood vessels in the dermis, particularly the dermal papillae, dilate (called **vasodilation**), bringing more blood closer to the surface. The extra blood also delivers more heat, and therefore the area feels extra warm. These effects, plus swelling of the area, are classic signs of **inflammation** (see *wound infections*, page 207). Sterile inflammation, i.e. not caused by a microorganism, can be the result of a blow or scratch to the skin surface. It can also occur if the skin is subjected to an external heat source, such as a fire, since heat causes blood vessels to dilate. Skin redness from vasodilation occurs often from psychological causes, e.g. embarrassment, stress, anger or from excessive physical activity. The skin sheds the heat generated during these scenarios (see Chapter 1). Pathological causes of redness include infections of the skin (e.g. wound infections; see page 206) or from the immune response to an external toxin, as in allergies, e.g. a reaction to an insect sting

- **Pallor** is the opposite of redness, i.e. it is caused by reduced blood supply to the skin. The skin's blood vessels constrict (called **peripheral vasoconstriction**) or the blood pressure falls, as in **shock**, and less blood gets to the skin (see Chapter 1). Pallor may precede **cyanosis** (see page 111) if the skin's blood supply continues to be constricted. Severe pallor and cold skin indicate a very low blood pressure and poor cardiac output. In shock, efforts must be made to restore blood pressure to a point where adequate blood supply to the vital organs is maintained. Restoring normal skin colour and temperature after pallor is an indication that blood pressure has been restored sufficiently to supply the skin and therefore the vital organs. Low blood pressures will cause a lack of blood to the brain with reduced levels of consciousness (see Chapter 11), and this becomes a priority for treatment. **Fainting** is an example of sudden loss of blood pressure resulting in pallor and loss of consciousness (see Chapter 11, page 242). Pallor will also occur with low skin temperatures since exposure to cold constricts the local peripheral blood vessels. Under these circumstances the reduced blood supply, usually to the extremities, may be accompanied by some degree of cyanosis.

### Lesions and rashes

Lesions of the skin are usually small, discrete, localised areas of change in the skin structure. Skin lesions come in many forms, identified in Table 10.2. Many are minor, asymptomatic and harmless, while some may progress to become a serious problem.

*Table 10.2* Skin lesions

| Skin lesion | Description |
| --- | --- |
| Bulla (blister) | Similar to vesicle (see below) but larger (greater than 5 mm diameter) and fluid filled. |
| Cyst | An encapsulated cavity lined with epithelium within the skin, containing semi-solid material or fluid. |
| Macule | Localised patch of different skin colour, either darker or lighter than the surrounding skin. Some are normal (e.g. freckles), others indicate skin changes. Usually less than 1 cm in diameter. |
| Mole (nevus) | A lesion formed from melanocytes accumulating at the basal epidermal layer forming a macule. Migration into the dermis causes the area to become nodular and palpable (Table 10.3). |
| Nodule | Larger than a papule (i.e. larger than 5 mm in diameter), they can be solid or a fluid-filled raised lump within any skin layer. |
| Papule | Small, solid raised lump less than 5 mm in diameter (e.g. a wart). |
| Plaque | A palpable, slightly raised, flat-topped patch of skin, more than 1 cm in diameter but usually below 5 mm in height. |
| Pustule | A visible collection of pus within a blister formation on the skin surface. |
| Scale | A thick layer of keratin loosely attached to the skin that can detach easily. |
| Ulcer | An open cavity or erosion (i.e. a circumscribed area of skin loss) extending into the dermis or deeper. |
| Vesicle | A small blister (less than 5 mm in diameter) filled with clear fluid occurring within or below the skin. |
| Wheal | A patch of dermal erythaema, slightly raised with oedema, seen in urticaria (page 214). |

**Rashes** (or eruptions) are usually more widespread than lesions and are often composed of many individual lesions, such as pustules accompanied by red areas known as **wheals** (Table 10.2). They are often part of the symptoms of a systemic infectious disease (e.g. chickenpox) or may be the only initial symptom of an insect or plant sting (e.g. nettle rash). They are likely to itch due to local **histamine** release, and scratching may cause the skin to break down, i.e. causing local skin trauma, which complicates the problem and may introduce infection. It is better to use a local antihistamine cream.

### Skin trauma

#### Wounds and bruises

Skin is tough, but being exposed directly to the environment means it is subject to many types of injury. Trauma can create breaches in the protective outer skin barrier which could easily lead to infection if care is not taken to prevent this.

**Wounds** may be closed or open. A closed wound is called a **bruise**. There is no actual breach in the skin but the effect of the trauma is to damage dermal blood vessels, causing bleeding into the dermis and below. In a bruise (also known as **contusion** or **ecchymosis**), the blood spreads out gradually from the traumatised area as a sheet. Blood can spread beyond the limits of the injury and usually drains to lower parts in response to gravity. Although the blood is not lost from the body, it is *lost from circulation*, and extensive bruising can lead to shock if there is enough blood loss into the dermis and subdermal tissues. The elderly are especially prone to bruising due to fragile capillaries, and extensive bruising in the elderly, e.g. following a fall down stairs, can cause shock. Bleeding often continues after the initial trauma, and this blood can be trapped in the tissues as a **haematoma**, which may solidify into a blood clot. A haematoma may form a palpable lump under the skin and takes longer to disperse than a bruise.

Resolving a bruise can take from 5 to 20 days or more, depending on the extent of the bruise and the presence of any haematoma. The red cells in the tissues break down to release haemoglobin which undergoes the same changes seen in jaundice (Figure 8.13 and see page 172). The difference is that these changes are happening in the dermis and surrounding tissues, and the colour changes (**biliverdin** green to bilirubin yellow, Figure 8.13) can be seen within the skin. The final stage of the bruise, i.e. the disappearance of the yellow colour, occurs as the bilirubin is removed from the skin for transport to the liver.

Open wounds can be from superficial to deep, causing many kinds of tissue damage. The type of wound depends on the cause – e.g. the instrument actually entering the skin – and the energy involved. Sharp instruments, e.g. a needle or a knife point in a stabbing injury, cause **puncture wounds** which are limited in width and amount of bruising. They can go deep causing trauma to underlying structures, including internal bleeding. Knife cuts create **lacerations** and **abrasions** occur when skin is scraped or eroded, e.g. when dragging along the ground. With blunt instruments, such as a hammer, the depth of injury depends on the force applied. They can cause damage to bones, organs, blood vessels and nerves when sufficient force is used. Flesh may be lost (**avulsion**) and an internal structure, e.g. a bone fragment, may be lost through the wound (**evulsion**). Low energy impacts cause less depth of wound but widespread bruising. Bleeding from open wounds depends on the blood vessels damaged. All wounds will bleed from capillary damage. Serious bleeding occurs when a vein or artery is damaged. Arterial bleeding is indicated by the pressure and will spurt out or flow very quickly. This requires urgent digital pressure on the wound to stop the flow, raising the injured limb if possible and urgent transportation to hospital. Extensive wounds may cause enough tissue disruption and bleeding such that tissue may even die, causing areas of necrotic tissue. **Necrosis** (tissue death) usually happens some days after the trauma; the skin area turns darker and eventually becomes black (sometimes called **gangrene**). Skin in this condition is non-viable tissue and must be surgically removed before the wound will heal.

Wound healing[2] is a process that depends entirely on the provision of a number of factors and the prevention of infection (Figure 10.3). Factors affecting wound healing are:

- *Age*: Wound healing slows with age. Younger individuals should heal minor wounds within 5 to 10 days or so, but this may become longer, in the elderly. Some wounds may take several weeks to show improvement. This is due to slower tissue growth, i.e. slower rate of cellular division – or **mitosis** – and reduced blood supply to the skin.
- *Nutrition*: This provides protein to build the new tissues, vitamins and minerals for enzyme function and carbohydrates for energy. Water is required for replacement of intracellular and extracellular fluid and removal of wastes.
- *Good blood supply*: Good **tissue perfusion** is required to deliver oxygen and nutrients to the wound and remove the wastes. Poor tissue perfusion delays healing and could cause non-healing.
- *Adequate immune response*: This critical to healing success. Microorganisms gain entry to the body via a wound if the defences are poor. Wound infection slows or prevents the healing process. Infection from wounds can spread to other tissues (e.g. lymphatic nodes) or even become systemic. Infection may be a cause for wounds to breakdown and reopen.
- *Existing disease*: Diseases such as diabetes or cancer may interfere with wound healing – either directly or indirectly – and may cause wounds to break down.
- *The extent of the wound*: Severe wounds with tissue loss may not heal without surgical intervention. The aim is to try, as much as possible, to get the wound edges together and ensure adequate blood supply. It may mean suturing or skin grafts where necessary. The best results occur if 100% skin coverage can be achieved.
- *Wound stress*: This occurs if the wound edges are constantly being moved or pulled apart, e.g. over a moving joint. Wound movement disrupts healing, so it is better if they rest without movement. Stress also occurs with pressure on the wound, e.g. from a bandage or dressing that is too tight or sutures that are pulled too tight. Pressure will exclude blood from the wound site.
- *Factors occurring at the wound site*: A foreign body in the wound, e.g. a splinter of wood, will aggravate the tissues and could hold the wound open. This delays healing and increases the risk of infection. Wet wounds delay healing and provide the ideal environment for infection. Dressings should be kept dry and not too tight and should not rub on the wound.
- *Radiotherapy and chemotherapy*: In patients undergoing cancer treatment these factors may affect wound healing by causing delays in cell division.
- *General stress*: Stress causes raised cortisol levels in circulation, and this reduces the permeability of capillary walls. Reduced permeability slows the rate in which oxygen and nutrients are delivered to the wound, delaying healing.

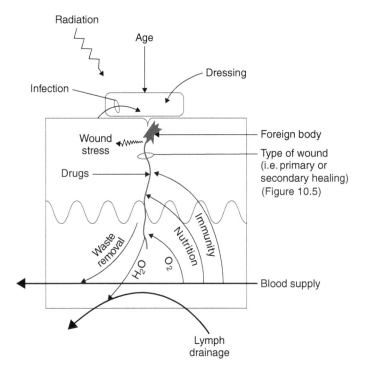

*Figure 10.3* The factors affecting wound healing. Blood supply brings nutrients, water, oxygen and immune cells to the wound site. Blood and lymph remove wastes. The wound will heal best with primary healing, i.e. when the wound edges are together. Detrimental factors include local infection, age, drugs, wound stress, foreign bodies and the nature of the dressing.

After bleeding has stopped, wound healing occurs in three main stages (Figure 10.4).

1 The **inflammation phase** begins shortly after the trauma and lasts up to 10 days under normal healing conditions. Inflammation and infection are different. Infection is an important cause of inflammation, but the inflammation identified here exists without infection, i.e. sterile inflammation, as a consequence of the activity by the immune system. Inflammation benefits both the immune system and the healing process by bringing more blood to the wound site. The body triggers *vasodilation* around the wound. Increased blood supply delivers more immune cells and proteins, oxygen and nutriments and water to the wound. It is also the cause of the symptoms of inflammation:

   * redness ('rubor') due to the additional blood
   * swelling ('tumor') due to the additional fluid leaking from the capillaries into the tissues
   * heat ('calor') due to more blood bringing more heat to the site
   * pain ('dolor') due to the swelling pressing on nerve endings.

   To this could be added *loss of function* because inflammation can interfere with the normal activity of the part involved. The inflammation phase starts the healing process and provides an immune cover to prevent infection.

2   The **proliferation phase** begins two or three days after the trauma and continues until the wound is completely healed. It involves **granulation**, where the structural protein **collagen** is produced from cells called **fibroblasts**, creating a matrix within which many blood vessels grow. This rich blood supply, i.e. highly vascular, makes granulation tissue very red in colour and grows quickly. It fills the dermis in the wound and is then covered by a new epidermis produced by **epithelialisation**.[3] A new layer of stratum germinativum (see page 197) covers over the granulation tissue, and from this a new epithelium grows.

3   The **maturation phase** is the period of wound maturity. It starts about 12 days after the trauma and continues indefinitely. Two events occur during this period:

- First is **remodelling** of the collagen, reducing scarring and giving the wound strength. It means converting type I to type III collagen, a strengthening process that requires vitamin C. It prevents breakdown of newly healed wound, i.e. giving the wound *tensile strength*).
- Second is **capillary regression**, i.e. reduction of the blood supply to the granulation tissue, so further growth stops preventing overgrowth. This also helps to reduce the impact of any scar tissue by making scars pale, not red.

Healing of wounds is more efficient if the edges are held together (often with sutures) without movement for the duration of the healing process (Figure 10.5). This is called *primary healing* and is the fastest way to heal a wound. It also carries the lowest risk of infection and other complications, and it usually heals with little or no scarring.

*Secondary healing* occurs when there is tissue loss, and the wound edges cannot be brought together causing gapping (Figure 10.5). *Tertiary healing* occurs in the deepest and most extensive wounds. Healing of these wounds take much longer than by primary, and they carry higher risk of infection and scarring. Skin grafts, often taken from other areas of the same patient, are used to provide adequate skin coverage.

One of the worst wound complications is infection, which should be avoided. Wound infections are usually bacterial and are often caused by organisms existing as harmless **commensals** on the skin surface. If they gain entry through the wound they become **pathogens**, i.e. cause infection. The risk is made worse by a wet or damp wound environment, which encourages bacterial growth. It is better to use dry dressings and to change them if

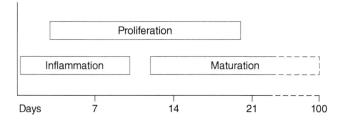

*Figure 10.4* The stages of wound healing. Inflammation begins soon after injury. Increased blood supply brings more oxygen, nutrients and the immune defences. The proliferation stage sees the growth of new cells that heal the wound from the dermis upward. The maturation stage, which goes on indefinitely, completes the process by maturing the collagen and increasing the tensile strength, which prevents the wound from being pulled apart.

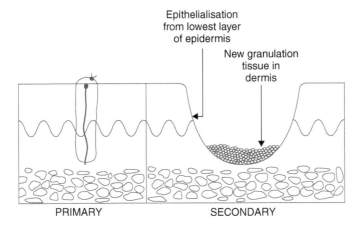

Figure 10.5 Different types of wound healing. Primary healing means the wound edges can be held together, perhaps with sutures (as shown). This form of healing is the best process since it is the fastest, incurs the least risk of infection and heals with very little scarring. Secondary healing involves tissue loss, leaving a wound open to the dermis or deeper tissues. Here, healing is much longer and involves a higher risk of infection and scarring. Skin grafts may be needed to provide adequate skin coverage and a better outcome.

they get wet. Dressings should not be kept on the wound for any longer than is necessary as they can, after a while, encourage a wound environment that favours bacterial growth.

The symptoms of a wound infection are:

1 Pain in the wound and extreme tenderness in the wound area.
2 Swelling of the tissues in and around the wound site.
3 Redness of the whole area, coupled with extra warmth.
4 An **exudate**, which is an infected discharge coming from the wound. Non-infected wounds may leave a normal healthy yellow stain, derived from protein-rich fluid leaking from the capillaries, on dressings. This fluid contains substances required to keep the wound clean and fight infection. Infected wounds produce excessive exudate discharge called pus, a fluid containing a mix of bacterial cells (alive and dead), immune cells and proteins. This infected exudate may have an unpleasant smell.
5 Failure of the wound to heal properly. Such failure can be of any degree, from delayed healing to total wound breakdown.

### Pressure sores (decubitus ulcers)

**Pressure sores** (called **decubitus ulcers**) are caused by continuous pressure on a localised skin site for many hours or days. They occur as a complication of long periods of bed rest or immobility in a chair. The patient is unable to move for themselves and relies on their carer for frequent relief of pressure. The most common sites where persistent pressure occurs depends on the patient's position, e.g. the buttocks and shoulders in those laying on their back (Figure 10.6).

Pressure sores are closed wounds which, if left untreated, become open wounds as necrotic tissue breaks down. They start with patches of *blanchable*[4] *redness* (**erythema**,

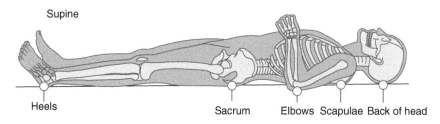

Supine

Heels     Sacrum     Elbows   Scapulae   Back of head

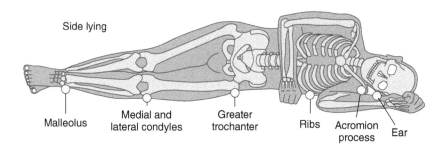

Side lying

Malleolus   Medial and lateral condyles   Greater trochanter   Ribs   Acromion process   Ear

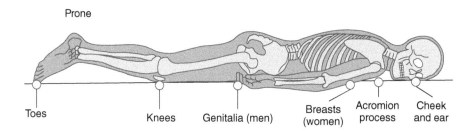

Prone

Toes     Knees    Genitalia (men)   Breasts (women)   Acromion process   Cheek and ear

*Figure 10.6* Sites where pressure can cause open sores. The sites are dependent on skin contact with a firm surface, usually skin over a bony prominence, thus shutting down the blood supply to that patch of skin for a significant time period.

also called a **reactive hyperaemia**). This warning sign indicates where the pressure is happening and alerts the carer to implement the appropriate prevention. If the pressure is not relieved, it progresses to *nonblanchable redness*, then *decubitus dermatitis*, then *decubitus ulcer*, leading to *black necrotic eschar*, i.e. a patch of dead skin that can slough off. Pressure sore formation is accelerated and made worse if the patient is lying in a bed contaminated with urine or faeces. Soiling of skin coupled with pressure results in an open skin lesion characterised by inflammation and surface moisture called **incontinent-associated dermatitis** (**IAD**).[5] This lesion is a high infection risk. The situation must be prevented if possible or corrected quickly with pressure relief, removal of acidic urine or faeces and an application of a skin protective barrier (Voegeli 2017).

Some scales have been developed to identify the risk of pressure sores occurring in clinical practice. These include the **Braden Scale** (mostly in the USA), the **Norton Scale** and the **Waterlow Scale** (Baxter 2008; Lewko *et al.* 2005). They consist of specific factors that are different for each scale, such as age, activity, mobility, hydration, incontinence, mental ability and nutrition. These are assessed on a numerical scale for each individual patient. The total indicates the overall risk for that individual. Their use varies across the health service and it is unclear how much they contribute to pressure prevention in clinical practice (Research Protocol 2019). They are a means of formally documenting which patients are of greatest risk.

Observations of the skin are best done at the time of bathing the patient, since these are the times when most of the skin area is exposed. Relief of pressure is paramount, combining change of position with pressure-relieving aids. Early ambulation out of the bed or chair, whenever possible, is the best preventative measure. If no relief of the pressure is forthcoming, the wall of capillaries in the affected area becomes disrupted and platelets aggregate, causing **microthrombi**, i.e. very small blood clots, which further block blood flow. The result is tissue **anoxia** (i.e. lack of oxygen), which leads to **necrosis**. Dead (necrotic) tissue breaks down due to the activity of **proteolytic enzymes**, i.e. enzymes that break up proteins and **macrophages**, i.e. cells that engulf and remove dead tissue. This is when the closed wound becomes open, with an increased risk of infection. The presence of infection and further pressure makes this wound very difficult to heal. Events should never get this far if preventative measures are implemented quickly.

### Burns and scalds

A burn is a thermal trauma to the skin caused by contact or exposure to high temperature. Scalds are contact with a wet source of high temperature, e.g. boiling water or steam. Burns are classified according to skin depth, i.e. a *superficial epidermal* burn with damage to the epidermis only; *superficial dermal (partial thickness)* burn involving the upper dermis; *deep dermal (partial thickness)* involving the deeper dermis; and *full thickness* burn involving the entire skin, subcutaneous tissues and perhaps even deeper structures (Figure 10.7).

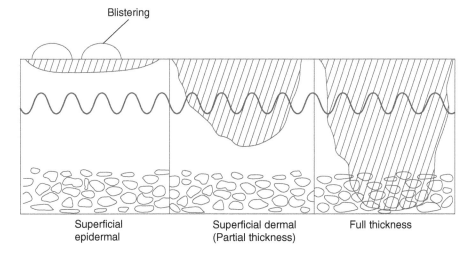

*Figure 10.7* Classification of burns. *Superficial epidermal* burns involve the top layers of epidermis only (e.g. sunburn). *Superficial dermal* (or partial thickness) burns are deeper, extending into the upper part of the dermis. *Deep dermal* burns (also partial thickness) extend into the lower parts of the dermis. *Full-thickness* burns extend through all the skin layers into the subcutaneous tissues or even internal structures. The burn is the shaded area (After NICE 2020).

The serious nature of a burn depends less on depth but more on the surface area of skin burnt. A large body area of superficial burn is far more serious than a small body area of deep burn. Burns of large body surface area disrupts more skin function than small areas of deep burn, particularly control of fluid loss through the skin. Life-threatening shock from uncontrolled fluid loss through large areas of burn is a major factor in the management of those burns. The other factors involving large areas of burn are pain control (see Chapter 12) and reducing the risk of infection. Therefore it becomes important to estimate the total surface area of the burn. One way to do this, the '**rule of nines**' is shown in Figure 10.8.

Burns appear as red (erythema) areas, sometimes with fluid filled blisters forming. These blisters are caused by fluid leaking from damaged and dilated blood vessels, i.e.

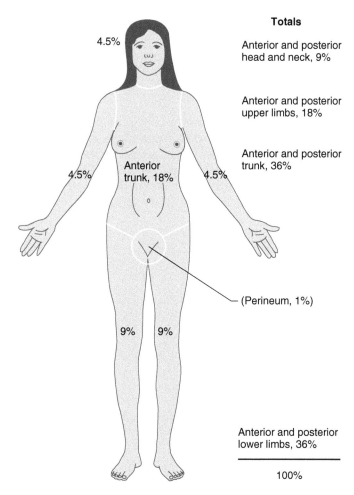

*Figure 10.8* The 'rule of nines' area of burn estimator. The body is divided into areas as follows: front and back of head = 9% (4.5% front and back); trunk = 36% (18% front and back); upper limbs = 18% (4.5% front and back times 2 limbs); lower limbs = 36% (9% front and back times 2 limbs). This adds up to 99%, the remaining 1% being the perineum. The majority of the percentage area (99%) is easily divisible by 9, hence the rule of nines. Doctors can estimate the often patchy nature of burns using this guide.

derived from blood plasma, the fluid then getting trapped beneath the tough outer layer, the stratum corneum. As more fluid leaks out, the stratum corneum gets further stretched into a balloon of fluid and may rupture. Blisters illustrate just how quickly fluid is lost through burns, and this is why, scaled up over a large surface area, fluid loss from burns can be substantial and become the cause shock.

In first aid:

- burns should be cooled rapidly with tepid water to stop the burning process and to ease pain
- never use *'lotions, potions or mother's notions'*, and this also exclude fats such as butter and even burn creams
- following the cool water, apply a sterile (if available) or clean dressing. If no dressings are available, use freshly laundered linen
- if required, continue to use cool water to ease pain
- seek medical advice as soon as possible. In extensive burns, urgent removal to hospital is essential to treat potential shock and pain and to prevent infection.

The healing of burns is similar to that of wounds. Superficial burns heal by epithelialisation, which replaces the lost epidermis. Deeper burns heal by granulation tissue to replace the damaged dermis, followed by epithelialisation. Collagen formation may be involved. New collagen becomes more prevalent in deeper burns and provides strength to new tissues. New collagen may sometimes cause contractions and scarring, two serious disfiguring complications of burns.

Infection is a major issue in burns, and larger burn areas are at greater risk than small burns. Large burns may need:

- strict sterile techniques
- skin coverage, even if temporary, should be achieved as soon as possible to reduce infection risk, reduce pain and to give a better outcome
- **autographs,** i.e. skin taken from the patient's own unburnt area
- **allographs**, i.e. skin used as a temporary biological dressings from an animal source to cover the burn
- antibiotic drugs
- isolation of the patient to prevent widespread infection in large-area burns
- dead and burnt tissue, i.e. non-viable tissue, must be surgically removed as this is a potential source of infection that may delay or prevent healing.

## Important skin diseases

It is beyond the scope of this book to describe all the skin disorders that occur, so this text provides an overview of the pathology of five important skin disorders; acne, urticaria, eczema, psoriasis and malignant melanoma.

### Acne

Teenage acne (**acne vulgaris**) is linked to hormone changes, mostly the **androgens**, i.e. **testosterone** and **dihydrotestosterone** in boys. These male hormones increase both the size and activity of the sebaceous glands. It does occur in females but is more common and more severe in males. Sebaceous glands become blocked by excess sebaceous material and keratin, and they swell as trapped sebum accumulates. They usually get infected with the bacterium *Propionibacterium acnes*. The skin of the face – and sometimes the trunk and limbs – develops a patchy cover of inflamed spots, which form pus when infected.

### Urticaria (hives)

Urticaria is patches of raised, red skin (called *wheals*; Table 10.2), usually due to a **type I hypersensitivity**, i.e. a reaction to contact with an allergen (Chapter 15, page 330). The allergen may be a drug, a specific food, insect or nettle sting or exposure to heat or cold. Oedema of the upper dermis from leaking capillaries causes swelling. The trigger is the release of histamine from **mast cells**, the histamine causing the local symptoms of inflammation. It typically lasts for less than 24 hours but may persist longer (Chapter 15).

### Eczema (eczematous dermatitis)

This is an inflammatory disease of the skin causing patchy areas of itchy redness, each patch having indistinct borders. Oedema forces the keratinocytes apart and creates a spongy effect. This eczema patches can break open, especially from scratching, and this allows for the oedematous fluid to leak out, which then dries to form a crust over the lesion. T-cell lymphocytes infiltrate the area and often histamine release from mast cells exacerbates the irritation (Krasteva *et al.* 1998). The lesions can form anywhere, but mostly on the trunk and limbs. Acute outbreaks happen at any time and may be related to stress. The term *eczematous dermatitis* incorporates a number of distinct conditions, all with very similar pathology but different causes. These include **contact dermatitis**, caused by skin contact with an allergen, e.g. a chemical, **atopic dermatitis** (*atopy* means prone to allergy) – probably caused by an inherited gene and usually running in families – and **primary irritant dermatitis**, caused by trauma to skin such as rubbing.

### Psoriasis

This is characterised by pink, well-demarcated plaques that have a loose surface layer of silvery white scales formed from the shedding of the epidermis. The plaques commonly form over joints, especially elbows and knees, on the scalp and the lower back but can form anywhere. It affects the nails in about 30% of cases, causing the nails to change colour to a dark brown and become thickened, pitted with some degree of separation from the nail bed. Psoriasis is an **autoimmune disease**, i.e. a disorder occurring when the immune system causes disruption in a body system, in this case the integumentary system (Sanchez 2010).

Several genes are known to be involved in the disease. One major gene mutation is the CARD14 mutation in the **HLA** gene cluster called *PSORS1* (psoriasis susceptibility gene 1). **Human leukocyte antigen** (**HLA**) genes on chromosome 6 code for cell surface proteins involved in immunity. CARD14 mutation codes for proteins which raise the production of NF-KB which then increases inflammatory factors. This resulting inflammation triggers a response from the immune system, notably **B-cells** and **T-cells**, **neutrophils** and other chemical agents, e.g. **tumour necrosis factor**, various **interleukins** and **interferon gamma**. The condition is usually inherited, i.e. it runs in families, but it mostly requires environmental factors, e.g. skin trauma or infections, to trigger the disease (McCance and

Heuther 2019). *PSORS1* is found at locus[6] 6p21 (Figure 10.9). Other genes linked to pso-riasis are *PSORS2* (locus 17q25) and *PSORS4* (locus 1q21).

There is a rapid increase in the rate of epidermal cells production in the stratum ger-minativum and faster movement of these cells through the epidermis to the stratum cor-neum, i.e. typically three to four days (see page 199). This causes the epidermis to thicken (called **acanthosis**). Abnormally dilated blood vessels within the dermal papillae cause the erythema, and they bleed easily if the skin is disturbed.

### Malignant melanoma

This is a cancer of the pigment-producing cells, the melanocytes (see page 199), mostly within the skin. The cause of melanoma involves multiple factors, including genetics and excessive exposure to ultraviolet (UV) light, especially ultraviolet A (UVA). Those having fair or red hair and pale skin have a higher risk of developing the disease than darker-skinned people. An aggregation of melanocytes in the skin is called a **nevus** (or **mole**; Table 10.3). Most nevi are no problem, but occasionally one may change to become

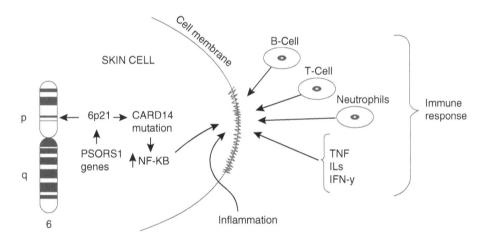

*Figure 10.9* Human leukocyte antigen (HLA) gene cluster *PSORS1* (locus 6p21) in skin cells as a cause of psoriasis. The mutation of the specific gene CARD 14, within *PSORS1*, causes an increase in NF-KB production, which then activates other genes leading to inflammation. A response from numerous immune factors, e.g. neutrophils, B-cells and T-cells and chemical agents such as interleukins (IL), tumour necrosis factor (TNF) and interferon-gamma (IFN-γ) results in psoriasis.

*Table 10.3* The ABCDE of nevi (mole) changes that require medical attention

| | |
| --- | --- |
| A | Asymmetrical in shape |
| B | Border irregularity |
| C | Colour variation |
| D | Diameter larger than 6 mm |
| E | Elevation |

*Table 10.4* Red and amber flag warnings of deteriorating skin conditions

℞  **Red Flag = Serious situation which needs urgent medical attention.**

℞  **Amber Flag = Important to get a medical assessment as soon as possible.**

| Flag warning | Details |
|---|---|
| ℞ **Red Flag** | **Full thickness burns anywhere, and burns of the face, hands, feet, perineum and genitalia.**<br>**Electrical, extreme cold thermal burns or chemical burns.**<br>**Large area burns.**<br>**Wounds involving arteries, bones, tendons or nerves or causing loss of function.**<br>**Infected wounds or burns.**<br>**Non-blanching rash when pressed.**<br>**Urticaria coupled with increasing symptoms of allergy or anaphylaxis.** |
| ℞ **Amber Flag** | **All wounds or burns that fail to heal in 14 days.**<br>**Rash in pregnancy or immunosuppressed patients.**<br>**Rapid increase in a skin nodule.**<br>**Change in shape, colour or texture in pigmented skin lesion (Table 10.3).** |

(After Hill-Smith and Johnson 2021, with permission)

malignant (cancerous). Any changes in a nevus, e.g. changes in size, colour or shape, should be reported to a doctor as soon as possible (Tables 10.3 and 10.4).

**Key points**

*Structure and function of skin*

- Skin has an outer epidermis and a deeper dermis.
- Epidermal cells migrate slowly towards the surface.
- Melanocytes are pigmentation cells in the epidermis.
- The dermis has two main layers.
- The dermis contains areolar connective tissue and patches of adipose fat tissue.
- The dermis has hair follicles, sweat glands, nerve endings and blood vessels.
- Subcutaneous (i.e. below the dermis) layer has adipose and fibrous tissue.
- Skin functions include part of the temperature control system, a sensory organ, barrier against infection, an excretory organ and vitamin D production.

*Skin observations*

- Skin observations involve colour, lesions, rashes, trauma and abnormal temperatures.
- Skin colour changes include cyanosis (blue), jaundice (yellow), erythema (red) and pallor.
- Rashes (or eruptions) are more widespread than lesions, being composed of many small individual lesions.

*Skin trauma*

- Trauma creates breaches in the skin barrier that can become infected.
- Wounds may be closed (bruise) or open.

- Open wounds penetrate the skin from superficial to deep, and can cause internal injury and blood loss.
- Arterial bleeding requires urgent compression to stop the bleeding plus emergency transportation to hospital.
- Wounds can be cleaned but not left wet.
- Wound dressings should be sterile or clean, non-abrasive and renewed daily.
- Wound healing occurs in three phases: inflammation, proliferation and maturation.
- Primary healing is the fastest and best way to heal a wound.
- Pressure sores (decubitus ulcers) are caused by long periods of continuous pressure.
- A burn is a skin trauma caused by high temperatures.
- A large area of burn is more serious than a single deep burn.
- Large burn areas leak tissue fluid resulting in fluid imbalance and shock.
- Large burn areas increase risk of infection and severe pain.
- The area of burnt skin can be estimated using the 'rule of nines'.
- Superficial burns heal by epithelialisation; deeper burns heal by granulation tissue followed by epithelialisation.

### Important skin diseases

- Acne occurs when sebaceous glands become blocked causing swelling as trapped sebum accumulates, and they become infected with *Propionibacterium acnes*.
- Urticaria are red, raised patches of skin, caused by a type I hypersensitivity.
- Eczema (dermatitis) is an inflammatory disease of the skin with itchy, red areas.
- Eczema includes contact dermatitis, i.e. skin reaction with an allergen and atopic dermatitis, which may be a genetic disorder.
- Psoriasis causes pink, well-demarcated plaques that have a loose, shedding surface layer of silvery white scales.
- It involves the rapid production and transition of cells from the lowest epidermal layers to the skin surface.
- Abnormal blood vessels in the upper dermis bleed if the skin is disturbed.
- Psoriasis is an autoimmune disease.
- Malignant melanoma is a cancer of the epidermal melanocytes.
- Exposure to excessive ultraviolet light A (UVA) is a key risk factor.

### Notes

1 The epidermis is mostly blood-free, except the basal stratum germinativum, a good reason why epidermal cells are largely dead – they migrate away from their blood supply.
2 Wound management is a major topic which falls outside the scope of this book. Different strategies for different wound scenarios can be found on the NICE website (NICE 2021).
3 The epidermis is stratified squamous keratinised epithelium.
4 Blanchable means it turns white when pressed but rebounds red when the pressure is removed.
5 IAD assessment tools are available and discussed in Voegeli (2017)
6 Locus is the chromosomal site where the gene is found, e.g. 6p21 means the sixth chromosome, 'p' is the short arm and 21 is the banding number along the arm.

### References

Anoop T. and George K. (2011) Differential clubbing and cyanosis. *New England Journal of Medicine*, 364(7): 666.
Baxter S. (2008) Assessing pressure ulcer risk in long-term care using the Waterlow scale. *Nursing Older People*, 20(7): 34–38.

Hill-Smith I. and Johnson G. (2021) *Little Book of Red Flags*. National Minor Illness Centre, Bedfordshire.

Krasteva M., Choquet G., Descotes J. and Nicolas J.F. (1998) Physiopathology of eczema. *La Revue Du Praticien*, *48*(9): 945–950.

Lewko J., Demianiuk M., Krot E., Krajewska-Kułak E., Sierakowska M., Nyklewicz W. and Jankowiak B. (2005) Assessment of risk for pressure ulcers using the Norton scale in nursing practice. *Roczniki Akademii Medycznej w Bialymstoku Annales Academiae Medicae Bialostocensis*, *50*(Suppl. 1): 148–151.

Lock-In, I. (2006) Investigation of jaundice. *Medicine*, *30*(October): 11–13.

McCance K.L. and Heuther S.E. (2019) *Pathophysiology: The Biological Basis for Disease in Adults and Children* (8th edition) Elsevier, St. Louis, Missouri.

NICE (National Institute for Health and Care Excellence) (2020) https://cks.nice.org.uk/topics/burns-scalds/diagnosis/assessment/ (Accessed 1st February 2023).

NICE (National Institute for Health and Care Excellence) (2021) https://cks.nice.org.uk/topics/lacerations/management/ (Accessed 1st February 2023).

Research Protocol (2019) *Pressure Ulcer Risk Assessment and Prevention: A Comparative Effectiveness Review*. Effective Health Care Program, Agency for Healthcare Research and Quality, Rockville, MD. Last reviewed December 2019. https://effectivehealthcare.ahrq.gov/products/pressure-ulcer-prevention/research-protocol (Accessed 13th March 2023).

Sanchez A.P.G. (2010) Immunopathogenesis of psoriasis. *Anais Brasileiros de Dermatologia*, *85*(5): 747–749.

Voegeli D. (2017) New insights on incontinence-associated dermatitis. *Independent Nurse*, 5 June: 18–21.

# 11 Neurological observations (I)

## Consciousness

### Introduction: *the hard problem*

Consciousness is a problem, referred to as *the hard problem*, because it cannot be currently explained. No one understands how brain cells create the subjective experience of consciousness, i.e. how the chemical activity of the brain produces a concept of reality. But this is important to the medical and nursing professions, and there are some known facts.

Consciousness is a *state of awareness* of the environment coupled with the ability to have some *control* over that environment. Awareness and control are closely linked. Without awareness, brain activity becomes *subconscious*, i.e. activity without the individual's knowledge or control.

*Awareness* involves communication of environmental stimuli to the brain via the **sensory nervous system** and the **special senses**, such as vision and hearing. The brain is almost entirely encased within the skull – cut off from the outside world – and can only appreciate the world through sensory stimuli. Consciousness also means being aware of your own thoughts, i.e. the process of **cognition** (mental activity).

*Control* is meaningful interaction with the environment, mostly through the **motor nervous system**, based on an understanding of the environment and what that interaction will achieve. Awareness and control are both lost in unconscious patients.

DOI: 10.4324/9781003389118-11

Measuring consciousness is another aspect of *the hard problem*. To try to overcome this difficulty, a unit to measure consciousness was suggested, called the **phi**, which 'captures the extent of consciousness. . . . The larger the phi, the richer the conscious experience' (Koch 2015: 84).

### Connectivity and consciousness

It appears that no single part of the brain is responsible for consciousness, but several parts of the brain, working together, somehow creates the phenomenon. Multiple brain areas linked and working together is called *connectivity*. The main areas involved in the connectivity of consciousness are the **cerebral cortex** (notably the **parietal lobe** and the **prefrontal cortex, PFC**), the **corpus striatum** and the **thalamus** (Figure 11.1). **Meta-consciousness** is the term used to identify the brain's ability for awareness of being aware (Young 2021).

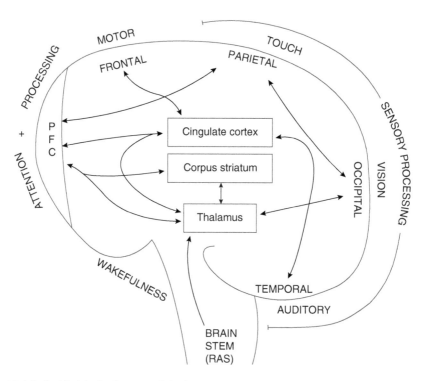

*Figure 11.1* Left side block diagram of the brain areas in connectivity of consciousness. The three main systems are: 1. Wakefulness, i.e. the brain stem, notably the reticular activating system (RAS), and the thalamus, that keeps the brain awake; 2. Attention and processing, i.e. the frontal lobe, notably the prefrontal cortex (PFC) and motor area; 3. Sensory processing, i.e. the parietal, occipital and temporal lobes processing touch, vision and auditory respectively. The subcortical areas i.e. the thalamus, corpus striatum and cingulate cortex, process and integrate the stimuli with memory, emotions, anticipation and motor activity.

## The cerebral cortex

A major brain area involved in consciousness is the **cerebral cortex** (Figure 11.2).

The cerebral cortex is separated into two halves, the left and right hemispheres. These are connected deeper down by the **corpus callosum**, through which communication between the two hemispheres occurs. Each hemisphere is further divided into *lobes*. The **frontal lobe** is anterior to the **parietal lobe**, the **temporal lobes** are to the side and at the back is the **occipital lobe** (Figure 11.2). The surface of each lobe is folded into ridges (called **gyri**) to increase the total surface area. This allows more grey matter (neuronal cell bodies) to be packed into the limited skull cavity.

Individual parts of the cortex are involved in specific conscious experiences. The right frontal lobe appears to house a primary centre for the concept of *self*, i.e. a conscious understanding of one's self. The parietal lobe processes the sensory information from the body, e.g. touch, pain etc, known as **somatic sensations** (soma = body).

The occipital lobe processes sensations of vision, and the temporal lobe processes sensations of hearing. All these sensations become fully conscious as the result of further processing in other areas of the brain, notably through the **prefrontal cortex** (**PFC**). The PFC is at the front of the brain and incorporates the **orbitofrontal cortex** and the **anterior cingulate cortex** (Figure 11.3). These areas carry out higher executive functions such as *planning* and *attention* and add some aspects of *emotion* to the conscious experience.

The cells of the cerebral cortex are arranged in a strict pattern according to function; thus, it becomes possible to map the brain surface using Brodmann numbers, as shown in Figure 11.4 and Table 11.1.

These functional areas are all related to the activities we identified with consciousness, i.e. *control*, motor function of the frontal lobe areas, *awareness*, sensory functions of the parietal, temporal and occipital lobe areas and *cognition*, frontal lobe and other **association areas**. Association areas exist between the main functional areas of the cortex and are essential for making sense of the sensory stimuli arriving at the cortex. They contain memories developed from previous sensory experience that are used for comparing with

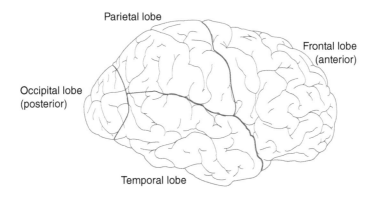

*Figure 11.2* The cerebral cortex from the right side showing the major lobes.

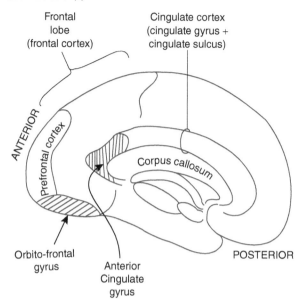

*Figure 11.3* Internal view of the brain showing areas in the brain important for processing consciousness: the frontal and prefrontal cortex and the cingulate cortex.

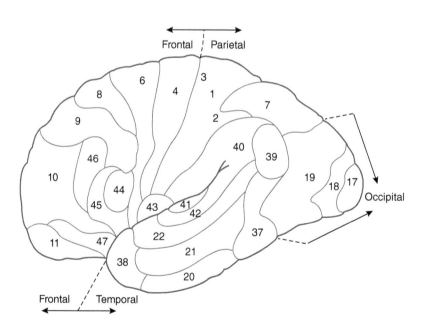

*Figure 11.4* Map of the left cerebral cortex according to cell function. Each area has a Brodmann
number (Table 11.1).

*Table 11.1* Brodmann numbers as shown in Figure 11.3

| Brodmann number | Notes |
| --- | --- |
| 1, 2, 3 | Primary somatosensory cortex in the parietal lobe |
| 4 | Primary motor cortex in the frontal lobe |
| 6 | Premotor cortex in the frontal lobe |
| 7 | Somatosensory association cortex (i.e. the visual-motor area, e.g. location of objects in space) in the parietal lobe |
| 8 | Part of the frontal lobe, including the frontal eye fields |
| 9 | Part of the dorsolateral prefrontal cortex (along with area 46) |
| 10 | Anterior most part of the prefrontal cortex |
| 11 | Orbitofrontal cortex in the frontal lobe |
| 17 | Primary visual cortex in the occipital lobe |
| 18 | Secondary visual area in the occipital lobe |
| 19 | Associated visual area in the occipital lobe |
| 20 | Inferior temporal gyrus in the temporal lobe |
| 21 | Middle temporal cortex in the temporal lobe |
| 22 | Superior temporal gyrus in the temporal lobe (part of Wernicke's area, processing language) |
| 24 | Anterior cingulate cortex (not shown in Figure 11.4, see 11.3) |
| 29 | Posterior cingulate cortex (not shown in Figure 11.4, see 11.3) |
| 37 | Fusiform gyrus in the temporal lobe (visual and language processing) |
| 38 | Temporopolar area in the anterior temporal lobe |
| 39 | Angular gyrus (part of Wernicke's area, processing language) |
| 40 | Supramarginal gyrus (part of Wernicke's area, processing language and many other functions) |
| 41 | Auditory area in temporal lobe |
| 42 | Primary auditory area in temporal lobe |
| 43 | Area subcentralis, includes part of the primary gustatory area (taste) |
| 44 | Part of Broca's area (with area 45) in the frontal lobe (verbal speech area) |
| 45 | Part of Broca's area (with area 44) in the frontal lobe (verbal speech area) |
| 46 | Part of the dorsolateral prefrontal cortex (along with area 9) |
| 47 | Inferior prefrontal cortex of the frontal lobe (language processing) |

new stimuli. Association areas must learn sensory stimulations and store them as memories for future use.

There are important association areas in the following lobes.

1  The parietal lobe sensory association area, which processes somatic sensations
2  The occipital lobe sensory association area, which processes visual sensations from the **visual cortex**
3  The temporal lobe sensory association areas, which process sensations of hearing from the **auditory cortex** (Figure 11.4).

Even within the main specialised functional areas of the **motor cortex** (frontal lobe) and **sensory cortex** (parietal lobe), the cells are carefully arranged in a layout that matches the body plan (Figure 11.5).

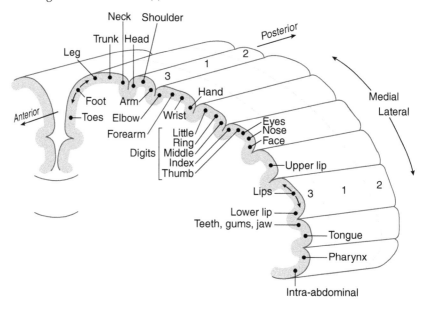

*Figure 11.5* The sensory cortex (Brodmann areas 1, 2 and 3), showing the layout of cells according to the areas of the body from which they receive transmissions. Notice the large areas involved in sensation of the lips (a very sensitive area) and the large areas for the fingers and hands compared with the feet and toes.

### Subcortical areas affecting consciousness

Connectivity with some *subcortical* regions of the brain, i.e. below the cortex, is required for a complete conscious experience, e.g. the **corpus striatum** and the **thalamus**, which adds further emotional processing (Figure 11.1).

The brainstem supplies the cerebral cortex with essential information that makes consciousness possible and maintains the state of awareness (Koch 2017). The brainstem has around 40 separate nuclei, each with a different role. Some of these roles relate to consciousness. One such nucleus (the **rostral dorsolateral pontine tegmentum**) has a pathway that passes to two higher centres: the **left ventral anterior insula** (**AI**) and the **pregenual anterior cingulate cortex** (**pACC**), thus forming a network (Figure 11.6; Fischer *et al.* 2016).

Lesions in the rostral dorsolateral pontine tegmentum are associated with coma, so this brainstem centre is essential for arousal and maintenance of consciousness, and if this network is disrupted the patient lapses into a coma. The two higher centres (i.e. AI and pACC) contain cells called **von Economo neurons** (**VENs**),[1] which are also known as **spindle neurons** because of their characteristic long spindle shape. Unlike other neurons, they have one dendritic extension at each end (Figure 11.7). They also vary in size between 50% and 200% larger than other neurons.

Spindle neurons are also found in the **dorsolateral prefrontal cortex** (Figure 11.6, Table 11.1). These cells appear to be fast-acting and form part of the emotional pathway between the **amygdala**, i.e. part of the limbic system that processes basic emotions and the frontal cortex, which provides sophisticated responses to emotions. The AI and pACC areas are involved in responding to social cues, the sense of self and emotions such as love, grief and anger. The reason for their distribution within a pathway that maintains

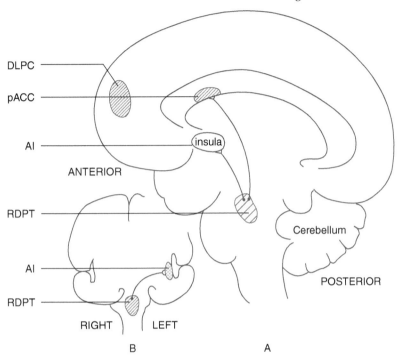

*Figure 11.6* The rostral dorsolateral pontine tegmentum (RDPT) has connections with both the left ventral anterior insula (AI) and the pregenual anterior cingulate cortex (pACC) in relation to maintaining consciousness. The dorsolateral prefrontal cortex (DLPC) is also shown. The DLPC, AI and pACC all contain spindle neurons (Figure 11.7). (A) Left lateral view (shown in section). (B) Anterior view (in section).

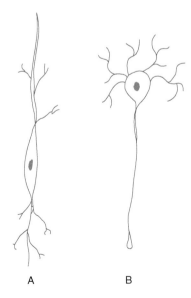

*Figure 11.7* Different types of neuron. (A) von Economo (or spindle) neuron. (B) Normal neuron.

consciousness has not been established. They may have a function directly linking conscious awareness of social cues with rapid changes in behaviour (Williams 2015).

Another brainstem area involved in consciousness and the sleep-wake cycle is the **reticular formation** (**RF**).[2] These small nuclei inhibit any sensory stimuli that are irrelevant or repetitive from proceeding to the higher conscious areas. Important, strong or unusual sensory stimuli are allowed to pass and will help to maintain a state of alertness. The RF contains the **reticular activating system** (**RAS**), which also has an alerting effect as part of the sleep-wake cycle.

Awareness requires the delivery of sensations coming into the brain from the body to the relevant sensory areas. Such stimuli must first pass to the **thalamus**, a sensory relay station above the brainstem that directs sensations the correct cerebral area. Information must go to the correct designated area. The thalamus is therefore the brain's *server* (as on a computer network), directing the *emails* (stimuli) to the correct *terminal computer* (sensory cell). What is amazing is that nature designed human computers with server systems some 4 million years or so before the first computer was invented.[3]

### Neurons

How the neurons in these areas generate a concept of reality is the real *hard problem*. What is known is that processing takes just thousandths of a second, which makes consciousness virtually instantaneous.

Neurons have a cell body and a long process, the **axon**, extending for varying distances away from the cell body (Figure 11.8). **Dendrites** are shorter cell body

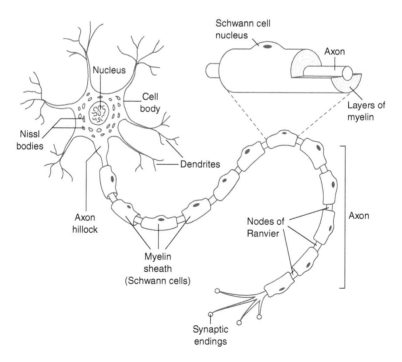

*Figure 11.8* The neuron. The cell body shows a nucleus surrounded by Nissl bodies. The axon starts at the axon hillock and terminates at the synaptic endings. Myelin covers the axon in segments with gaps between, called the nodes of Ranvier. An enlarged myelin segment is shown. Myelin is laid down in layers by cells called Schwann cells.

processes connecting cells together. Dendrites are **afferent** (= *towards*) because they convey impulses *towards* the cell body; axons are **efferent** (= *away from*) because they convey impulses *away from* the cell body. The axons are mostly **myelinated**, i.e. covered by a fat (lipid) layer, the **myelin sheath**, the purpose of which is to speed up nerve impulse transmission from about 2 metres per second (unmyelinated) to as much as 120 metres per second (myelinated). **Neuroglia** (often shortened to **glial cells**) do not convey nerve impulses, but they provide other structural or chemical functions that are essential for brain activity.

The human brain has about 100 billion neurons, with about 50 to 80 times more neuroglia. Most glial are **astrocytes**, named after their star shape, which have vital chemical and nutritional roles to perform in the brain.

Neuronal myelin sheaths are layers of fat, making the axons appear white. Neuronal cell bodies, being free from myelin, appear grey. **Grey matter** consists of cell bodies packed together, e.g. on the surface of the cortex, whereas **white matter** consists of axons packed together as they extend deeper into the brain (Figure 11.9).

Neurons connect to each other through **synapses**, microscopic gaps between one axon and what lies beyond, which could be a cell body or dendrites or another axon (Figure 11.10).

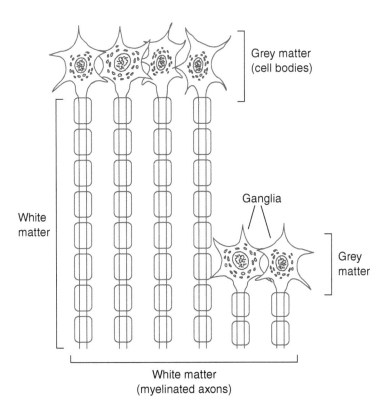

*Figure 11.9* Neurons in clusters form grey matter (cell bodies) and white matter (axons). Ganglia are cell bodies (patches of grey matter) separated from the main group of cell bodies.

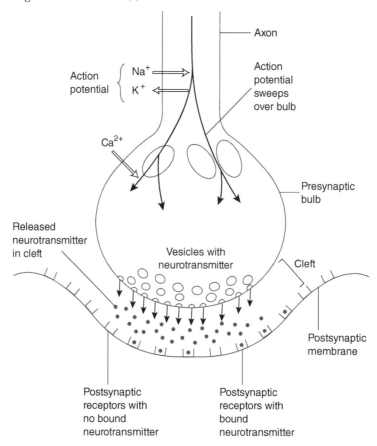

*Figure 11.10* Action potentials and the synapse. An action potential (or impulse) consists of a sodium (Na⁺) inflow into the axon (depolarisation), followed by a potassium (K⁺) out flow from the axon (repolarisation), followed by a return of the ions (refractory). This happens all the way down the axon to the presynaptic bulb. At the bulb the inflow of ions changes from sodium (Na⁺) to calcium (Ca²⁺). This causes vesicles to release a neurotransmitter into the cleft, i.e. the gap between the presynaptic and postsynaptic membranes. The neurotransmitter binds to receptor sites on the postsynaptic membrane. Neurotransmitters effect the cell beyond the postsynaptic membrane.

## Neurotransmitters

Some neurons may have up to 100,000 synaptic connections each with other neurons. Synapses require a **neurotransmitter** to fill the gaps during the passage of an impulse. The neurotransmitter binds to receptors on the other side of the synapse causing a change in the **post-synaptic membrane**. In many cases this change is a new impulse in the next neuron. There are many different neurotransmitters, the main one in the cerebral cortex being **glutamate**. Glutamate is **excitatory** in almost every site it is used, i.e. it generates a new increase in neuronal activity when released at the synapse. Glutamate is produced as part of a chemical cycle that also generates another neurotransmitter called **gamma-aminobutyric acid** (**GABA**; Figure 11.11).

GABA is largely **inhibitory**, i.e. it binds to receptors that prevent any changes in the postsynaptic membrane, so it reduces (inhibits) brain activity. The brain has both excitatory and inhibitory abilities because this allows the brain to operate at a moderate level most of the time, with the option of increasing or decreasing brain activity as the need arises. By carefully regulating the chemical cycle that produces both the excitatory and inhibitory neurotransmitters, the brain can fine-tune glutamate or GABA production to meet its activity needs (Carlson and Birkett 2017).

The 40 or so brainstem nuclei use various neurotransmitters at their synapses. There are a range of receptors for each neurotransmitter, and so it is not currently possible to assign consciousness to any specific neurotransmitter. It all depends on which receptor it binds to, and it is likely that a combination of neurotransmitters and receptors are involved. The rostral dorsolateral pontine tegmentum projects **acetylcholine**-producing fibres to the higher centres, and acetylcholine is a neurotransmitter known to have a general alerting (excitatory) effect.

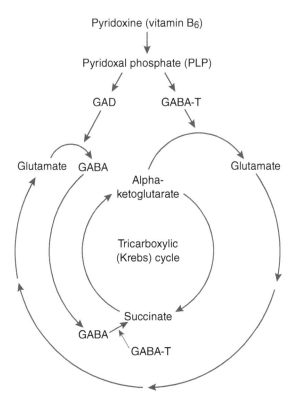

*Figure 11.11* The gamma-aminobutyric acid (GABA) and glutamate (glutamic acid) cycle. The Krebs cycle (Chapter 1, Figure 1.3, page 4) provides alpha-ketoglutarate as the starting point for glutamate, which returns to the Krebs cycle as GABA. The enzymes are GABA transaminase (GABA-T) and glutamic acid decarboxylase (GAD). Vitamin B6 (pyridoxine) is important for these enzymes to function.

*Brainstem reflexes*

The brainstem has control of several reflexes. The **pupillary reflex** controls the pupil size and reaction to light. The **corneal reflex** causes the lids to close sharply when the eye surface is touched (see Chapter 13). The **gag reflex** occurs when a stimulus is applied to the back of the throat inducing a sensation of retching (wanting to vomit; see Chapter 9). A sensory input passes to the vomit centre in the medulla triggering a motor response from the muscles of the throat and upper digestive tract. Like most brainstem reflexes it is protective, attempting to prevent unwanted substances from entering the stomach by inducing vomiting (Chapter 9, Figure 9.4).

## Observations of consciousness

There are various degrees of consciousness, i.e. a spectrum of consciousness from fully conscious at one end to a deep state of unconsciousness, known as **coma**, at the other. The various points on this spectrum are the **altered states of consciousness** (Figure 11.12). Notice that **sleep** does not appear on the same spectrum. Sleep is an altogether different state and should not be confused with unconsciousness. Sleep is distinguished from unconsciousness by several characteristics:

- Sleep is a natural body requirement; unconsciousness is an abnormal state, indicating pathology exists, often within the brain itself.
- Sleep has recognised brain areas that control its onset and duration. Whilst *consciousness* has control centres, *unconsciousness* has no controlling brain areas and appears to be a loss of function of those areas responsible for consciousness.
- Sleep has a distinct normal circadian pattern of activity occupying about 8 hours out of every 24 hours. Being abnormal, unconsciousness should never happen.
- In sleep, the subject is rousable, but in a state of unconsciousness the subject cannot be roused (depending on the depth of the unconsciousness; Figure 11.12).
- Sleep has a typical normal pattern of brain activity that can be observed using an **electroencephalograph**, a machine for measuring and displaying the electrical output of the brain that produces an **electroencephalogram** (**EEG**). Unconsciousness has no typical EEG pattern and may even show abnormal patterns.

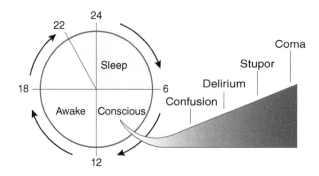

*Figure 11.12* The consciousness-coma continuum and the sleep-wake cycle. The sleep-wake cycle is normal, but the coma continuum is due to pathology.

It becomes important to assess the level of consciousness in a patient for two reasons. First, the point that the patient occupies on the spectrum of consciousness is important since this has a bearing on the management of the patient's condition and prospects for a successful recovery, i.e. the patient's **prognosis**. Second, it is very important to know whether the patient is moving along the spectrum, either by regaining consciousness or, more urgently, to know whether the patient is deteriorating by going deeper into coma. Assessing consciousness is difficult because the patient may be unresponsive, and only close observation of specific signs can provide any evidence of the conscious state.

**Coma scales** are recordings of specific signs that can be assessed and will give some evidence of the conscious state and any changes in it. Terminology has been developed to assess the position of a patient on the consciousness spectrum using specific symptoms that may be present in any combination (Figure 11.12; modified from Hickey 2013):

- **fully conscious**: awake, alert, orientated in time and place, understands spoken words, reads written words, expresses ideas verbally, responds to the environment.

Then the *altered states of consciousness* are:

- **confusion**: disorientated in time, place or person, memory lapses, short attention spans, difficulty in following instructions, possibly hallucinations or false perceptions, agitation and bewilderment
- **lethargy**: orientated but very slow in motor activity and speech, low level of mental activity, high accident risk
- **obtundation**: very drowsy, rousable only when stimulated, verbal responses are very limited, attempts to follow only very simple commands, high accident risk
- **stupor**: generally unresponsive except to vigorous verbal or touch stimuli, attempts at eye opening or incomprehensible sounds may be the only response, responds to pain, minimal spontaneous movements, very high accident risk
- **coma**: no response to verbal or touch stimuli, no verbal sounds, response to pain stimuli as follows:

  - **light coma**: purposeful withdrawal from pain, gag, corneal and pupillary reflexes intact
  - **medium coma**: non-purposeful responses to pain, variable brainstem reflex responses, some being absent
  - **deep coma**: unresponsive to pain, brainstem reflexes absent.

The specific signs are assessed by the carer delivering a sensory stimulus to the patient and then observing the response. The grade recorded on the coma scale will depend on the patient's best response to that stimulus. Auditory stimuli are usually tried first. These are sounds beginning with a normal speaking voice, e.g. asking the patient a question such as 'What is your name?' If there is no response give a louder command e.g. 'Open your eyes!' or a clap of the hands. Such auditory stimuli enter the brain via the **vestibulo-cochlear nerve** (**cranial nerve VIII**, also known as the **auditory nerve**) and directly excite neurons of the auditory cortex within the temporal lobe (Figure 11.4 and Table 11.1). If there is no response to auditory signals, this is noted, then **tactile stimuli** are tried. These are touch-related somatic sensations, e.g. gently shaking their arm, which pass via **spinal nerves** to the **spinal cord**. On arrival in the brainstem, they pass upwards to the thalamus, which then relays the stimulus on to the appropriate part of the parietal lobe's somatic sensory cortex (Figure 11.5). Thus, speech and touch pass by different routes to different areas of the cerebral cortex. It may be necessary to increase the somatic stimulus from touch to pain. Almost every conscious person responds to **painful stimuli** in some form or another; it is a powerful stimulus of cerebral cortex function. Pain is associated with injury, and it is very important to use a method of pain application that causes no tissue damage. The practice of rubbing the sternum with the knuckles of a clenched fist should stop since large haematomas and extensive bruising over the front of the chest has occurred. It is better to apply pressure to the fingernails and toenails, which are hard, dead tissue and therefore will not be damaged. The response to pain is *motor*, i.e. a reaction from the frontal lobe motor cortex causing movement of the limbs. Even a verbal response to pain is motor in origin, albeit from the brain's motor speech area (called **Broca's area**), in the frontal lobe. Such a reaction would, however, probably mean that the patient was conscious. The somatic motor responses can be called **purposeful responses** if they show limb withdrawal from the pain or attempts to push the carer's hand away, i.e. they show signs of trying to stop the pain, so the pain is registering as conscious. The limb movements may cross the body's midline. **Non-purposeful responses** are limb movements without any attempt to stop the pain or withdraw from it and do not cross the midline. **Unresponsive** is a feature of the deepest comas. Pain is handled by the nervous system somewhat differently from all other stimuli. Both the cord and the thalamus have their own ways of managing pain (see Chapter 12).

*The Glasgow Coma Scale*

Several coma scales have been developed. The **Glasgow Coma Scale** has been the most widely adopted (Figure 11.13). This assessment defines coma as three conditions: the patient is unable to open the eyes is unable to obey commands and is unable to speak. Eye opening, motor response to both verbal commands and painful stimuli and the ability to speak are the specific signs adopted for assessment (Figure 11.13). The patient is assessed by applying various stimuli and observing for a response. Reliability between different observers is good, making this a valid tool for the universal assessment of consciousness (Juarez and Lyons 1995).

Another method for assessing consciousness is the **AVPU** system. It stands for alert, voice, pain, unresponsive, and it means that the patient is in one of the following states:

- fully awake (A)
- responding to speech (V)
- responding only to painful stimuli (P)
- not responding to any stimuli (U).

This system incorporates the same broad parameters as the Glasgow scale (e.g. verbal and painful stimuli), but being simpler means it may be more appropriate for use in emergency situations.

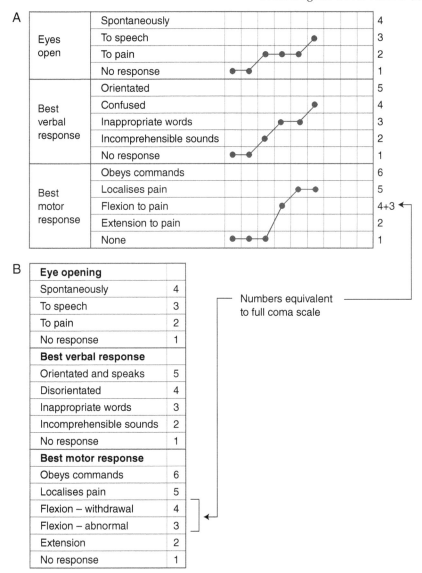

A

| Eyes open | Spontaneously | 4 |
| | To speech | 3 |
| | To pain | 2 |
| | No response | 1 |
| Best verbal response | Orientated | 5 |
| | Confused | 4 |
| | Inappropriate words | 3 |
| | Incomprehensible sounds | 2 |
| | No response | 1 |
| Best motor response | Obeys commands | 6 |
| | Localises pain | 5 |
| | Flexion to pain | 4+3 |
| | Extension to pain | 2 |
| | None | 1 |

B

| Eye opening | |
|---|---|
| Spontaneously | 4 |
| To speech | 3 |
| To pain | 2 |
| No response | 1 |
| **Best verbal response** | |
| Orientated and speaks | 5 |
| Disorientated | 4 |
| Inappropriate words | 3 |
| Incomprehensible sounds | 2 |
| No response | 1 |
| **Best motor response** | |
| Obeys commands | 6 |
| Localises pain | 5 |
| Flexion – withdrawal | 4 |
| Flexion – abnormal | 3 |
| Extension | 2 |
| No response | 1 |

Numbers equivalent to full coma scale

*Figure 11.13* The Glasgow Coma Scale, partly completed to show a patient regaining consciousness.

## Major causes of unconsciousness

### Epilepsy

A **seizure** is an abnormal pattern of electrical discharge in the brain resulting in neuronal activity that renders the brain in some state of altered consciousness. Some seizures appear as a **convulsion** (or fit), where they are usually unconscious and show abnormal rapid muscle activity. **Epilepsy** is a chronic disorder in which convulsions are the major feature. The affected person may go through a convulsive phase (having fits), but there are various types of epilepsy known (Table 11.2).

The cause is often a small area of damaged or disturbed brain tissue, the **epileptogenic focus**, which may or may not be detectable or operable. The focus, which is highly excitable, acts as a trigger by causing an abnormal burst of electrical impulses both sideways (laterally) into adjacent cells and along the axons to all parts lower down. On reaching the muscles these excessive impulses cause repeated rapid contraction of the muscles (Figure 11.14). The focus is overactive and can discharge impulses very easily. Part of the reason for this hyperactivity is a lack of **gamma-aminobutyric acid** (**GABA**) at the focus (see page 229), which results in a loss of the inhibitory system, and **glutamate**, the excitation neurotransmitter, then becomes dominant. Other chemical changes such as an abnormal influx of calcium ($Ca^{2+}$) and disturbances to glucose and protein metabolism at the focus cause excitability. The lateral spread of the abnormal burst of impulses across the brain surface gets other cerebral cells involved, and the person goes unconscious for the duration of the fit, about three to five minutes. Breathing, the heart cycle and blood pressure remain, since they are not conscious activities and are controlled by brain areas lower down in the brainstem. The course of events during a convulsion – or **grand mal** fit – starts with collapse, then rigidity (the tonic phase), then convulsion (the clonic phase) and finally full recovery (Table 11.3; Blows 2022).

Minor fits (called **petit mal** or **absences**) involve a short period of staring into space with fumbling followed by complete recovery. This is not complete unconsciousness but a state in which the brain is incapable of all normal conscious responses and goes into *pause* or *standby* mode.

Possible post-epileptic complications include **status epilepticus**, where the patient has repeated fits, and **twilight states**, when the patient may wander aimlessly for hours or days, not knowing who or where they are (Blows 2022: 341).

### Strokes

Strokes – or **cerebrovascular accidents** (**CVAs**) – are sudden, usually unpredictable, disruptions to the blood supplying the brain. This blood loss causes a rapid alteration of

*Table 11.2* The various types of epilepsy

| | |
|---|---|
| Grand mal | Major convulsive fit in several phases (Table 11.3). Complete loss of consciousness with no memory of the event. |
| Petit mal (absences) | Minor fit. Brief episode of staring vacantly (loss of touch with reality) during which objects held are dropped. Recovery in seconds. |
| Jacksonian | Twitching in one point in the body spreading to all other parts and causing loss of consciousness. |
| Focal | Twitching in one point in the body (e.g. mouth or digit) without spread or loss of consciousness. |
| Psychomotor | Sudden disturbance of behaviour with perhaps hallucinations. Temporal lobe epilepsy is one form. |
| Myoclonic | Sudden involuntary muscle jerking occurring like a shock, often in the arms of known epileptics. |
| Post-traumatic | After severe brain injury. It involves all epileptic types except petit mal. |
| Status epilepticus | Repeated epileptic fits, often one after another, can last for hours before consciousness is regained. |

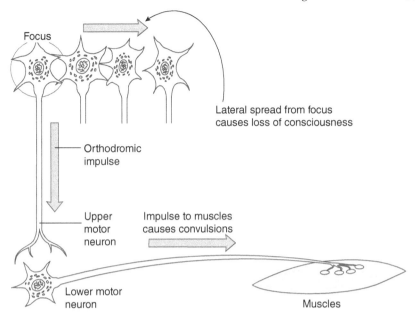

*Figure 11.14* Events that occur during a fit. The epileptogenic focus spreads abnormal impulses laterally to cause the cerebral surface cells to lose consciousness. Rapidly repeating impulses travelling down the focal axon to the lower motor neurone cell in the spinal cord, causes impulses to be sent out to the muscles, which then respond with strong, erratic, rhythmic contractions.

*Table 11.3* Stages of a grand mal seizure

|   | Stage | Notes |
|---|-------|-------|
| 1 | Aura | A warning of impending fit. Not always present or recognised. May take the form of flashing lights or other hallucinations. |
| 2 | Tonic | Lasts up to 30 seconds. Full muscle tone causes gross rigidity, including respiratory muscles, causing breathing to stop. |
| 3 | Clonic | Lasts up to 45 seconds or so. The convulsion phase, with gross twitching and thrashing of limbs. Breathing is spontaneous. |
| 4 | Recovery | Clonic convulsion stops and the patient 'sleeps' off the effects for up to 15 minutes or so. Should waken with no memory of the event. |

consciousness. The stroke is the result of either bleeding into the brain itself (**intracerebral bleed**) or sudden obstruction of the blood vessels leading to the brain (**cerebral thrombosis** or **embolus**).

The blood supply to the brain begins as blood leaves the left side of the heart via the aorta (see Chapter 2). A series of arteries branch off from the aorta carrying blood upwards to the head (Figure 11.15). The **brachiocephalic** and **common carotid** arteries distribute blood towards the neck; the internal carotid arteries take blood up to the **circle of Willis** in the base of the brain (Figure 11.16).

Blood also arrives there from the **vertebral arteries**, branches of the **subclavian** arteries that pass up through the cervical (neck) vertebrae (Figure 11.15). The circle of Willis therefore has four blood supplies, i.e. two vertebral and two internal carotid arteries. Six main arteries leave the circle, i.e. two **posterior**, two **middle** and two **anterior cerebral arteries**. The circle of Willis is the major blood distribution point for the entire brain (Figure 11.16).

Strokes often occur as a result of one or both of two factors: (1) the systemic blood pressure is too high (*systemic hypertension*; see Chapter 3) or (2). arterial disease, such as **arteriosclerosis**. This can cause narrowing of the vessels leading to **thrombosis**, i.e. blood clot formation in the artery, or **emboli**, i.e. blood clots moving from elsewhere and blocking

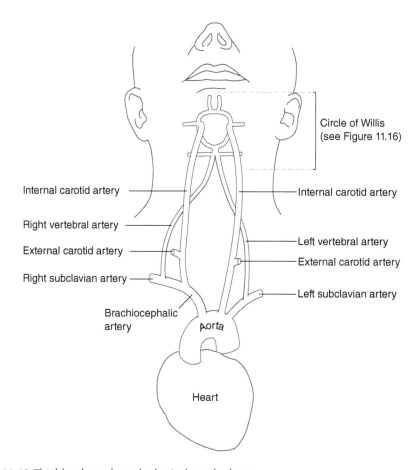

*Figure 11.15* The blood supply to the brain from the heart.

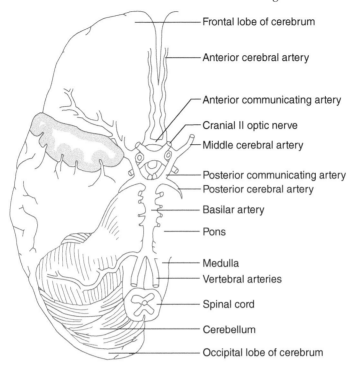

*Figure 11.16* The arteries of the circle of Willis distributing blood to the brain.

the artery. The sudden loss of blood supply causes areas of the brain to cease functioning with a potential loss of neurons. These areas may become necrotic (i.e. dead), known as **cerebral infarcts** (similar to *myocardial infarcts*; see Chapter 3) if the blood supply is not restored. In either case, be it bleeding or obstruction, the effect is similar (i.e. sudden collapse, varying degrees of altered consciousness – including sometimes coma – and severe head pain if the patient is conscious). Weakness (**hemiparesis**) or paralysis (**hemiplegia**) are often experienced by the conscious patient down one side of the body. This occurs on the opposite side to the stroke lesion due to the crossing over (**decussation**) of most of the motor pathways in the brainstem. Other signs may be present, such as speech loss (**aphasia**; see FAST, Table 11.5). The signs depend entirely on where the CVA has occurred in the brain, how big the lesion is and what neurons and pathways are affected. If a small area of cerebral cortex is involved, consciousness may be retained throughout or return quickly if lost previously. Large areas of cortex involved may mean prolonged coma from which the patient may not recover. Some strokes may result in loss of life. Recovery is also dependent on the degree of brain damage sustained. Some survivors who regain consciousness may make a full recovery, whereas others may be left with some degree of **neurological deficit** (i.e. permanent symptoms, such as one-sided weakness or speech loss).

### Head injury

In head injury, unconsciousness is caused by either shaking of the brain (**concussion**), damage to the brain or pressure on the brain (**compression**). The difference between them is critical, i.e. the difference between full, partial or no recovery. Because the brain is a soft organ inside a hard skull, it can suffer the *jelly in a tin* effect when the head is struck. Imagine a ready-to-eat jelly placed in a tin with the lid on. If the tin is dropped from only waist height, the tin will survive more or less intact. But will the jelly? Head injuries are either caused by a **deceleration trauma**, i.e. the head is moving but suddenly stops as it hits an immovable object or an **acceleration trauma** where the head is stationary but is caused to move suddenly and violently when struck by a fast-moving object. Because the brain is basically floating in **cerebrospinal fluid** (**CSF**) (see Figure 11.18), brain movement is always slightly behind the skull movement. If the moving skull stops suddenly the brain carries on briefly and collides with the inside of the skull. Similarly, if the stationary skull moves suddenly the brain lags behind and again collides with the skull. The first collision causes an injury to one part of the brain, e.g. at the front, followed by an *equal but opposing reaction* causing the brain to move in the opposite direction, creating a second injury directly opposite to the first, e.g. at the back. This is known as the **contracoup injury** (Figure 11.17; McCance and Heuther 2019).

The problem is that the top surface of the brain, i.e. the surface exposed to the inside of the skull, is the cerebral cortex, the part involved in consciousness. So, in either scenario, consciousness is likely to suffer. Some protection to this surface is afforded by the **meninges**, which cover the surface of the brain and cord (collectively called the **central nervous system** or **CNS**) and by the jacket of watery fluid within the meninges (the **cerebrospinal fluid**, or **CSF**; Figure 11.18).

The meninges are three CNS coverings: from the inner to the outer layers, they are the **pia mater**, the **arachnoid mater** and beneath the skull the **dura mater**. A small, dry space, the **subdural space**, exists between the dura mater and the arachnoid mater below, but a larger CSF-filled space, the **subarachnoid space**, exists between the arachnoid mater and the pia mater below. Cerebrospinal fluid (CSF) provides most of the cushioning effect around the brain. It is produced within the **ventricles** of the brain from blood plasma. It circulates around the brain and cord and is returned to the blood via the **arachnoid villi** extending from the arachnoid mater. This fluid is constantly being renewed, and a relatively constant pressure of CSF must be maintained. The hardness and roundness of the skull, plus the CSF cushion and, perhaps, surprisingly *the hair* all help to prevent

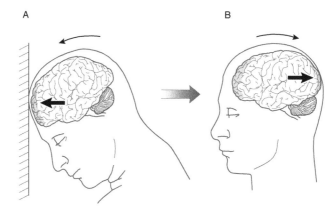

*Figure 11.17* Contracoup trauma to the brain in head injury. (A) The initial injury to the front of the brain when the head is thrown forward and hits a solid object. (B) The secondary injury.

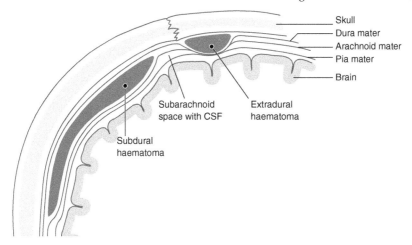

*Figure 11.18* The meninges, showing the sites within the three layers of a subdural and an extradural haematoma. CSF: cerebrospinal fluid.

brain injury during minor head collisions. It takes a hard blow to the skull to cause the involvement of consciousness, e.g. injuries sustained while travelling at speed. This demonstrates the need for external protection, i.e. helmets, seat belts and head rests, to prevent deceleration injury for various high-risk forms of transport and activities.

The skull has a limited internal space, most of which is filled with the brain. This, together with the blood and CSF volumes circulating through the brain, cause an internal pressure within the skull, the **intracranial pressure** (or **ICP**), which is normally anything up to 15 mmHg. About 80% of this pressure is caused by the brain, and the remaining 20% is shared between the blood and CSF volumes. **Raised intracranial pressure** (or **RICP**), i.e. any pressure persistently sustained over 20 mmHg, is caused by anything that abnormally demands space inside the skull, i.e. a **space-occupying lesion**, or **SOL**. SOLs can be many things, such as brain tumours, excessive CSF volume (**hydrocephalus**) and bleeding inside the skull. After brain shaking (**concussion**; see page 237), small capillary bleeds into the cerebral cortex may occur (*brain bruising*, or **contusion**). The blood lost may build up if bleeding continues or if a larger blood vessel is damaged, and this puts pressure on the brain (**compression**). The process leading to RICP is often continuous, and the casualty's condition deteriorates with loss of consciousness. The site where the bleeding occurs inside the skull and meninges is important. The most common sites associated with head injuries are the **extradural**[4] **haematoma**, i.e. blood in the *extradural space*, between the dura and the skull (see more later) or in the **subdural haematoma**, i.e. blood in the subdural space (Figures 11.18 and 11.19).

The *extradural space* does not normally exist. The space has to be created by the lesion, which must therefore be a high-pressure bleed to force the separation of the dura from the skull. This means it must be an arterial bleed, e.g. the **middle meningeal artery**. This injury is less common than the venous bleed that causes the subdural haematoma, i.e. four subdural bleeds to every extradural bleed. They are even rarer in the elderly because the dura gradually fuses on to the skull with increasing age, making the creation of an extradural space almost impossible. The main difference, apart from the site and blood vessel involved, is speed of onset of symptoms. The extradural haematoma is *rapid*,

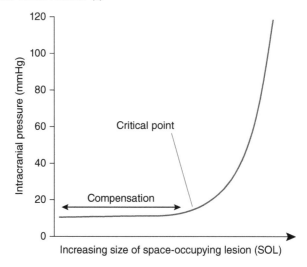

*Figure 11.19* The sudden rise in the intracranial pressure (RICP) occurs when the brain compensatory mechanism fails. This critical point must be watched for very carefully.

i.e. life-threatening symptoms can occur within a few minutes, compared with the *slower* subdural haematoma, which causes problems over several hours or even days. This indicates two things:

1  The need for a scan or a 24-hour stay in hospital for head injuries to exclude the extra-dural haematoma. If the subdural develops at home after that, there is time to get the patient back to hospital.
2  The need for continuous observation since the patient may deteriorate rapidly and die if vital symptoms of an extradural are missed.

The symptoms of RICP fall into two categories:

1  **General symptoms**: those that indicate the presence of RICP but give no clue to the exact site of the pressure on the brain
2  **Local** (or **focal**) **symptoms**: those that indicate both the presence and the site of pressure on the brain.

*General symptoms* are **headache** (which is worse on wakening), **nausea, vomiting, altered state of consciousness** (see page 230, Figure 11.12), **blurred vision, respiratory irregularities** and **papilloedema** (see Chapter 13, page 283). **Slow pulse rate (bradycardia)** and **raised blood pressure** may occur late as the patient deteriorates and should not be relied on.
*Focal symptoms* are:

• unilateral (one sided), ipsilateral (on the same side as the injury) **fixed dilated pupil** followed later by bilateral fixed dilated pupils
• nystagmus (Chapter 13, Figure 13.13)
• visual field defects (Chapter 13, page 271)
• fits (page 233)
• aphasia (loss of speech)

- ataxia (unsteady walking)
- hemiparesis and/or hemiplegia (Chapter 14, page 300)
- specific sensory losses.

These symptoms will develop at different speeds depending on several factors. For extradural and subdural haematomas, the factors include which blood vessel is bleeding, the location of the bleed and the brain's compensatory mechanism. These compensatory mechanisms allow for a certain increase in the space occupying lesion (SOL), i.e. the bleed, without undue change in the intracranial pressure (ICP).

As the SOL grows with further bleeding, the pressure it exerts is compensated at first by a *reduction* in the blood volume entering the skull and the CSF volume produced. These account for 20% of the ICP (see page 239), and this percentage could drop to accommodate the growing SOL. This compensation only lasts for a while, after which the ICP will rise sharply because the brain then comes under pressure (Figure 11.19). This is the critical point, i.e. the change from compensation to decompensation, where the resultant RICP may prove fatal if it is not noticed urgently. Increasing RICP will displace the brain, forcing it downwards and/or sideways, referred to as **herniation** of the brain structures, with associated tearing of membranes and crushing of nerves. As the brainstem is forced downwards, it impacts on the **foramen magnum**, the large opening in the base of the skull through which the spinal cord emerges. This impaction blocks the flow of CSF through the opening and puts pressure on the vital centres of the brainstem: the cardiac and vasomotor centres (Chapter 3) and the respiratory centre (Chapter 5). This is a life-threatening situation, called **coning**, and it is far better avoided by accurate observation. The treatment for RICP is generally a surgical opening made into the skull, called a **burr hole**, to let the haematoma out. This vital procedure, combined with accurate neurological observation, can save the patient's life. ICP is regularly monitored in those patients who are at risk of RICP. This can be done by placing a probe within the skull connected to an external monitor (Chitnavis and Polkey 1998).

Head injuries may also result in a fractured skull. The symptoms of this may be obvious very soon after the accident, and they may get worse quickly. These symptoms include:

- an open wound on the scalp with varying degrees of blood loss. It may be the site of a fracture below the wound
- bleeding into the eye socket (the orbit), i.e. a **periorbital haematoma**, which may be either unilateral or bilateral, causing the soft tissue in and around the socket to swell and making the lids difficult to open. The area around the eye becomes blackened
- blood or clear fluid (cerebrospinal fluid, CSF) coming from one or both ears
- bruising behind the ear
- clear fluid (CSF) coming from the nose
- post traumatic deafness.

Any suspect skull fracture requires urgent removal to hospital (Table 11.5).

*Other causes of loss of consciousness*

There are many other causes of unconsciousness. Here are a few important examples:

1 Lack of oxygen, either in the air or through strangulation, choking, drowning or airway obstruction
2 Various poisons and toxins

3  Central nervous system infections, such as **meningitis** (inflammation of the meninges) or **encephalitis** (inflammation of the brain substance).
4  Intoxication by alcohol or drug abuse or drug overdose
5  Electric shock
6  Loss of blood pressure, temporarily as in **fainting** (also known as **syncope**) or more profound as in severe shock
7  Metabolic disorders, such as **diabetes** (see Chapter 8), where both high and low blood sugar levels induce coma in response to instability in the blood insulin level.

**Fainting** is possibly the most common cause of unconsciousness, the one most people may suffer or encounter. The temporary drop in blood pressure causes a transient loss of blood supply to the brain, which then causes the brain to go unconscious. It is usually temporary because it tends to treat itself. The problem is caused by the brain being *vertically* above the heart, which then has the job of pumping blood *uphill*, against gravity, to the brain. This requires a good arterial blood pressure, and if the left ventricle fails to deliver this blood, the brain suffers. It is normally self-treating because fainting causes the person to collapse and this puts the brain *horizontally in line* with the heart, and the pressure then required to supply blood to the brain is much reduced. In short, fainting does away with gravity. Now the left ventricle can happily supply blood to the brain at the new lower pressure, and the brain recovers. The fall can cause injury since the head (and therefore the brain) has furthest to fall. The casualty must remain flat until the ventricular pressure is high enough to supply the brain once more in the upright position. If the person faints while pinned in an upright position, i.e. unable to fall to the ground, such as standing in a tightly packed train on a long, hot journey, the drop in blood pressure results in the blood being unable to flow uphill to reach the brain. If the person is unable to fall down, the brain is starved of blood for longer.

### The anaesthetic drugs

Anaesthetic drugs may be **local** or **general**. Local anaesthetics cause loss of sensation, including pain, at the site where they are administered. They do not affect consciousness. General anaesthetics (Table 11.4) cause loss of consciousness and therefore loss of awareness.

They can be given by inhalation or by intravenous routes. Some general anaesthetics also provide a degree of pain relieve after consciousness has returned, i.e. they have an analgesic effect (see Chapter 12).

Currently, it is not possible to say exactly how most of the general anaesthetic drugs create unconsciousness. Lipid solubility is a common feature of these drugs and correlates well with their anaesthetic properties, i.e. the more lipid-soluble, the greater their power of anaesthesia. One theory suggests that they may get incorporated into cortical neurone cell membranes, which are themselves lipid-based. Distortion of these membranes by the drugs may disrupt ionic movement across the membrane and cause the neurone to fail temporarily. However, growing evidence is now supporting the notion that general anaesthetics block the passage of neuronal impulses necessary for conscious connectivity (Figure 11.1, see page 220). They do this by targeting specific proteins in the cell body membrane or at the pre- and postsynaptic membranes (Figure 11.10). These proteins then fail to move or function properly and connectivity is lost. Different drugs appear to act in different ways and may often need to be used in combination (Table 11.4). This makes isolating the mechanism of function in any single drug difficult to achieve.

Of concern are the post-operative problems that may be linked to anaesthetics, especially in the elderly. These include **post-operative delirium** (temporary disorientation, hallucinations and memory losses) and **post-operative cognitive dysfunction** (**POCD**; learning difficulty, memory losses and short attention spans). While there is no direct evidence that these are caused by the drugs, there is circumstantial evidence that the anaesthetics may be involved (Anderson 2017).

*Table 11.4* General anaesthetics

| Drug | Possible side effects | Use and other notes |
|------|----------------------|---------------------|
| Etomidate | Depresses breathing, nausea, hypotension, skin reactions. | Given by injection. |
| Propofol | Depresses breathing, nausea, hypotension, arrhythmias, headache. | Given by injection. |
| Desflurane | Blood clots, conjunctivitis, abdominal pain, malaise. | Volatile liquid halogenated inhalation vapour. |
| Isoflurane | Skin reactions, dyspnoea, delirium, mood changes. | Volatile liquid halogenated inhalation vapour. |
| Nitrous oxide | Addiction, disorientation, dizziness, euphoria, nausea. | Inhalation gas. |
| Sevoflurane | Drowsiness, fever, confusion, asthma attack. | Volatile liquid halogenated inhalation vapour. |
| Thiopental sodium | Arrhythmias, poor appetite, cough, skins reactions. | Slow intravenous injection |

*Table 11.5* Red and amber flag warnings of deteriorating consciousness

℞ **Red Flag = serious situation which needs urgent medical attention**.

℞ **Amber Flag = important to get a medical assessment as soon as possible**.

| Flag warning | Details |
|--------------|---------|
| ℞ **Red Flag** | **Sudden drowsy, fainting, confusion or seizure for unknown reason.** <br> **Fainting in a fixed upright position, i.e. unable to lay the patient flat; get the patient flat urgently.** <br> **Fainting with symptoms or a known past history of diabetes or heart condition.** <br> **Symptoms of stroke: F.A.S.T. = sudden Facial or Arm weakness on one side; rapid Speech impediment; Time for urgent medical care.** <br> **Symptoms associated with a head injury:** <br> • **loss of consciousness** <br> • **drowsiness** <br> • **confusion** <br> • **convulsion** <br> • **amnesia for longer than 5 minutes** <br> • **increasing or persistent headache** <br> • **vomiting** <br> • **unilateral or bilateral fixed dilated pupils** <br> • **bleeding or clear fluid from the ear** <br> • **periorbital bleeding** <br> • **history of anticoagulation medication, illicit drug or alcohol consumption.** |
| ℞ **Amber Flag** | **Fainting that does not recover consciousness after 15 minutes.** <br> **Fainting in patient with known hypotension** (Chapter 3). <br> **Signs of epilepsy.** |

(After Hill-Smith and Johnson 2021, with permission)

**Key points**

*The nature of consciousness*

- The cerebral cortex, particularly the prefrontal cortex, is part of a network of connectivity in the brain to achieve alertness and maintain consciousness.
- Awareness of the environment and control of activities are qualities of consciousness.
- The cortex is made up of nerve cells called neurons.
- Neurons have a cell body with dendrites and an axon that is often myelinated.
- Grey matter is cell bodies packed together and white matter is axons packed together.
- Neurons connect to each other through synapses. These tiny gaps require a neurotransmitter, the most important of which for consciousness is glutamate.
- The left and right hemispheres of the cortex are further divided into lobes: the frontal, parietal, temporal and occipital lobes.
- The motor cortex is in the frontal lobe and the sensory cortex is in the parietal lobe. The cells are carefully arranged in a layout that matches the body plan.
- Sensations coming into the brain from the body must first pass to the thalamus, a sensory relay station that sends sensations on to the correct part of the cerebral cortex.

*Unconsciousness assessment*

- Consciousness can be considered as a spectrum, from fully conscious at one end to coma at the other. The various points on this spectrum are the altered states of consciousness.
- Painful stimuli are achieved by applying pressure to the fingernails and toenails, which are dead tissue and therefore will not be damaged. The response to pain is motor, i.e. limb movements.
- Purposeful responses are signs of trying to stop painful stimuli; non-purposeful responses are limb movements without any attempt to stop painful stimuli.
- The Glasgow Coma Scale is the most widely adopted scale. This defines coma as unable to open the eyes, unable to obey commands and unable to speak.

*Epilepsy*

- The cause of epilepsy can be a small area of damaged or disturbed brain tissue, the epileptogenic focus.
- The grand mal fit involves collapse, tonic rigidity, clonic convulsions and then full recovery.
- Minor fits (petit mal or vacancies) are short periods of aimless staring with fumbling, followed by complete recovery.

*Strokes*

- Strokes, or cerebrovascular accidents (CVAs), are sudden, unpredictable disruptions to the blood supply to the brain, bleeding into the brain (intracerebral bleed) or sudden arterial obstruction (cerebral thrombosis or embolus).

*Head injury*

- Unconsciousness in head injury is caused by shaking of the brain (concussion), damage or pressure on the brain (compression, e.g. raised intercranial pressure).
- Some protection to the brain is afforded by the meninges, the pia mater next to the brain, the arachnoid mater and, beneath the skull, the dura mater and by the cerebrospinal fluid or CSF.
- The development of unconsciousness with an extradural haematoma is rapid, e.g. within minutes, compared with the slower subdural haematoma, which takes several hours or days.
- The symptoms of raised intracranial pressure (RICP) are general, i.e. those that indicate RICP is present but do not identify the site or focal, i.e. those that indicate both RICP and the site of pressure. A slow pulse rate and raised blood pressure may occur late and should not be relied on.
- Coning, i.e. death by the medulla impacting on the foramen magnum, is avoidable with accurate observation.
- Symptoms of possible fractured skull fracture includes, unilateral or bilateral periorbital bleeding, blood or cerebrospinal fluid coming from the ears or cerebral spinal fluid coming from the nose and post-traumatic deafness.

*Fainting*

- Fainting is a common cause of unconsciousness caused by a temporary drop in blood pressure with loss of blood supply to the brain.
- It can be self-treating because collapse puts the brain level with the heart and the pressure required to supply blood to the brain is much less.
- If a person faints while pinned in an upright position, i.e. unable to fall, it could be fatal.

**Notes**

1 Constantin von Economo (1876–1931) was an Austrian neurologist and psychiatrist.
2 Reticular means it appears as a network of fibres.
3 This '*Nature first*' concept also applies to many other things in biology, including the wheel!
4 Extra means *outside of*. . . . In this case its outside the dura mater between the dura and the skull. This space does not normally exist and must be created by the bleed. The dura gets fixed firmly to the inside of the skull with increasing age.

**References**

Anderson A. (2017) The risk of going under. *Scientific American*, *28*(2): 61–65.

Blows W.T. (2022) *The Biological Basis of Mental Health* (4th edition). Routledge, Abingdon.

Carlson N.R. and Birkett M.A. (2017) *Physiology of Behavior* (12th edition). Pearson Educational, Harlow, Essex.

Chitnavis B.P. and Polkey C.E. (1998) Intracranial pressure monitoring. *Care of the Critical Ill*, *14*(3): 80–84.

Fischer D.B., Boes A.D., Demertzi A., Evrard H.C., Laureys S., Edlow B.L., Liu H., Saper C.B., Pascual-Leone A., Fox M.D. and Geerling J.C. (2016) A human brain network derived from coma-causing brainstem lesions. *Neurology*, *87*(23): 2427–2434.

Hickey J. (2013) *The Clinical Practice of Neurological and Neurosurgical Nursing* (7th edition). Lippincott Williams & Wilkins, Philadelphia, PA.

Hill-Smith I. and Johnson G. (2021) *Little Book of Red Flags*. National Minor Illness Centre, Bedfordshire.

Juarez V. and Lyons M. (1995) Interrater reliability of the Glasgow Coma Scale. *Journal of Neuroscience Nursing*, *27*(5): 283–286.

Koch C. (2015) Closing in on consciousness. *New Scientist: The Collection*, *2*(1): 84–85.

Koch C. (2017) The footprints of consciousness. *Scientific American Mind*, *28*(2): 53–59.

McCance K.L. and Huether S.E. (2014) *Pathophysiology: The Biological Basis for Disease in Adults and Children* (8th edition). Elsevier, St. Louis, Missouri.

Williams C. (2015) The consciousness connection. *New Scientist: The Collection*, *2*(1): 87–89.

Young E. (2021) Is consciousness detectable in the brain? In Consciousness expanded (part 8). *New Scientist*, 10 July, *251*(3342): 41–42.

# 12  Neurological observations (II)

Pain

- Introduction
- Nature and causes of pain
- Pain pathways
- Observation of pain
- Genetic influence over pain
- Pain in children
- Pain management
- Key points
- Notes
- References

## Introduction

Observing pain is one of the most difficult assessments to make, but it is important to get pain assessment as accurate as possible. One way of assessing a patient's pain is to ask them. But this type of assessment is not measurable, so there is no hard data upon which pain treatment can be based. People have different pain thresholds, and staff could interpret a patient's pain while unconsciously adding their own pain perceptions. This becomes evident when carers say things such as, 'Come on, it can't hurt that much!' Pain observations are an attempt to overcome these problems (D'Costa 2011).

## Nature and causes of pain

There are three physiological types of pain:

1 **Nociception**, caused by actual or potential tissue injury or irritation
2 **Neuropathic pain** caused by nerve damage (Meijler 2006)
3 **Nociplastic pain** caused by the brain's pain centres becoming overactive (Lawton 2022). Every individual adds an emotional (or **affective**) component to their pain which is derived from complex neuroanatomy. It amounts to a *pain network* in the brain which is poorly understood.

DOI: 10.4324/9781003389118-12

*Nociceptive pain*

Nociception is pain caused by everyday injuries or disease, (e.g stings, burns etc) and is important for localising the site of the pain. There are several types of nociception:

- **Acute pain** has recently occurred and is of relatively short duration. It identifies that something is wrong and needs attention, and it can protect the individual against further tissue injury, such as withdrawing quickly from burning.
- **Chronic pain** has a longer duration, lasting for more than 3 months (Wood 2002; Osborne-Crowley 2022). Chronic pain changes some synaptic connections in the brain in a manner that makes the brain's pain centres more sensitive to future pain or continues the pain long after any tissue damage is healed. This brain centred cause of pain is known as *central sensitisation*. It can be referred to as **intractable pain** which is chronic pain with no detectable reason causing it, and it may never have had any physical cause. It can result from a combination of physical effects, emotional trauma and memory of previous injury. It is very difficult to treat such pain when no cause can be found (Osborne-Crowley 2022).
- **Inflammatory pain** is caused by inflammation which is caused by local trauma or irritation, e.g. infections, stings and mechanical or thermal injury (Figure 12.1). The immune system could not function adequately without inflammation. The increase in capillary wall permeability that occurs in inflammation causes more water to leak into the tissues from blood plasma, along with proteins and white blood cells. Extra protein in the tissue fluid attracts more water from the capillaries. This causes a local **oedema** (see page 129).

**Pain mediators**, i.e. chemicals causing pain, are released at the site, notably **histamine**, **prostaglandins** and **bradykinins** (Figure 12.2). These bind to receptor sites on **nociceptors**,

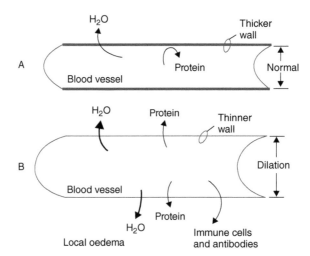

*Figure 12.1* Inflammation. (A) The non-inflamed blood vessel is normal width and has a wall thick enough to prevent inappropriate leakage of blood contents into the surrounding tissues. (B) In inflamed tissues, blood vessels are dilated and the walls are stretched and thinner, and leakage of water, proteins, immune cells and antibodies can take place. Protein that has escaped into the tissues attracts further water out of the blood, causing local tissue oedema. This oedematous swelling puts pressure on nociceptors (pain receptors). Pain is generated by this swelling and locally released pain mediators (Figure 12.2).

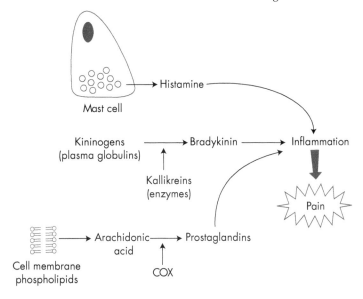

*Figure 12.2* Pain mediators. Histamine is released from mast cells (found in most tissues), bradykinins are derived from the plasma globulins kininogens, and prostaglandins are formed from arachidonic acid.

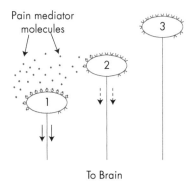

*Figure 12.3* Pain mediator molecules bind to nociceptors (1, 2 and 3). Number 1 has bound a lot of molecules and sends rapid impulses to the brain, and pain is experienced. Number 2 has fewer molecules and sends a slower rate of impulses, which the brain interprets as irritation. Number 3 has no molecules and sends no impulses to the brain.

which are pain nerve endings. Two types of nociceptors occur: **mechanoreceptors** and **polymodal receptors**. Mechanoreceptors are pain receptors that respond to mechanical injury, while polymodal receptors caused pain from many types of tissue injury.

Conscious perception of pain requires certain criteria. First, sufficient chemical mediators must bind to the nociceptors to raise the level of stimulation to the **pain threshold** point or beyond. Threshold means the amount of chemical stimulation necessary to generate strong enough impulses from the nociceptors that are recognised as pain by the brain. With less chemical binding, i.e. below threshold level, weaker impulses can still be generated from the nociceptor, and these are recognised by the brain as **irritation**. **Itching** is one form of irritation caused by mediators binding to nociceptors in concentrations below that needed to activate the pain threshold level (Figure 12.3).

Second, once the threshold is exceeded, the nature, severity and duration of pain are dependent on the intensity of neuronal firing from the nociceptor and any pain blocking mechanisms occurring higher up the pathways (see *pain pathways*). If the nociceptor firing is weak, i.e. just above threshold level, the pain will be less than if the firing intensity increased. It is a simple relationship; the greater the intensity of impulses generated, the greater the perceived pain.

## Pain pathways

Pain impulses pass to the brain via the peripheral **sensory nervous system**. There are two major types of sensory nerve pathways that carry impulses to the brain. These are 'Aδ' **fibres** and '**C' fibres**. The '**A' fibres** (fast fibres) are divided into subtypes, '**Aα' (A alpha)**, '**Aβ' (A beta)** and '**Aδ' (A delta)**, of which the Aδ fibre carries pain. Aδ fibres are the slowest of the fast fibres, i.e. they convey impulses at speeds up to 30 metres per second. '**C' fibres** are much slower than this, up to 2 metres per second. The speed difference is caused by the thickness of the fibres and the degree of **myelination** (Chapter 11, Figure 11.8) the fibre has. Myelin is the fatty covering along the axon of neurons that are involved in impulse conduction. The better the myelination (as in 'A' fibres), the faster the impulse will travel. 'C' fibres are unmyelinated and transmit impulses at the slowest speeds. 'C' fibres carry about 80% of pain impulses to the brain. Nociceptors at the peripheral end of the 'Aδ' fibres are found in the skin (see Chapter 10) and mucous membranes, where they are the first to warn the brain against sudden, sharp pain due to trauma. Compare that to nociceptors of 'C' fibres, which are also in the skin but are found in most other body tissues.

The pathway from the periphery to the brain is a *three-neuronal system*, i.e. the impulse must pass through *three* **sensory neurons** to get from the nociceptor to the brain (Figure 12.4).

- *Neuron 1* passes from the nociceptor into the posterior part of the **spinal cord**. It is a specialised neuron, having the cell body on a branch just outside the cord. This cell body is called the **posterior root ganglion** (**PRG**). Placing the cell body near the cord protects it against injuries. Death of this cell body would result in loss of the neuron and the skin would lose sensation
- *Neuron 2* synapses with the first neuron in the cord, the axon first crossing the midline before passing up the cord to part of the brain called the **thalamus**. The crossover in the cord (called a **decussation**) means that impulses from the left of the body will continue up the right-hand side of the nervous system, and vice versa
- *Neuron 3* synapses with neuron 2, the axon passing from the thalamus to the **sensory cortex** in the parietal lobe of the **cerebrum**.

**Synapses** are connections between neurons (Chapter 11, Figure 11.10). Synapses use chemicals called **neurotransmitters** to bridge a gap that the synapse creates. These gaps (called the **synaptic cleft**) and the neurotransmitters there are essential in pain transmission (Figure 12.4).

### The spinal cord

The posterior spinal cord is the site of the first synapse, i.e. between neurons 1 and 2. This connection permits the formation of a pain **reflex arc** (Chapter 14, Figure 14.11, page 297) and **cross reflex** (Chapter 14, Figure 14.12, page 298). In the simple reflex arc, a

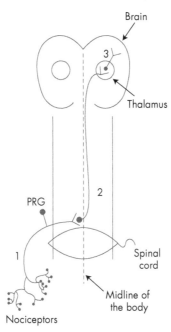

*Figure 12.4* All sensations, including pain, use a three-neuronal system from periphery to the brain. Neuron 1 extends from the nociceptor in the periphery to the cord (PRG = posterior root ganglion, the cell body of neuron 1). Neuron 2 crosses the midline in the cord and extends to the thalamus. Neuron 3 relays the impulses from the thalamus to the cerebral cortex of the brain.

connector (or association) neuron connects the sensory neuron at the back of the cord to the motor neuron at the front of the cord (i.e. the **lower motor neuron, LMN**). This mechanism then allows pain impulses to trigger another impulse in the corresponding motor neuron in the cord, which then causes muscles to contract and withdraw the affected part away from the source of pain. This arc is also the location for a pain-blocking process called the **gate control theory** (Figure 12.5).

The gate control theory of pain is shown in Figure 12.5. In the centre of the spinal cord is an area of nerve cell bodies (**grey matter**). Part of this grey matter is a collection of neuronal cell bodies called the **substantia gellatinosa** (or 'jelly substance'). This can be activated by Aδ fibre stimulation but deactivated by C fibre stimulation. Pain impulses arrive first via the faster 'A' fibres of neuron 1, and these impulses pass on up to the brain via neurone 2. At the same time, 'A' fibre impulses activate the substantia gellatinosa. This blocks all further 'A' and 'C' fibre impulses, and the 'gate' is closed to pain (Figure 12.5). Slower pain impulses passing along 'C' fibres arrive a little later. They cannot pass through this 'gate', but 'C' fibre stimulation switches off the substantia gellatinosa, thus opening the 'gate' to pain impulses. In reality, the so-called gate will be neither fully opened nor fully closed but will fluctuate between the two states, depending on which fibres have the greater stimulus at any given moment. Anything that promotes 'A' fibre stimulus will help to block pain at the spinal cord level, and this may be how mechanisms such as **transcutaneous electrical nerve stimulation** (**TENS**) or **acupuncture** could work. The 'gate control' mechanism and the reflex arc are significantly influenced by the higher

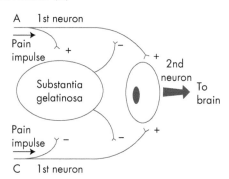

*Figure 12.5* The gate control theory. The first sensory neurons (from the periphery to the spinal cord) are both A (fast) and C (slower) fibres. Both carry pain impulses and both stimulate (+) the second neuron in the cord. The A fibre also activates the **substantia gelatinosa (SG)** with stimulatory (+) synapses. The SG then blocks impulses along both the A and C fibres using its own negative (−) inhibitory synapses. This closes the gate to pain impulses reaching the second neuron (a prerequisite for impulses going to the brain). C fibre stimulation shuts down the SG using negative (−) inhibitory synapses and therefore opens the gate to pain by switching off the SG (−) synapses and allows impulses to reach the second neuron. Generally, the 'gate' is neither fully open nor fully closed but varies between the two states and can be influenced by impulses from the brain.

intellectual centres of the brain. Impulses descending from the **brainstem**, the **hypothalamus** and especially from the cerebral cortex all modify the events at the cord level. The brain does this because factors such as emotions, culture, personal beliefs and memory are all involved in the total pain experience. In Chapter 11, pain was used in the assessment of consciousness (see page 232), but it is not always reliable to determine if the pain response is cortical or spinal (i.e. automatic). Descending neurons from the brain create synapses in the cord that use a variety of neurotransmitters such as **enkephalins**, **endorphins** and **dynorphins** (see page 261) to block further pain transmission up the cord (Clancy and McVicar 1998).

### The thalamus

Impulses entering the brain pass through the **brainstem** and on to the **thalamus**. The thalamus passes the impulse to the third sensory neuron, which conveys it to the appropriate part of the body plan in the sensory cortex (parietal lobe; Figure 12.4 and Chapter 11, Figure 11.5, page 224).

The thalamus can modulate pain stimuli from the cord through its projections down the cord. It can also discriminate between different pain sensations and it can change the individual's mood and motivation in relation to pain. The thalamus also communicates with the **motor cortex** of the cerebrum (in the **frontal lobe**) and thus influences movement in response to the pain (called a **thalamic response**; Figure 12.6).

Both synapses in the three-neuronal system, i.e. in the cord and in the thalamus, have motor connections facilitating movement responses to pain. This is vital as such motor responses save lives and further injury.

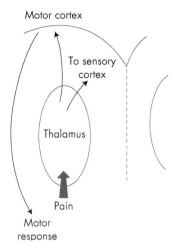

*Figure 12.6* Thalamic response to pain. Pain impulses are not only passed from the thalamus to the sensory cortex, but also, by including the motor cortex, the thalamus can initiate a motor response to pain.

### The cerebral cortex

The nociceptive impulses arrive at the sensory cortex of the parietal lobe, part of the cerebrum, via neuron 3. This is a major part of the conscious brain, where the individual will become fully aware of the pain as a noxious and unpleasant sensation. By then, both the pain blocking mechanisms and the motor movement responses to pain at the spinal and thalamic level would have been activated and reduced the pain intensity. The cells of the sensory cortex are laid out in a plan representative of the body layout (Chapter 11, Figure 11.5, page 224). Having been 'relayed' from the thalamus, the pain impulses will arrive at that part of the cortex that represents the area of the body from where the pain has originated. Thus, pain impulses arising from the abdomen, for example, will arrive in the cortex area that specialises in the abdomen. The crossover (decussation) of the sensory neuron 2 in the cord means that pain impulses from the left of the body will arrive in the right cortex and vice versa. The conscious nature of the cortex allows for the individual to make decisions about the pain. This is very different to the unconscious responses found at cord or thalamic levels that are less sophisticated and are only there to save life and prevent further injury.

Pain sensation is only fully conscious when it reaches the brain, but we recognise the pain as arising from the body part affected. In the previous example, the pain impulses arising from the abdomen are not conscious and therefore not recognised as pain, until they reach the brain. Yet as soon as they arrive in the brain we actually 'feel' the pain in the abdomen, not the brain. This is because there is part of the cortex where the brain cells are representatives of the abdomen. When these brain cells receive pain impulses, they make the person aware of pain in the abdomen, *not* in the brain. The brain *itself* does *not* feel pain! Surgeons have operated on the brains of *conscious* patients. Tissues around the brain require anaesthesia, but the brain itself cannot 'feel' pain. If the surgeon stimulated that part of the cortex representing the abdomen, the patient feels the sensation in the abdomen. The brain makes you aware of pain arising from all other parts of the body except itself. The cerebral cortex could not be both the *initiator* – i.e. the nociceptor – and the *receiver* of pain impulses at the same time!

**Observation of pain**

It is not difficult to identify when a person is in pain; they can usually tell you, and they may show the signs of pain (Figure 12.7). But how *much* pain are they suffering, i.e. is it quantifiable, and is it getting better or worse? Pain is an individual (or subjective) concept; what is mild pain to one person could be severe to another. How much does conscious or subconscious exaggeration of the pain or other factors such as memory and emotions enter the equation?

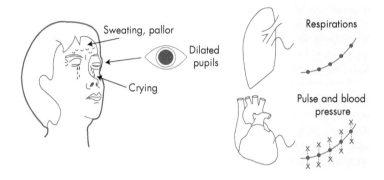

*Figure 12.7* The signs of pain. The pulse, blood pressure and respiration rates rise. The pupils dilate, and the person may show sweating and pallor and they may cry.

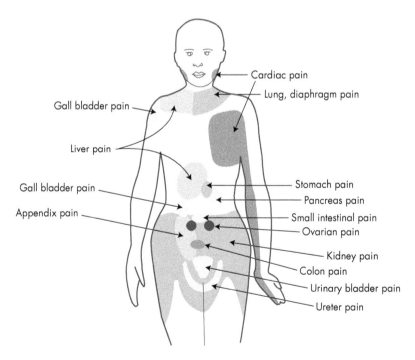

*Figure 12.8* Areas of referred pain and the organs the pain is derived from. Redrawn from Gubrud *et al.* (2019).

Pain assessment requires judgement concerning the following factors:

1 Pain site, i.e. where is the pain? Not all pain occurs at the site of the pathology. **Referred pain** occurs some distance away from the cause (Figure 12.8). Pain impulses travel along nerve pathways and sometimes gives the brain a false impression of where the pain is originating from
2 Pain intensity, which is very subjective and will vary between individuals and at different times in the same individual
3 The nature of the pain, i.e. is it sharp such as caused by a knife, or a dull ache or burning?
4 Is the pain associated with specific activities, such as eating, vomiting or urinating or with a specific movement or position?
5 Duration of the pain, i.e. is it sudden or acute, or is it chronic?

In an attempt to be as objective as possible about such a subjective phenomenon, **pain assessment scales** have been devised.

Pain assessment scales fall into three categories:

1 **Verbal descriptor scales** use words that may be appropriate to describe pain ranked in order of severity, e.g. *no pain, slight pain, moderate pain, severe pain, agonising pain*. Patients indicate the word most applicable to their pain, and a numerical ranking alongside the words would aid in charting the response (Figure 12.9). The word list may provide limited choice when applied to some patients' pain, but it is easy to score. The McGill Pain Questionnaire is more extensive which identifies 78 *descriptors* (or terms) for pain, each with an associated score that can be added up. Included are pain location and intensities (Demming 2022)

| Description | Score |
| --- | --- |
| No pain | 0 |
| Slight pain | 1 |
| Mild pain | 2 |
| | 3 |
| Moderate pain | 4 |
| | 5 |
| Severe pain | 6 |
| More severe pain | 7 |
| Very severe pain | 8 |
| | 9 |
| Worst possible pain | 10 |

*Figure 12.9* Verbal descriptor scale for pain.

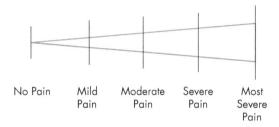

No Pain     Mild       Moderate    Severe      Most
            Pain       Pain        Pain        Severe
                                               Pain

*Figure 12.10* Visual analogue scale for pain.

2 **Visual analogue scales** consist of a line representing a pain continuum, with descriptive word 'anchors' at both ends. An example is the continuum that stretches from *no pain* at one end of the line to *pain as bad as it could be* at the other end. Patients must indicate where along this line their pain ranks. Additional words may be added along the line to aid the patient in their choice (Figure 12.10). They are relatively easy to use and don't rely heavily on the choice of wording. However, they may not be suitable to all patients, particularly the elderly or confused or those with educational disabilities

3 **Pain behaviour scales** are based on the understanding that patients in pain demonstrate certain behaviour patterns. These behaviour patterns are most likely to consist of:

- *verbal responses to pain*, e.g. crying or swearing
- *pain-related body language*, e.g. holding affected area or rubbing
- *specific facial expressions*
- *certain behaviour changes*, e.g. seeking analgesia or medical attention
- *changes in conscious level*
- *pain-related physiological responses* e.g. mild pain causes a rise in blood pressure, severe pain causes a drop in blood pressure.

These scales can be used on patients with communication problems, but they are more time-consuming and complex than the previous scales, and they remove the patient's own subjective assessment (Manchester Triage Group 1997).

4 **Biometric scales**, where biological (or physiological) parameters which can be measured accurately are used to show changes caused by pain. It builds on the *signs of pain* shown in Figure 12.7. Biometrics such as pulse rate, blood pressure, pupil size, sleep pattern disturbance and even brain function are being investigated to see how changes in these parameters can be used to assess pain levels. With regard to brain function, this involves brain scans taken on subjects while both experiencing pain and not in pain. From these scans prediction of the level of pain experienced may be possible. The software is more than 80% accurate in predicting pain from the brain scan changes identified. This may become the standard method for determining pain levels (Brown *et al.* 2011). Biometrics are now being incorporated into miniature technology, i.e. small enough to be built into wrist watches which will give the wearer continuous 24-hour readings through the skin contact (Demming 2022). Variations of these scales may be seen in clinical practice where they have been combined or modified to suit specific needs.

*Genetic influence over pain*

The gene ***TRPV***$_1$[1] has been linked to pain. The TRPV$_1$ protein that the gene encodes is found in nociceptor synapses. This protein creates a greater sensitivity to heat, i.e. both temperature heat and the hot sensation experienced with **capsaicin**, the chemical that makes chillies taste 'hot' (Sutherland 2022). The same protein has been shown to increase sensitivity to other chemical irritants such as **allicin**[2] and **mustard oil**. Generally, the increased sensitivity to pain (called **hyperalgesia**) that is caused by the $TRPV_1$ protein is not present all the time but is induced by the presence of pain mediators seen in inflammation (Figure 12.1) such as various prostaglandins and bradykinin (Figure 12.2).

### Pain in children

Recognising pain in children is not easy, especially in babies and young children. There are some clues that can suggest the child is in pain. Babies are likely to cry, but they may be crying for other reasons. If they remain crying while attempting to feed or when they are being held and comforted, then this may be due to pain. Their cry caused by pain may be different from crying caused by anything else. They may hold or rub the painful part or draw up their legs if the pain is in the abdomen. The child may be old enough to explain their pain, its location and severity. There may be other symptoms with pain, such as vomiting, pallor, breathing difficulty or reluctance to use a limb. Chronic pain may cause the child to become quiet, unwilling to move and withdrawn. Digestive pain may occur during peristalsis, which means it would occur at regular times every few minutes, with periods of no pain between. Observing the child when in pain will not only indicate the presence of pain but will give important clues that the doctor can use as part of the medical diagnosis, and therefore implement the appropriate treatment.

### Pain management

Drug therapy is central to pain management. **Analgesia** (an = without, algesia = increased sensitivity to pain, thus 'without sensitivity to pain') is the absence of pain *without* causing loss of consciousness or loss of touch sensation. Two major groups of analgesic drugs: the **opioids** and the **non-steroidal anti-inflammatory** (**NSAI**). They work in different ways, not only in the mechanism of action but also in the location of action within the nervous system. NSAI drugs act in the tissues where pain originates, i.e. they work *peripherally*, while opioids work in the brainstem and spinal cord, i.e. they work *centrally*.

#### *Non-steroidal anti-inflammatory (NSAI) analgesic drugs (Table 12.1)*

**Linoleic acid** is a natural fat-based component of the diet which is converted to **arachidonic acid**, an important part of cell membrane **phospholipids**. Arachidonic acid can be recovered from cell membranes when required, since arachidonic acid is the basic substance (or **substrate**) from which other substances are made (Figure 12.2).

One class of these other substances is **prostanoids**, chemicals that include **prostacyclins**, **prostaglandins** and **thromboxanes**. These act similarly to hormones, mostly locally but sometimes systemically. Unlike hormones, these will only be produced if required. When they are produced, they bind to specific receptors causing tissue changes, similar to hormones but generally close to where they are produced. Prostacyclins cause local **vasodilation**. Thromboxane $A_2$ does the opposite, causing **vasoconstriction**. Prostaglandins have many local and widespread effects, including **prostaglandin E** (**PGE**) which is pro-inflammatory and is an important pain mediator, increasing the sensitivity of nociceptors to other pain mediators, i.e. lowering the threshold to pain (see page 249). It also causes fever (see *antipyretic drugs*, Chapter 1, Figure 1.15, page 18).

Production of these from arachidonic acid requires the enzyme **cyclo-oxygenase** (**COX**) (Chapter 1, Figure 1.15), which occurs in two forms: **COX-1** and **COX-2**. COX-1 is found in most cells for much of the time, i.e. it is *constitutive*, forming part of the constituents of the cells. COX-2 is found in inflammatory cells when activated during inflammation, i.e. it is *induced*, being produced only when required. **Non-steroidal anti-inflammatory** (**NSAI**) drugs (Table 12.1) work by blocking (or inhibiting) COX-1 in peripheral tissues, including the site of pain. The best-known drug in this group is **aspirin** (**acetylsalicylic acid**), which causes irreversible blockage of COX-1, preventing the formation of the prostaglandin pain mediators.

*Table 12.1* The NSAI analgesic drugs

| Drug | Some possible side effects | Uses and other notes |
|---|---|---|
| Acetylsalicylic acid (Aspirin) | Oral use: Dyspepsia, gastric bleeding, skin reactions, tinnitus,[3] vertigo. | Mild to moderate pain and migraine. It has anticoagulation properties and can cause bleeding. With or without codeine. With or without paracetamol. |
| Aceclofenac | Diarrhoea, nausea, dizziness, skin reactions. | Pain and inflammation. |
| Celecoxib | Cough, diarrhoea, dyspnoea, fluid retention, skin reactions. | Pain and inflammation associated skeletal disorders. |
| Dexketoprofen | Diarrhoea, nausea, vomiting, anxiety, dizziness, skin reactions. | Mild to moderate pain. |
| Diclofenac potassium | Poor appetite, diarrhoea, dizziness, nausea, vertigo. | Mild to moderate pain. |
| Diclofenac sodium | Poor appetite, diarrhoea, skin reactions, vertigo, vomiting. | Pain and inflammation. With or without misoprostol. |
| Etodolac | Blood disorders, confusion, constipation, drowsiness, nausea, insomnia, tremor, nervousness, skin reactions. | Pain and inflammation. Extensive list of possible side effects. |
| Etoricoxib | Constipation, dizziness, hypertension, palpitations, skin reactions, oedema. | Pain and inflammation. Risk of serious side effects in the elderly. |
| Felbinac | Gastrointestinal disturbance, skin and photosensitivity reactions, bronchospasm. | Pain in musculoskeletal conditions. |
| Flurbiprofen | Blood disorders, drowsiness, diarrhoea, fatigue, vertigo, skin and photosensitivity reactions, bronchospasm. | Pain and inflammation. Extensive list of possible side effects. |
| Ibuprofen | Gastrointestinal disturbance, skin reactions. | Pain and inflammation. |
| Indometacin (Indomethacin) | Blood disorders, poor appetite, confusion, anxiety, cardiac problems, nausea. | Moderate to severe pain. Extensive list of possible side effects. |
| Ketoprofen | Diarrhoea, skin reactions, nausea. | Pain and inflammation. Low incidence of side effects. |
| Mefenamic acid | Blood and bone marrow disorders, drowsiness, dyspnoea, insomnia, skin reactions, tinnitus, nausea. | Pain and inflammation. Extensive list of possible side effects. |
| Meloxicam | Constipation, vomiting, gastrointestinal disturbance. | Pain and inflammation. |
| Nabumetone | Constipation, tinnitus, gastrointestinal disturbance. | Pain and inflammation in skeletal conditions. |

| Drug | Some possible side effects | Uses and other notes |
|---|---|---|
| Naproxen | Blood disorders, drowsiness, dyspnoea, skin reactions, tinnitus, nausea, vertigo, gastrointestinal disturbance, visual disturbance. | Pain and inflammation in musculoskeletal conditions. With or without esomeprazole. Extensive list of possible side effects. |
| Piroxicam | Hypoglycaemia, confusion, palpitations, blurred vision, | Pain in musculoskeletal conditions. |
| Sulindac | Acute psychosis, blood and gastrointestinal disorders, visual disturbance, vomiting. | Pain and inflammation. Extensive list of possible side effects. |
| Tenoxicam | Constipation, nausea, skin reactions, vomiting, fatigue. | Pain and inflammation. |
| Tiaprofenic acid | Blood disorders, drowsiness, dyspnoea, skin reactions, visual disturbance, vertigo. | Pain and inflammation. Extensive list of possible side effects. |

**Indomethacin** (a derivative of **indole acetic acid**) inhibits COX-1. **Diclofenac** (derived from **phenyl acetic acid**) and **naproxen** (derived from **proprionic acid**) inhibit COX-1 and COX-2 equally. **Nabumetone** (derived from **naphthylacetic acid**) blocks COX-2 specifically. Naproxen and nabumetone are used mainly for skeletal pain. Selectivity for COX-2 means that nabumetone improves gastric tolerance when given by mouth, gastric intolerance being a problem for the COX-1 inhibitors.

These drugs are also **anti-inflammatory** and reduction of inflammation is important in pain relief. The NSAI drugs are often marketed as tablets that have a combination of several drugs and sometimes have **caffeine** as this may enhance their analgesic property.

NSAI drugs are good for controlling mild pain, but severe pain requires a stronger analgesia.

*Non-opioid analgesics*

**Paracetamol** (**acetaminophen**), is a popular analgesic. It acts in the periphery (i.e. the tissues) and centrally in the brain and cord. In the brain the mechanism of action is complex and still unclear. It interrupts a number of pain nociceptive systems from the spinal cord, through the thalamus and onto the cerebral cortex.

In the tissues paracetamol is a weak inhibitor of both COX-1 and COX-2. Some metabolites of arachidonic acid caused by the action of COX are **hydroperoxides**, and these further stimulate COX to produce more cytokines. Paracetamol blocks this feedback pathway, inhibiting COX indirectly by stopping the activity of hydroperoxides. Paracetamol is particularly active in the brain, where it has an analgesic and antipyretic effects, i.e. reducing high body temperatures (Chapter 1). It has no anti-inflammatory effects (Waller *et al.* 2009).

**Nefopam hydrochloride** is taken orally and treats moderate pain. It has anti-nociceptive effects (blocks pain transmission), and anti-hyperalgesia effects (i.e. reduces the perception of pain) when active in the brain and spinal cord.

*The opioid drugs (Table 12.2)*

**Opium**, the natural product of the opium poppy plant, is a powerful analgesic and psychoactive drug. It is used in pain management and sedation. It was used in the last century

*Table 12.2* The opioid analgesics

| Drug | Some possible side effects | Uses and other notes |
|---|---|---|
| Buprenorphine | Anxiety, diarrhoea, tremor, depression. | Moderate to severe pain. Opioid receptor partial agonist.[4] |
| Co-codamol | Blood disorders, irritability, restlessness. | Combination of codeine phosphate and paracetamol. Moderate to severe pain. |
| Codeine phosphate | Hypothermia, mood changes, postural hypotension. | Moderate to severe pain. Alone or with paracetamol (as co-codamol). |
| Diamorphine hydrochloride (Heroin hydrochloride) | Mood changes, postural hypotension. | Acute pain. |
| Dihydrocodeine tartrate | Painful urination, mood changes, postural hypotension. | Moderate to severe pain. With or without paracetamol. |
| Dipipanone hydrochloride with cyclizine | Blood disorders, dry throat, mood changes, tremor, hypotension, blurred vision. | Acute pain. |
| Fentanyl | Hyper or hypotension, respiratory disorders, visual disturbance. | Chronic intractable pain. |
| Hydromorphone hydrochloride | Anxiety, poor appetite, sleep disturbance. | Severe pain in cancer. |
| Meptazinol | Diarrhoea, gastrointestinal discomfort, hypotension. | Moderate to severe pain. |
| Morphine | Mood changes, poor appetite, insomnia, gastrointestinal discomfort. | Acute and chronic pain. |
| Oxycodone hydrochloride | Anxiety, diarrhoea, insomnia, malaise, poor appetite, memory loss. | Moderate to severe pain. With or without naloxone. |
| Pentazocine | Blood disorders, chills, mood changes, fainting, muscle ache, seizures. | Moderate to severe pain. |
| Pethidine hydrochloride | Painful urination, hypotension, hypothermia. | Acute pain. |
| Tapentadol | Anxiety, poor appetite, diarrhoea, sleep disturbance, tremor. | Moderate to severe pain. |
| Tramadol hydrochloride | Fatigue, postural hypotension, dyspnoea. | Moderate to severe pain. With or without paracetamol. With or without dexketoprofen. |

as **tincture of opium** (i.e. **laudanum**), which contains **morphine**, an opium derivative. Laudanum is not used now, but morphine is still used, along with other opium drug derivatives.

The opioids work *centrally*, i.e. within the central nervous system (CNS). They bind to special receptors within the brain and cord to provide analgesia at the spinal cord level (**spinous analgesia**) or brainstem level (**supra-spinous analgesia**, i.e. above the spine). There are three main receptors in the CNS that bind opioid drugs: the **mu (μ)**, **kappa (κ)** and **delta (δ)** receptors. These are **metabotropic**, i.e. thy change the metabolism of the cell (Blows 2022: 61–63). The mu receptor is found mostly in the brainstem and is mostly associated with supra-spinous analgesia, respiratory depression, euphoria and drug dependence. Morphine mostly binds to this receptor. The kappa receptor is found in the upper spinal cord and provides spinous analgesia by blocking substance P (see later mention). The importance of the delta receptor in pain control is not fully known, although its analgesic effects are less than those of the mu receptor.

The substances that bind naturally to opiate receptors are called **ligands**. All nervous system receptors have their own particular ligand. For the mu, kappa and delta receptors, the *natural* ligands are **endorphins**, **enkephalins**, **dynorphins** and **endomorphines**. Some less well-known small peptide ligands are known, such as **dermorphins** and **morphiceptins**.

Endorphins are the largest peptide molecules. Various forms are **alpha-endorphin (α)**, **beta-endorphin (β)** and **gamma-endorphin (γ)**. They are produced in the brain in response to severe pain and provide analgesia for four hours or so.

Enkephalins are smaller peptide molecules in two types: **met-enkephalin** (met = **methionine**) and **leu-enkephalin** (leu = **leucine**). They occur in the ratio of about 4 met to 1 leu. They are produced in response to mild pain and provide analgesia for around two minutes.

**Substance P** (also known as **neurokinin-1**) was identified as a facilitator for the passages of pain impulses across the synapse between neurons 1 and 2 of the pain pathways (page 250). Substance P is a pain mediator at spinal cord level. By binding to kappa receptors in the spinal cord, enkephalin inhibits the release and function of substance P, reducing pain impulses at the spinal cord level (page 251).

Dynorphins are small peptide molecules of two types: **dynorphin A** and **dynorphin B**. Endomorphins are also two types of small peptide molecules: **endomorphin-1** and **endomorphin-2**.

Receptors that naturally bind these ligands also bind the opioid drugs. These are:

1 **Morphine** is a major analgesic for pain relief. It does cause respiratory depression (page 106), nausea, vomiting and constipation as side effects. Morphine also causes a state of euphoria and some forms of mental detachment (Blows 2022), which is useful in reducing the psychological response to pain.

   Morphine has variable absorption when taken by mouth and undergoes considerable **first-pass metabolism** (Chapter 15, page 312) in the liver, making injection more efficient as a route of administration. The metabolism of morphine in the liver results in a metabolite called **morphine-6 glucuronide**, which has a greater analgesia than morphine. **Morphine-3 glucuronide** is also produced but it has no analgesic effect. Morphine glucuronides are excreted through the urine and through the biliary system to the bowel, from where the morphine component is largely reabsorbed. The duration of activity for morphine is about 3 to 4 hours.

2 **Diamorphine** (**heroin**) is an analgesic that is converted to morphine in the body, although diamorphine is more active as an analgesic than morphine. Diamorphine crosses the blood-brain barrier better than morphine and enters the brain faster, especially when given intravenously (IV). This makes it attractive as a drug of illicit use. Diamorphine is active in the body for about 2 hours.

3 **Pethidine** provides rapid but short-lasting analgesia. It is less potent than morphine, even in higher doses, but it is less constipating. Long term control of severe pain is better with other drugs than pethidine. Pethidine is metabolised in the liver to **norpethidine**, a metabolite with hallucinogenic and convulsant properties.

4  **Codeine** is made from morphine (codeine is **3-methylmorphine**) but is better absorbed when given by mouth than morphine, although it has only about 20% of the analgesic effect. Codeine is effective for treating mild to moderate pain but is not advisable for long-term use due to it causing constipation. It causes little euphoria, is rarely addictive.

5  **Fentanyl** is similar to, but shorter-lasting, than morphine and is available in transdermal skin patches for the prevention of '*breakthrough*' pain, i.e. transient periods of pain occurring whilst on other analgesics. **Hydromorphone** has a similar efficacy to morphine but with fewer side effects, especially nausea and vomiting.

Opioid dosage must be accurately calculated to combine a complete pain-free state without excessive drug administration. Finding the right dosage level is called **titration**. Opioid drug titration is defined as *calculating the least amount of the drug required in circulation to achieve full analgesia*. Opioid titration relies on feedback from the patient on their pain status, and this is where a pain assessment scale is of value. If they are still in pain, then they require more analgesia. Each additional dose is less than the previous doses, and these 'top-up doses' are given until a pain-free state is achieved.

Side effects of opioids must be considered, especially **respiratory depression**, i.e. reduced breathing caused by opioid drugs binding to respiratory centre receptors in the brainstem. Respiratory depression is particularly dangerous in the elderly due to reduced lung capacity and in those with pre-existing respiratory disease. Drug addiction would not normally apply to this situation. Giving opioids to treat pain is less likely to cause addiction unless the drugs are used for many weeks or months. Opioid addiction occurs when the drugs are administered to individuals who are already pain-free.

In those patients where further treatment options are not an option, the term **palliative care** is used. Palliative care indicates the management of symptoms, such as pain and nausea, so that the patient can live their remaining life in comfort. Drug addiction is not a concern, but care must be taken to prevent respiratory depression or accidental drug overdose.

### The analgesic ladder and adjuvant therapy

In 1986 the **World Health Organization** (**WHO**) introduced the concept of a 3-step approach to pain management in cancer, known as the 'analgesic ladder' (Figure 12.11; Anekar and Cascella 2022, Vargas-Schaffer 2010).

- *Step 1*: The baseline treatment to start with is a *non-opioid* drug, e.g. a **non-steroidal anti-inflammatory** agent, with or without **adjuvant therapy** (see more later). Such non-opioid drugs include aspirin, paracetamol or ibuprofen.
- *Step 2*: If pain persists or increases, an **opioid drug** suitable for moderate pain is introduced, with or without the NSAI drug or adjuvant therapy. Such opioid drugs include codeine, dihydrocodeine, pentazocine, dipipanone (not suitable for palliative care) and oxycodone.
- *Step 3*: If pain continues to persist or increase, a stronger opioid drug is introduced, i.e. one reserved for severe pain. These are morphine, diamorphine, pethidine, methadone or fentanyl (see page 261). The addition of the NSAI and adjuvant therapy remains an option. This is pursued until the patient is pain-free.

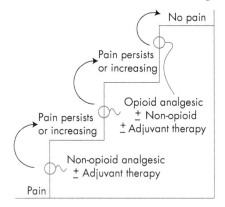

*Figure 12.11* The 1986 original 3-step analgesic ladder. If pain persists or increases, the next level of analgesia must be attained.

Source: Redrawn from Tobias and Hochhauser (2010)

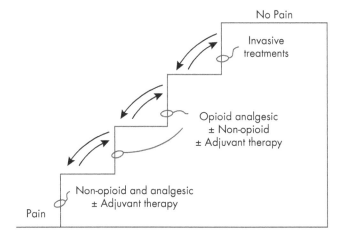

*Figure 12.12* Revised analgesic ladder. A new fourth level involves invasive steps to control pain, plus the concept of reversing the process back to earlier steps if the pain reduces.

In all cases, drugs must be given:

- in a dose sufficient to induce a pain-free state
- regularly, not on demand
- with a warning about potential side effects
- in conjunction with adjuvant therapy as required.

A modified 4-step analgesic ladder was proposed that would take the process in both directions and possibly include invasive surgery (Figure 12.12; Anekar and Cascella 2022).

**Adjuvant therapy** – or co-analgesics – include a range of drugs that are not associated with analgesia but indirectly aid with pain relief. They include tricyclic antidepressants (e.g. amitriptyline and nortriptyline), serotonin and norepinephrine reuptake inhibitors

(SNRIs; e.g. duloxetine and venlafaxine), anticonvulsants (e.g. gabapentin and pregabalin), topical anaesthetics (e.g. lidocaine patches), corticosteroids and cannabinoids.

Non-drug treatments for pain consist of a range of possibilities, from simple massage techniques to surgery. The following is a summary of therapies available:

1  Local **radiotherapy**, which can relieve symptoms, including pain.
2  **Epidural infusion** of local anaesthetic, given slowly via an infusion pump. Infusions are into the **epidural space**, a space outside the **dura mater** (page 238), and they may be continuous or intermittent. Effectiveness is only for a few weeks, after which tolerance becomes a problem. It is good for acute pain control without paralysis or disturbance of the autonomic nervous system.
3  **Transcutaneous electrical nerve stimulation** (**TENS**) is an electrical apparatus for delivery of a small charge across the skin surface for pain relief. It is effective, being used in midwifery during labour. The analgesic effect comes on about 20 minutes after starting and continues for a significant period after use. There are no important side effects. Limitations of use are:

   • not to be used near the eye or over the heart if the patient has had a heart complication
   • not to be used on the head or neck in epileptic patients
   • used with caution in pregnancy and under medical advice
   • not to be used near cardiac pacemakers, electrocardiographs (ECG) or electroencephalogram (EEG) machines when these are in use as TENS can interfere with their function. How TENS works is not known, but it may induce the closure of the spinal gate to pain (see *gate theory of pain*, page 252).

4  Massage and **aromatherapy**.
5  **Acupuncture**, the Chinese art of inserting needles to relieve pain. Like TENS, the way acupuncture works is unknown, but it may prevent the flow of pain impulses through the gate control mechanism. It may also release hormones from the endocrine system, stimulate the immune system, release antibodies and increase the body's resistance to inflammation (L. Zhang-Lheureux, personal communication).
6  **Psychological support**, i.e. staying with the patient, comforting them, distracting their attention away from the pain, e.g. reading to them. Distraction, like television or favourite games, are particularly useful with children in pain.
7  **Nerve block** is carried out by injecting parts of the sensory nerves (e.g. the **dorsal root**) or sympathetic nerves with phenol or alcohol, thus blocking pain sensations. The destruction of the nerve by the chemical is irreversible, so the procedure is not carried out until other avenues have been tried.
8  **Surgery** is a last resort because it is also irreversible. The aim is to permanently divide the pain pathways and therefore stop the passage of pain impulses.

New approaches to pain control include drugs which sedate the brain pathways that would otherwise amplify the perception of pain, as well as reducing brain activity related to pain anticipation and treating depression which also amplifies pain.

*Patient-controlled analgesia (PCA)*

Self-administration of the potent opioids in hospitals and hospices has provided the patients with a more consistent pain relief. The analgesia is delivered by a PCA pump (or

*Table 12.3* Red and amber flag warnings of deteriorating pain condition

⚑ **Red Flag = serious situation which needs urgent medical attention.**

⚑ **Amber Flag = important to get a medical assessment as soon as possible.**

| Flag warning | Details |
|---|---|
| ⚑ Red Flag | **Severe abdominal pain made worse when coughing.**<br>**Sudden onset of chest pain, radiating down the left arm or into the jaw, with sweating.**<br>**Headache associated with fever, vomiting and/or photophobia, skin rash, hypertension or neck stiffness/pain.**<br>**Testicular pain.** |
| ⚑ Amber Flag | **Any unexplained abdominal pain, especially in pregnancy or associated with inability to pass urine.**<br>**Migraine lasting longer than 3 days with no response to treatment.**<br>**Neck pain with any neurological signs e.g. numbness or tingling in extremities.** |

(After Hill-Smith and Johnson 2021, with permission)

**syringe driver**) attached to an intravenous (IV) or subcutaneous line. This is a cannula in a vein (IV) or under the skin (subcutaneous), usually in the arm, connected to a delivery system. On the end is a syringe driver or PCA pump. The pump houses a syringe containing the analgesia, and by operating a switch the pump pushes a controlled dose of a drug along the line into the patient. Once operated by the patient, the pump usually provides a 'lockout' period, perhaps about five minutes, during which the patient cannot operate it again. After the 'lockout' period, the pump is again ready for use. Patients can therefore keep pain under control according to their own needs. The drug and dose are prescribed by the doctor and prepared by the pharmacy, so the nurse has only to set up the pump and change the syringe when empty.

A PCA regime may consist of intravenous morphine or subcutaneous diamorphine. Diamorphine is the drug of choice because its higher rate of solubility than morphine allows adequate dosages to be delivered in smaller fluid volumes.

Different clinical settings and consultants may set up PCA in different ways, and staff must become familiar with the regime and delivery method used in their area.

## Key points

- Acute pain is recently occurred and of short duration. Chronic pain has a longer duration.
- Intractable pain is chronic pain without a detectable cause.
- Localised pain is often caused by inflammation of the tissues involved.
- Pain mediators are released at the site, e.g. histamine, prostaglandins and bradykinins.

### Pain pathways

- Nociceptors are pain nerve endings occurring in two types: mechanoreceptors and polymodal receptors.
- Two types of sensory nerve pathways carry pain impulses to the brain: fast Aδ fibres and slower C fibres.

- The Aδ and C fibres are the first neurons of a 3-neuronal system from the periphery to the brain.
- The gate control theory describes a pain-blocking process in the spinal cord.
- The thalamic response to pain is to activate movement to overcome pain.

*Pain assessment*

- Pain assessment scales are: verbal descriptor, visual analogue, pain behaviour and biometric scales.
- Referred pain occurs some distance away from the site of the cause.

*Analgesia*

- Analgesia is the absence of pain without causing loss of consciousness or loss of touch sensation.
- Two major groups of analgesics are the opioids and the non-steroidal anti-inflammatory (NSAI).
- NSAI drugs act in the peripheral tissues, while opioids work centrally in the brainstem and cord.
- Opioid drugs bind to the mu (μ), kappa (κ) and delta (δ) receptors within the brain and cord.
- The opioid receptors mu, kappa and delta bind the naturally produced endogenous opioids: endorphins, enkephalins, dynorphins, endomorphines, dermorphins and morphiceptins.
- Morphine is the major potent opioid drug for pain relief. It can cause respiratory depression, nausea, vomiting and constipation.
- Opioid drug titration is defined as calculating the least amount of the drug required in circulation to achieve full analgesia.
- Respiratory depression is particularly dangerous in the elderly due to reduced lung capacity and in those with pre-existing respiratory disease.
- A 3-step approach to pain management is known as the 'analgesic ladder'.
- Adjuvant therapy is non-drug treatment for pain, e.g. TENS, acupuncture, aromatherapy, nerve block and surgery.
- Patient-controlled analgesia (PCA) is delivered by means of a PCA pump (or syringe driver) attached to an intravenous (IV) or subcutaneous line.

## Notes

1 $TRPV_1$ is *transient receptor potential cation channel subfamily V member 1* gene at locus 17p13.2. This means that the gene is on the short arm of the 17th chromosome at the 13.2 site.
2 Allicin (diallylthiosulfinate) is found in garlic, giving garlic its characteristic smell and taste.
3 Tinnitus: a constant sound in the ears, e.g. buzzing or ringing.
4 See Chapter 15 for the definitions of agonist, partial agonist and antagonist.

## References

Anekar A.A. and Cascella M. (2022) WHO analgesic ladder [Updated 2022 Nov 15], in *StatPearls* [Internet]. StatPearls Publishing, Treasure Island, FL. www.ncbi.nlm.nih.gov/books/NBK554435/ (Accessed 16th February 2023).

Blows W.T. (2022) *The Biological Basis of Mental Health* (4th edition). Routledge, Abingdon.

Brown J.E., Chatterjee N., Younger J. and Mackey S. (2011) Towards a physiology-based measure of pain: Patterns of human brain activity distinguish painful from non-painful thermal stimulation. *PLoS ONE, 6*(9): e24124. http://doi.org/10.1371/journal.pone.0024124 (Accessed 15th February 2023).

Clancy J. and McVicar A. (1998) Homeostasis: The key concept to physiological control (neurophysiology of pain). *British Journal of Theatre Nursing, 7*(10): 19–27.

D'Costa K. (2011) The ways we talk about pain. *Scientific American*. http://blogs.scientificamerican.com/anthropology-in-practice/2011/09/27/the-ways-we-talk-about-pain/?WT_mc_id=SA_CAT_MB_20110928 (Accessed 15th February 2023).

Demming A. (2022) How can you measure someone's pain? In pain, special report. *New Scientist, 256*(3413): 43–44 (Accessed 19th November 2022).

Gubrud P., Carno M. and Bauldoff G. (2019) *LeMone and Burke's Medical-Surgical Nursing, Clinical Reasoning in Patient Care* (7th edition). Pearson Education, Prentice Hall, NJ.

Hill-Smith I. and Johnson G. (2021) *Little Book of Red Flags*. National Minor Illness Centre, Bedfordshire.

Lawton G. (2022) The third type of pain, in pain, special report. *New Scientist, 256*(3413): 41 (Accessed 19th November 2022).

Manchester Triage Group (1997) Pain assessment as part of the triage process, in Mackway-Jones K. (ed.) *Emergency Triage*. British Medical Journal Publishing Group, London.

Meijler W.J. (2006) Nociception and sensitisation. *Nederlands Tijdschrift Voor Tandheelkunde, 113*(11): 433–436.

Osborne-Crowley L. (2022) What is chronic pain? In pain, special report. *New Scientist, 256*(3413): 42 (Accessed 19th November 2022).

Sutherland S. (2022) What is pain? In pain, special report. *New Scientist, 256*(3413): 38–39 (Accessed 19th November 2022).

Tobias J. and Hochhauser D. (2010) *Cancer and Its Management* (7th edition). Wiley-Blackwell, Oxford.

Vargas-Schaffer G. (2010) Is the WHO analgesic ladder still valid? Twenty-four years of experience. *Canadian Family Physician; Medecin de famille canadien, 56*(6): 514–517, e202–205.

Waller D.G., Renwick A.G. and Hillier K. (2009) *Medical Pharmacology and Therapeutics* (3rd edition). W.B. Saunders, Edinburgh and London.

Wood S. (2002) Special focus: Pain. *Nursing Times, 98*(38): 41–44.

# 13 Neurological observations (III)
## Eyes

- Introduction
- Visual disturbance
- Basic eye observations
- Further visual neurobiology
- Further eye observations
- Key points
- Notes
- References

## Introduction

Observations of the eyes can provide important information concerning pathological changes taking place in the brain. The eyes have both motor and sensory components.

### The visual system

The sensory component of vision is the pathway extending from the retina posteriorly into the brain. Light passes through the **pupil** at the front of the eye and falls on to the **retina** at the back (Figure 13.1). The light-sensitive retina at the back of the eye is the only part of the nervous system visible from the outside world.

The majority of light falls on that part of the retina that lies directly opposite the pupil: the **macula**, the central part of which is the **fovea**. The fovea has the greatest concentration of daylight-sensitive cells, the **cones**. The straight line from the pupil to the retina is known as the **visual axis**. Cones produce nerve impulses in response to daylight and colour, unlike the other type of light-sensitive cells, the **rods**, which create impulses in response to low light levels and black and white stimuli. Just off-centre to the macula, i.e. a little divergent from the visual axis, is the **optic disc** (Figure 13.2), the area where the retina attaches to the **optic nerve** (Figure 13.1). This nerve is the sensory pathway of vision from the eye: the second cranial nerve (cranial nerve II), which passes posteriorly through the rear of the orbit into the brain.

DOI: 10.4324/9781003389118-13

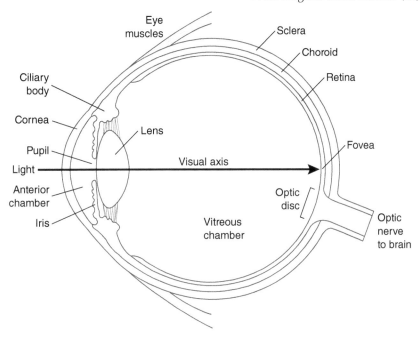

*Figure 13.1* Section through the eye.

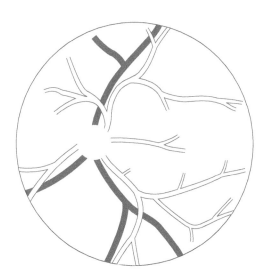

*Figure 13.2* View of the retina through an ophthalmoscope showing a normal optic disc.

The left and right optic nerves converge at the **optic chiasma** (Figure 13.3). By the definition of the word nerve, i.e. neurons *outside* the brain and cord, the visual neurons are called the optic nerves *only* from the retina to the chiasma. Neurons from the chiasma to the visual cortex are *within* the brain; therefore, they are *pathways* or *tracts*.

The optic chiasma is the point where 50% of the fibres cross to the opposite side (crossover = **decussation**) (Figure 13.3). The **temporal** (outer) half of each retina generates

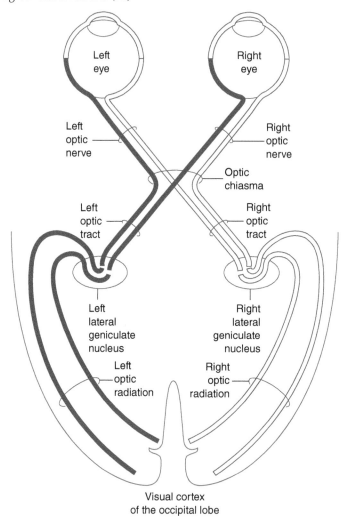

Left
eye

Right
eye

Left
optic
nerve

Right
optic
nerve

Optic
chiasma

Left
optic
tract

Right
optic
tract

Left
lateral
geniculate
nucleus

Right
lateral
geniculate
nucleus

Left
optic
radiation

Right
optic
radiation

Visual cortex
of the occipital lobe

*Figure 13.3* Superior view of the optic pathways.

impulses that remain *ipsilateral*, i.e. they remain on the same side as they originated from without crossing over, whereas the **nasal** (inner) half of each retina generates impulses that decussate, i.e. they cross to the opposite side in the chiasma. The result is that each half of the brain, both left and right, receives visual impulses from the temporal retina of the same side but also impulses from the nasal retina of the opposite side. But despite this, the brain interprets these signals as a normal complete visual image. From the chiasma backwards to the thalamus, the pathways are *inside* the brain and are therefore called the **optic tracts** (Figure 13.3). After the thalamus, the main pathways continue posteriorly as the **optic radiations**, and these terminate at the back of the brain in the **visual cortex** (the **V1 area**) within part of the **cerebrum** called the **occipital lobe** (Figure 13.3).

To become conscious to us, the visual stimulus must be further processed, first by the frontal lobe, then the prefrontal cortex, the anterior cingulate gyrus and finally the parietal lobe (Figure 13.4). The timing is virtually instantaneous, e.g. the visual cortex activates

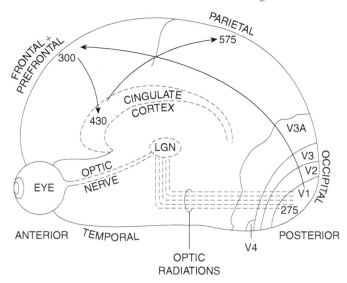

*Figure 13.4* Left side of the brain showing the pathways taken to achieve visual consciousness. Impulses from the retina of the eye arrive at the lateral geniculate nucleus (LGN) of the thalamus, then pass via the optic radiations to the visual cortex (V1) of the occipital lobe. From there, the impulses are sent to the frontal and prefrontal cortex, then to the anterior cingulate cortex and finally on to the parietal cortex. The numbers at each site indicate the time taken for the impulse to reach that site after arriving at the retina (measured in milliseconds, i.e. thousandths of a second).

within 275 milliseconds[1] (ms) of exposure to the visual stimulus. The frontal lobe activates at 300 ms, the cingulate cortex activates at 430 ms and the parietal lobe activates at 575 ms. In just over half a second, the visual stimulus becomes conscious. The retina converts light to nerve impulses that pass through the visual pathways subconsciously until they reach the visual cortex – and these other brain areas – after which we become aware of them. Of course, the visual pathways are crucial in the delivery of the impulses to the visual cortex initially, which is why **blindness** can occur from a disorder at any point along this pathway.

The area of vision we see before us constitutes the **visual field**, the centre of which falls on the visual axis and is therefore the point of our gaze. Nothing that exists outside the periphery of the visual fields can be seen without turning our eyes and head, i.e. adjustments to form new centres for our gaze.

### The motor system (movements inside and outside the eye)

The motor supply to the eye operates the three muscular aspects of vision: (1) muscle movements of the *whole* eye within the **orbit** (the eye socket); (2) the movement of the **iris** governing pupil size; and (3) the movement of the **lens** for the purpose of accommodation (focusing on objects at differing distances from the eye).

1 Movement of the whole eye is achieved by the six *striated* muscles attached to the *outside* of each eye. These muscles remain *within* the orbits. These muscles are controlled by several cranial nerves:

- **cranial nerve III**, the **oculomotor nerve**, part of which innervates four of the orbital muscles on both sides
- **cranial nerve IV**, the **trochlear nerve**, which innervates one orbital muscle on each side (the **superior oblique**)
- **cranial nerve VI**, the **abducens** nerve, which innervates one other orbital muscle on each side (the **lateral rectus**; Figure 13.5).

Cranial nerves are so-called because they come directly from the brain (i.e. *not* via the cord), with cranial nerves III, IV and VI arising in nuclei within the **brainstem** (III and IV in the **midbrain**, and VI in the **pons**). They operate a **reciprocal innervation** of the muscles (i.e. contracting one muscle while relaxing the muscle that moves in the opposite direction). This allows the eyes to both move in one direction at a time (i.e. the eye muscles are **yoked**, which means that their movements are tied together). Although this brainstem function is automatic, it can also occur at a conscious level from the cerebrum (see Chapter 11). In addition, the oculomotor nerve also operates striated muscle that elevates the upper lid.

2  Pupil size is a function of *smooth* muscle activity *inside* the eye. Pupils respond to light stimuli automatically; the smooth muscle is operated by the **autonomic nervous system** (**ANS**), which has both **sympathetic** and **parasympathetic** neurons. **Pupil constriction** is caused by the *parasympathetic* component of the oculomotor nerve,[2] which automatically innervates the iris **sphincter** muscles in response to bright light. In low light, the *sympathetic* nerves control the iris **radial dilator** muscles and automatically opens the pupil (i.e. **pupil dilation**). The sympathetic nerve supply to the smooth muscle of the iris comes from the upper thoracic spinal cord (T1 to T3, i.e. first to third thoracic vertebral level), part of the **sympathetic outflow** (Figure 13.6). Thus, the sympathetic nerve supply is a *spinal* outflow (cord and spinal nerves), while the parasympathetic nerve supply is a *cranial* outflow (medulla and cranial nerve III), a point of importance when considering pupil observations as part of head injury care.

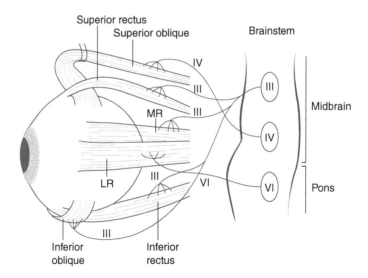

*Figure 13.5* The external (skeletal) eye muscles and their innervation from the brainstem nuclei of the cranial nerves III, IV and VI. LR: lateral rectus muscle; MR: medial rectus muscle.

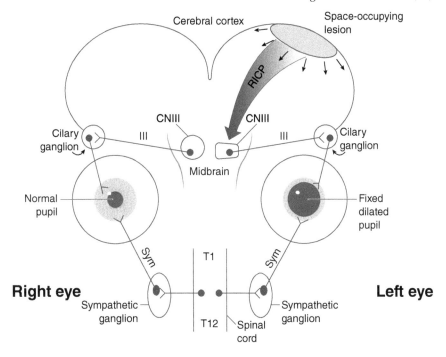

*Figure 13.6* Pupil size innervation in normal conditions (shown on the right side of the brain) and in head injury (shown on the left side of the brain). The parasympathetic supply that constricts the pupil comes via the third cranial nerve (III) from the cranial nerve III nuclei (CNIII) in the midbrain. They reach the pupil via the ciliary ganglion. The sympathetic (sym) supply to the eye that dilates the pupil comes from the thoracic spinal cord; the sympathetic emerges from the cord between vertebrae T1 and T12 via the sympathetic ganglion. Raised intracranial pressure (RICP) comes from a space-occupying lesion and compresses the nucleus on the same side, causing an ipsilateral fixed dilated pupil.

3  The *parasympathetic* component of the oculomotor nerve (cranial nerve III) also controls **accommodation**. This is the process of stretching or relaxing the suspensory smooth muscles that control the shape of the lens for the purpose of focusing on objects that are different distances from the eye. The **near point** is the closest an object can get to the eye and remain in focus, and the eye should be able to focus on an object from this point to infinity.

### Visual disturbance

Opacity of the lens, called a **cataract**, will prevent light from entering the posterior chamber of the eye. The lens is normally made from clear cells to allow light through, but they are unable to receive a direct blood supply since blood entering the lens would mean that we would see the world through a volume of blood, giving us a permanent red view of the world. This would obviously be disadvantageous for us as well as unpleasant, so these cells must remain crystal clear and acquire their nutrients and oxygen via a pass-along system. In this system, the cells at the edges collect what is needed from the blood and pass it, cell by cell, to all the others in the lens. Waste products flow in the opposite direction. Failure of this transport mechanism, as can occur in old age or exposure to prolonged radiation from the sun, leads to the milky opacity seen in cataracts. This is an observable sign that the cells are not getting adequate nutrients or oxygen and are dying. Cataracts are still a common cause of blindness, especially in developing countries, despite the fact that the relatively simple surgery of cataract removal can restore sight quickly.

**Glaucoma** is becoming better understood, not just as a disturbance of vision with acute eye pain caused by raised **intraocular pressure** (**IOP**), but by the fact that beneath these symptoms hides a neurodegenerative disorder affecting retinal cells and their axons (Vasudevan *et al.* 2011). Raised IOP (i.e. the fluid inside the front of the eye) builds up in volume and then stretches the front of the eye, and this a major risk factor in causing retinal degeneration. Patients complain not only of the severe pain, but of seeing distorted images surrounded by a halo of light. The urgent treatment is to administer drops to constrict the pupil (see page 276) to improve drainage of the front chamber of the eye. Long-term treatment may require laser or surgery to improve the drainage of the fluid. A good account of the treatment options can be found on the National Health Service website (NHS 2021).

Damage or death of cells in the retina, as may occur from looking directly at the sun or from detachment of the retina from the inner wall of the eye, can impair vision. Anything that interrupts the function of the optic nerve, such as pressure from a tumour or injury, will block impulses from the retina from reaching the brain. Inside the brain, similar tumour growths, bleeding (as in strokes) or trauma from head injuries can disrupt the pathways from the optic chiasma to the thalamus or from the thalamus to the visual cortex of the occipital lobe. The visual cortex itself can be affected by intracranial bleeds, infarcts or direct injury causing trauma to the cells that interpret what we see. It seems odd that loss of vision can be the result of a blow to the back of the head. Some blind patients report only a partial visual loss, which could be a reduction in the ability to see light across the entire visual field, or it may be a narrowing of the field itself. Defects of the visual fields can be detected on examination or reported by the patient. **Tunnel vision** is one such defect, where the peripheral aspects of the fields are gradually or suddenly lost; the patient only sees what is on or close to the visual axis.

## Basic eye observations

### Pupil size and reaction to light

The normal average pupillary size is about 3.5 mm, with a range from 2 to 6 mm diameter (Clark *et al.* 2006). A light shone into one eye should cause a fast constriction of the pupils in *both* eyes, a **direct reaction** in the pupil to which the light was applied and a **consensual reaction** in the opposite pupil. The opposite pupil reacts because some branches of the neuronal connections in the brainstem decussate, whereas others remain ipsilateral (Figure 13.7). The pupil size is partly governed by a **pupillary reflex**, an autonomic motor response to the sensory stimulus of light intensity falling on the retina. As noted earlier (see page 272), the reflex action to bright light is a circuit consisting of a sensory input from the retina (the optic nerve, cranial nerve II), the brainstem (midbrain) relay areas and a motor output to the pupillary muscles of the iris (the parasympathetic oculomotor nerve, cranial nerve III; Figure 13.7). Pupil size is also partly governed by optical needs; the pupil will constrict as part of the mechanism for regulating depth of focus, and under these circumstances the constriction is independent of light intensity.

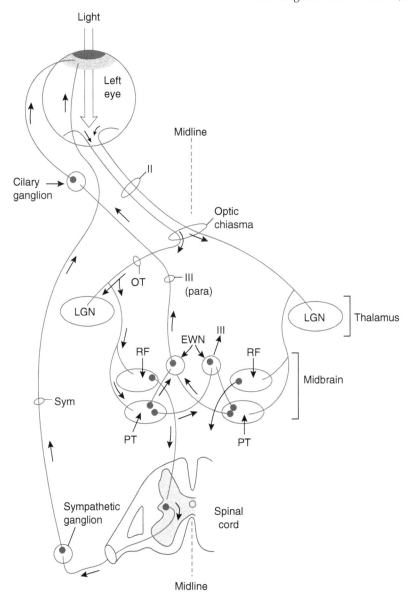

*Figure 13.7* Diagram showing detail of the pathways involved in establishing pupil size in response to light. Light enters the eye and impulses pass to the brain from the retina via the optic nerve (cranial nerve II). Medial retinal impulses cross the midline at the optic chiasma; lateral retinal impulses do not cross. Impulses then pass to the lateral geniculate nucleus (LGN) via the optic tracts (OT). Some impulses are redirected to the reticular formation (RF) and the pretectum (PT). From the pretectum, the impulses pass to the Edinger-Westphal nucleus (EWN), which is part of the cranial nerve III (oculomotor nerve) nucleus. This nerve provides parasympathetic (para) innervation to the pupil via the ciliary ganglion to cause constriction in bright light. From the reticular formation, pathways descend the spinal cord to the sympathetic output of the thoracic cord. From here, the pupil is supplied with sympathetic (sym) fibres that dilate the pupil in dull light. Only the left side is shown.

*Abnormal pupils*

Abnormal pupils are an important observation and require careful interpretation and sometimes urgent intervention. Blindness in one eye, due to causes involving the front of the eye or to the retina or the optic nerve, will mean the loss of the sensory component (the light) in the pupillary reflex response to light. Therefore, light shone in the blind eye will not affect either pupil size, but light will cause pupillary constriction in *both* eyes if it is shone in the good eye, provided the oculomotor nerve is functioning. Problems *inside* the brain that cause blindness are beyond the pupillary reflex, and the pupils should therefore still react to light.

In **pinpoint pupils** (i.e. **miotic pupils**; Figure 13.8A), pupil size is at its minimum (i.e. the pupils are just visible at 1 mm or less in diameter and are unlikely to constrict further to light). **Opiate drugs**, such as heroin, in large enough doses can cause this, and pinpoint pupils are a sign used to observe for opiate abuse. Alternatively, it may be caused by anything that obstructs the sympathetic supply to the eye, thus allowing the parasympathetic full control (e.g. spinal lesions with cervical nerve damage, causing **Horner's pupil**, or **Horner's syndrome**) (Figure 13.8D, see page 284) (Mojon and Stehberger 2005; Patel and Ilsen 2003). Pinpoint pupils may also be a feature of direct trauma to the orbit (eye socket) which is identified by other signs of orbital injury, such as bruising filling the orbit and causing swelling around the eye (a **periorbital haematoma**). Small pupils (i.e. smaller than 3 mm) are naturally going to occur in bright light and should be capable of further constriction if the light gets brighter. Bilateral small pupils that respond to light are sometimes seen in comas caused by a number of abnormal metabolic conditions, e.g. diabetic ketoacidosis or imbalance of blood electrolytes (Chapter 6), or they could be due to bilateral injury to the thalamus or hypothalamus (referred to as **bilateral diencephalic damage**). Small irregular pupils that do *not* react to light but do constrict on accommodation of close objects are called **Argyll Robertson** pupils and have long been associated with **syphilis** (a sexually transmitted infection often involving the brain) but can also be a feature of other brainstem disorders. Small or pinpoint pupils can result from the use of **miotic** drugs such as **pilocarpine** as a treatment for glaucoma (see page 274).

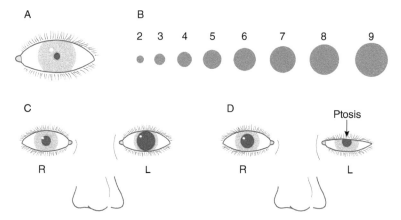

*Figure 13.8* Pupil sizes. (A) Pinpoint pupils. (B) Various sizes from 2 to 9 mm. (C) Unilateral fixed dilated pupil on the left seen in oculomotor nerve compression or damage due to raised intracranial pressure. (D) Horner's syndrome, with right dilated pupil and left ptosis.

*Table 13.1* Antimuscarinic drugs affecting pupil size

| Drug | Some possible side effects | Uses and other notes |
|---|---|---|
| Tropicamide | Eye erythema (redness), headache, blurred vision, nausea, fainting, eye pain. | Short-acting (6 hours) mydriatic eye drops used for fundoscopy. |
| Cyclopentolate hydrochloride | Some local and systemic side effects mostly seen in children and older adults, or from prolonged use. | Long acting (up to 24 hours) cycloplegic eye drops used in eye examination. |
| Atropine sulfate | Rare but occasional systemic side effects can occur. | Long acting (up to 7 days) cycloplegic eye drops used in eye examination. |

Normal average-sized pupils that, however, are *not* reacting to light indicate a failure of both components of the autonomic nervous system, and may be a feature of midbrain injury from **infarction** (a sudden loss of blood supply leading to an area of dead or dying tissue) or **herniation** (part of the brain forced out of position by internal pressure, usually downwards).

Dilation of the pupils (or **mydriasis**, 6–8 mm diameter) occurs normally in low-light conditions, but the pupils will constrict again on exposure to light (Figure 13.8). Pupil dilation can also be induced by the use of antimuscarinic **mydriatic** or **cycloplegic**[3] drugs for eye examination purposes, i.e. **fundoscopy**, the drugs dilate the pupil in order to view the back of the eye (see footnote 4; Table 13.1). **Tropicamide** is a parasympatholytic agent that dilates the pupils by blocking the parasympathetic muscarinic receptors, thus increasing the sympathetic stimulation to the eye. Cycloplegic drugs, e.g. **cyclopentolate hydrochloride** and **atropine sulfate**, are also antimuscarinic drugs that dilate the pupil by paralysing the muscles that constrict the pupil (see note 3).

Pupil dilation can also be caused by high-dosage of **amphetamines** (nervous system stimulants) and large pupils may also be due to direct orbital injuries (as with small pupils) if the trauma causes pressure on the third cranial nerve with concurrent loss of pupillary constriction.

Chapter 11 identified the abnormal changes in pupil size and reaction to light as a focal sign of **raised intracranial pressure** (**RICP**), but they could be due to other intracranial disorders. In head injury, these changes are initially a dilated pupil that is *unilateral* (on one side), *ipsilateral* (on the same side as the injury) and *fixed* (no response to light). Later (and this could be anything from minutes to hours), the fixed dilated pupil becomes *bilateral* (both sides) (Table 13.2). The time taken for the progression from unilateral to bilateral is dependent on the rate of increase in the **space-occupying lesion** (**SOL**; see Chapter 11) that is causing the increased pressure, e.g. the *extradural haematoma*, which progresses much faster than a *subdural haematoma* in head injuries (see Chapter 11). The observation made is twofold: first, identification of the size of the pupil on both sides so that equality of the left pupil with the right pupil can be assessed, and second, the pupil's reaction to light. Pupils that are widely dilated (9 mm or more in diameter) and fixed (not reacting to light) are a very serious observation, suggesting intracranial bleeding after head injury or some other SOL, such as a brain tumour or cerebral oedema and must be reported and acted upon urgently (Table 13.2). Raised intracranial pressure (RICP) from the developing SOL causes failure of the brainstem areas controlling pupil constriction

*Table 13.2* Red and amber flag warnings of deteriorating condition

℞ **Red Flag = serious situation which needs urgent medical attention.**

| Flag warning | Details |
| --- | --- |
| ℞ Red Flag | Fixed dilated pupils (unilateral then bilateral) that do not respond to light. Swelling and blackening of the eye sockets (orbits), unilateral or bilateral, such that it is difficult to open their eyes (Chapter 11). |

(After Hill-Smith and Johnson 2021 with permission)

or compression of the oculomotor nerve. This is often unilateral at first, becoming bilateral as the RICP increases, causing compression down on to the brainstem. Continued compression of the brain as the SOL gets larger will result in **coning**, a herniation of parts of the brain, especially the medulla, the lowest part of the brainstem. The herniation is usually downwards into the foramen magnum at the base of the skull. As the cardiac and respiratory centres are in the medulla, they will be compressed and both the heart and the lungs will stop functioning, with little chance of resuscitation. Fixed bilateral dilated pupils are also seen in the terminal stages of many conditions, including **cerebral ischaemia** (loss of blood supply to the brain) and severe **cerebral anoxia** (loss of oxygen to the brain), and indeed it is also the state seen after death has occurred.

### Further visual neurobiology

*Sensory pathways*

The optic tracts link the chiasma with parts of the thalamus (see Chapter 11, page 226) known as the **lateral geniculate nucleus** (**LGN**). About 10% of the visual stimulus passing along this optic tract connects with part of the **midbrain**, the **superior colliculus** (Figure 13.9).

The superior colliculus responds to retinal impulses by operating the muscles that are keeping the eye and head in a position to retain the viewed image on the fovea. It is therefore responsible for maintaining the eye's *gaze* on a subject, especially if that subject is moving. The superior colliculus is linked to the three cranial nerves operating the orbital muscles that move the eye (see page 272). These muscles are attached to the external surface of the eyeball (Figure 13.5). Gaze is a vital requirement for hunting and survival, and in lower vertebrates the superior colliculus is the main area to which *all* the retinal output goes. The fact that in humans only 10% of the pathway goes there suggests that it may be less important for us, although 10% of *human* retinal output is roughly the equivalent to the *entire* retinal output of a cat (Bear *et al.* 1996). Another area of the midbrain that receives light-induced impulses is the **pretectum**, the relay nucleus that has partial control over pupil size and some eye movements in response to light intensity. The pretectum is an intermediary link between the incoming sensory impulses from the retina and the outgoing motor impulses of the parasympathetic third cranial nerve (see page 275). Another area that receives light-induced impulses from the optic tracts is the **hypothalamus** via the **retinohypothalamic** tract (Figure 13.9). Through this pathway, the **sleep-wake cycle** is controlled by the light intensity falling on the retina and transmitted as impulses to the hypothalamus via the retinohypothalamic tracts. This cycle determines when the brain will sleep (in response to low light) and when it will awake (in response to greater light levels).

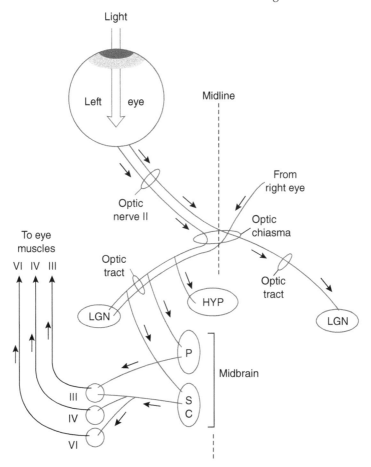

*Figure 13.9* Pathways in the brain that respond to light intensity. Nerve impulses passing down the optic nerve not only go to the lateral geniculate nucleus (LGN, on the visual pathway), but some pass to the hypothalamus (HYP), via the retinohypothalamic tract. The hypothalamus governs the sleep-wake cycle in response to light intensity. Some light also passes to the pretectum (P), which helps to control pupil size, and some goes to the superior colliculus (SC), which aids in eye movements via the cranial nerves III, IV and VI. Only the left side is shown.

The retina causes impulses to travel along the optic nerve (sensory) to the pretectum, then on to the **Edinger-Westphal nucleus**, which is part of **the third cranial nerve nucleus** in the midbrain (Figures 13.7 and 13.9). The Edinger-Westphal nucleus is the pupillary control centre and origin of the *parasympathetic* component of the oculomotor nerve. From here, the oculomotor nerve passes to the orbit, where a **synapse** occurs with the cell body of the second neurons, called the **ciliary ganglion**, before the nerve entering the iris. Neurons of the oculomotor nerve also pass from the ciliary ganglion into the **ciliary body** inside the eye, where they control suspensory *smooth* muscles that pull on the lens. The first neurons of the *sympathetic* outflow pass down the upper thoracic spinal nerves into the **sympathetic trunk** on each side of the spine and then pass up the trunk to synapse with the **superior cervical ganglion**, the cell body of the second neurons. From here, the second neurons pass up towards the head and follow the arterial pathway into the eyes.

*Motor system and eye movements*

Eye movements are essential to allow the subject of visual interest to remain on the fovea when it is stationary (**gaze holding**) or moving (**gaze shifting**) and also to respond quickly to new visual stimuli entering the visual fields. A rapid eye movement (or sudden attention change) in order to bring a new or peripheral object on to the fovea is called a **saccade**. Saccades are the fastest specialised form of *gaze shift* and can be vertical, horizontal or a combination of these. Vertical saccades are controlled by an area at the highest point of the midbrain, close to the thalamus, from where connections pass to the oculomotor and trochlear nuclei. Horizontal saccades are commanded from lower in the brainstem, close to the pons (Figure 13.10).

Bilateral lesions in either of these command areas, as may be possible in brainstem ischaemia or bleeds, can result in a loss of the corresponding saccade. Other gaze shifts include **smooth pursuit** (retains the image of a moving object on the fovea) and **vergence** (the eyes move in opposing directions to retain the image simultaneously on both foveae). These are conscious motor activities and are therefore controlled by specific areas of the

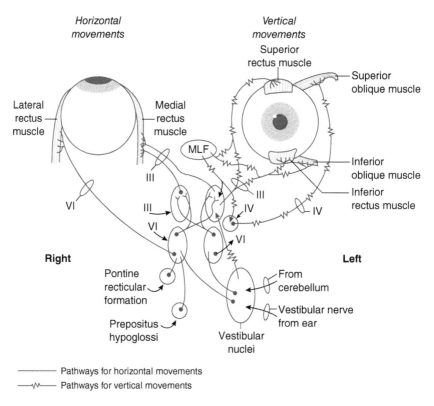

*Figure 13.10* Control of eye movements. The right side shows control of horizontal movements. Input to the cranial nerve VI nucleus is from the pontine reticular formation, the vestibular nuclei and the prepositus hypoglossi. The cranial nerve VI nucleus connects to the cranial nerve III nucleus on both sides. The left side shows control of vertical movements. Input to the cranial nerve III nucleus is from the cerebellum and vestibular nerve via the vestibular nuclei and from the medial longitudinal fasciculus (MLF), which also has direct output to the superior and inferior rectus muscles.

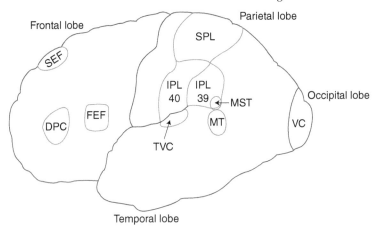

*Figure 13.11* Areas of the cerebral cortex involved in eye movement control. DPC: dorsolateral prefrontal cortex (area 46). FEF: frontal eye fields (parts of areas 4, 6, 8, 9). IPL: inferior parietal lobe (areas 39, 40). MST: medial superior temporal visual area (parts of areas 19, 37, 39). MT: mid-temporal visual areas (parts of areas 19, 37). SEF: supplementary eye fields (part of area 6). SPL: superior parietal lobe (areas 5, 7). TVC: temporal vestibular cortex (parts of areas 41, 42). VC: visual cortex (area 17).

cerebral cortex (Figure 13.11). Since they are in response to visual sensory stimuli, neuronal connections occur between the sensory visual cortex in the occipital lobe and the various ophthalmic motor centres of the parietal and frontal lobes. From these centres, motor pathways descend through the basal ganglia via the superior colliculus, the gaze control centre, with output to the cranial nerve nuclei in the brainstem that govern eye muscle movement. In general, nuclei in the midbrain (cranial nerves III and IV) control vertical gaze, whereas the nucleus in the pons (cranial nerve VI) controls horizontal gaze.

The **vestibulo-ocular reflex** (**VOR**) allows for fixation of the gaze on an object during head movement and involves vestibular information from the middle ear (balance) and ocular information from the eyes (vision) working together with the cerebellum to control balance during saccades and gaze holding. VOR is discussed in Chapter 15 (Figure 15.5, page 325).

### Further eye observations

*Abnormal eye movements*

Healthcare professionals may note abnormalities of both gaze holding and gaze shift in conscious patients (but to a much lesser extent in an unconscious patient who is unable to cooperate). Abnormal gaze holding can be seen in unilateral paralysis of each of the cranial nerves that control eye muscles, and these present with the characteristic symptom of the two eyes no longer functioning together (Figure 13.12). **Diagonal diplopia** (diplopia = double vision) is seen in unilateral **cranial nerve III palsy** (paralysis of one oculomotor nerve), where the eye *on the affected side* looks 'down and out' with ptosis (see page 282) and pupil dilation, while the other eye appears normal. Unilateral **cranial nerve IV palsy** results in a **vertical diplopia**, as the eye on the affected side becomes

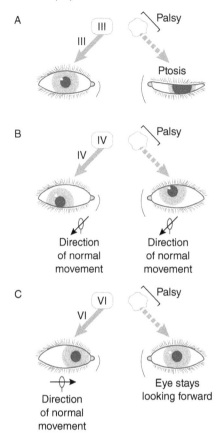

*Figure 13.12* Disturbance of eye positions in various cranial nerve palsy. (A) Cranial nerve III palsy causes the 'down and out' appearance of the affected eye with dilated pupil and ptosis of the lid. (B) Cranial nerve IV palsy causes the affected eye to have limited ability to look down when it is adducted (moved to face the nose). (C) Cranial nerve VI palsy causes the inability to abduct (move to face the ear) the affected eye when both eyes are commanded to look in that direction.

unable to look down when adducted (turned towards the nose). Unilateral **cranial nerve VI palsy** causes **horizontal diplopia** because the affected eye cannot be abducted (turned outwards; Figure 13.12).

Abnormal *gaze shift* may be seen when the patient is asked to follow the examiner's finger through a range of up, down, left and right movements. **Nystagmus** describes the involuntary rhythmic oscillations of the eyeball, a back-and-forth movement over which the patient has no control (Figure 13.13; Nebbioso *et al.* 2009). Nystagmus may occur in the horizontal, vertical, mixed or rotary directions. Two types of nystagmus have been identified: the more common *jerky* form, in which movements in one direction are faster (rapid saccade) than in the other direction or the *pendular* form, in which the movements in both directions are equal in speed. Nystagmus can be artificially induced in normal individuals by putting cold water into an ear, a procedure called a **cold caloric** test. It causes **vestibular** (= balance or equilibrium) stimulation by chilling the fluid within **the lateral semicircular canal**, part of the **labyrinth** (= cavity) of the inner ear, thus creating

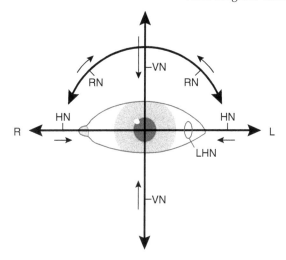

*Figure 13.13* The range of movements in nystagmus. Nystagmus has a slow movement phase (short, thin arrow) and a rapid return phase (long, thick arrow). The rapid phase arrows show the direction given for the horizontal nystagmus (HN), vertical nystagmus (VN) and rotary nystagmus (RN). It can also be a mix of these.

convection currents in this fluid. This tests the function of the pathway passing from the semicircular canals of the inner ear (the vestibular branch of cranial nerve VIII) to the brainstem and **cerebellum**, then on to the cranial nerve nuclei controlling eye movements (see page 326). The cerebellum controls balance (in response to semicircular canal activity) and both the speed and the coordination of eye saccades. **Labyrinthine vestibular nystagmus**, a rotary jerky form, may be caused by diseases of the inner ear. Other jerky forms can be caused by brainstem or cerebellar diseases or as the result of barbiturate overdose. Pendular nystagmus is usually a feature of **intraocular disease** (i.e. disorders of the retina or fluid pressures inside the eye).

### Papilloedema

**Papilloedema** is swelling of the optic disc due to oedema (Figure 13.14).

Using an **ophthalmoscope**, the retina is viewed[4] and the retinal blood vessels can be identified (Figure 13.2). These vessels spread out to all parts of the retina from a single point, the optic disc, just off-centre from the macula. The blood vessels are the **retinal arteries and veins**, the blood supply to this light-sensitive layer and they follow the optic nerve pathway between the brain and the eye. The veins are some 30% larger than the arteries, but like everywhere else, the retinal arteries carry blood at greater pressure than the veins. Papilloedema is usually caused by raised intracranial pressure (RICP; see Chapter 11). This is because the meninges surrounding the brain are continuous along the optic nerve to the optic disc, and any RICP will exist along the optic nerve and on to the disc itself. When pressure is applied to the blood vessels from RICP, the veins will tend to be occluded before the arteries, i.e. at an early stage of RICP. Blood passing along the vessels enters the retina easier via the arteries than it can leave via the veins. The RICP together with some venous congestion causes excess tissue fluid to accumulate, called oedema, at the point around the vessel entry, the optic disc. This obscures the normally obvious disc margins; they become distorted and swollen, with the disc becoming a reddish colour, i.e. visual proof of the

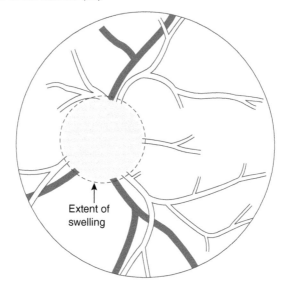

*Figure 13.14* The retina with papilloedema (swelling of the optic disc). The fluid accumulation obscures the ability to see the arteries and veins around the optic disc. Compare this with Figure 13.2.

existence of RICP. This becomes a very important visual check for RICP. It is not only carried out as part of the neurological examination of the patient but is also done to exclude the existence of RICP before a **lumbar puncture** (**LP**). A lumbar puncture is the introduction of a needle into the spinal canal below the level of **lumbar vertebra 2** (**L2**) in order to obtain a sample of **cerebrospinal fluid** (**CSF**). If RICP was present during a lumbar puncture, the sudden decompression of the cord by removing CSF could cause coning (see page 241).

*Ptosis*

The elevation of the upper eyelid is a function of the oculomotor nerve (see page 272) and incomplete opening of the upper lid is a condition called **ptosis** (or **lid lag**). It can be seen by observing the narrowed **palpebral fissure**, i.e. the gap between the upper and lower lids, when the patient is asked to open the eyes. Ptosis may be unilateral or bilateral and may be the result of oculomotor nerve or brainstem injury compression from trauma or disease, as in raised intracranial pressure. It could be part of several neurological disorders, e.g. Horner's syndrome,[5] where ptosis, constricted pupils and dry facial skin indicate the presence of a spinal cord lesion (Figure 13.7). Some drugs (e.g. the **benzodiazepines**, such as **diazepam**) may cause ptosis when given in sufficient dosage to induce sedation before minor surgical procedures.

**Key points**

*Visual anatomy*

- The optic nerve (cranial nerve II) is the sensory nerve of vision from the eye. It passes posteriorly from the retina into the brain.
- The left and right optic nerves converge at the optic chiasma.

- The optic tracts link the chiasma with the lateral geniculate nucleus (LGN), part of the thalamus.
- Ten per cent of the visual stimulus passing along this optic tract connects with the superior colliculus, part of the midbrain. This area operates the muscles that keep the eye fixed on an image, maintaining the gaze.
- The pretectum in the midbrain receives retinal impulses and has partial control over pupil size and some eye movements in response to light intensity.
- Posteriorly to the LGN, the optic radiations pass to the visual cortex, part of the occipital lobe of the cerebrum.
- Cranial nerve III (oculomotor) innervates four of the orbital muscles, cranial nerve IV (trochlear) innervates the superior oblique muscle, and cranial nerve VI (abducens) innervates the lateral rectus muscle.
- The third cranial nerve nucleus in the medulla contains the Edinger-Westphal nucleus, the pupillary constriction centre and origin of the parasympathetic component of the oculomotor nerve.
- The sympathetic supply to the iris comes from the upper thoracic spinal cord (T1 to T3) – part of the sympathetic outflow – and causes pupillary dilatation.
- The pupil size is partly due to a pupillary reflex, an autonomic motor response to the sensory stimulus of light intensity falling on the retina, and partly due to optical adjustments required for depth of focus.

### Pupils and drugs

- Miotic pupils are pinpoint, and mydriatic pupils are dilated. Miotic and mydriatic drugs can be used to close and open the pupils, respectively.
- Unilateral, followed by bilateral widely, dilated and fixed pupils may be due to intracranial bleeding after a head injury and must be reported urgently.

### Eye disorders

- A rapid eye movement or sudden attention change is called a saccade.
- Nystagmus is the rapid involuntary rhythmic back and forth movement (fast saccades) of the eyeball and may be due to vestibular (balance) disorder, intraocular diseases or barbiturate overdose.
- Diplopia is double vision.
- Papilloedema is swelling of the optic disc and is visual proof of the existence of RICP.
- Incomplete opening of the upper lid is a condition called ptosis (or lid lag).

### Notes

1 One millisecond (ms) is one-thousandth of a second.
2 The oculomotor nerve (cranial nerve III) has both motor fibres active on the muscles *outside* the eye (see page 272) and parasympathetic fibres active on muscles *inside* the eye.
3 Tropicamide contracts the iris dilator muscle, thus increasing iris dilation with corresponding widening of the pupil. Cycloplegic means the drugs paralyse (plegia = paralysis) the ciliary muscles (affecting the lens) but also paralyse the iris sphincter muscle and therefore cause pupil dilation (see also *blurred vision*, Chapter 15).
4 Known as a fundoscopic examination (fundoscopy) since the fundus is the deepest part of the eye and is part of the retina.
5 Syndrome = a collection of symptoms that tend to be present together.

## References

Bear M., Connors B. and Paradiso M. (1996) *Neuroscience: Exploring the Brain*. Williams & Wilkins, Baltimore, MD.

Clark A., Clarke T.N.S., Gregson B., Hooker P.N.A. and Chambers I.R. (2006) Variability in pupil size estimation. *Emergency Medicine Journal*, *23*(6): 440–441.

Hill-Smith I. and Johnson G. (2021) *Little Book of Red Flags*. National Minor Illness Centre, Bedfordshire, UK.

Mojon D.S. and Stehberger B. (2005) Diagnosis of Horner syndrome by pupil dilation lag. *Klinische Monatsblätter für Augenheilkunde*, *222*(3): 211–213.

National Health Service (NHS) (2021) www.nhs.uk/conditions/glaucoma/treatments/ (Accessed 16th February 2023, website due for update in February 2024).

Nebbioso M., D'Innocenzo D., Rapone S., Di Benedetto G. and Grenga R. (2009) Nystagmus in ophthalmology. *La Clinica Terapeutica*, *160*(2): 145–149.

Patel S. and Ilsen P.F. (2003) Acquired Horner's syndrome: Clinical review. *Optometry*, *74*(4): 245–256.

Vasudevan S.K., Gupta V. and Crowston J.G. (2011) Neuroprotection in glaucoma. *Indian Journal of Ophthalmology*, *59*(Suppl. 1): S102–S113.

# 14 Neurological observations (IV)

## Movement

- Introduction
- The neurology of movement
- Movement observations
- Movement losses
- Movement excesses
- The immobile patient
- Key points
- Notes
- References

## Introduction

Most movements, such as standing, walking and running, are learnt throughout child-hood, often by trial and error. Learning involves gaining neuronal connections (synapses) and neurotransmitter receptors at those synapses. Learning also requires sensory feed-back. A normal child will gain specific movement skills such talking,[1] playing a game or an instrument only after additional learning and practice. Movement does not come easy due to the complexity of the motor system.

## The neurology of movement

Muscle movement involves balance and posture, muscle tone, coordination and smoothing out of muscle activity, special skills such as synergy (see page 296) and the importance of sensory feedback. Apart from the conscious control over the obvious movements, there are many thousands of subconscious (or automatic) muscle changes and neuronal activities going on continuously, many of which make conscious movements possible.

Conscious muscle control begins with the **primary motor cortex** within the frontal lobe of the cerebrum. Cells here are the start of the **pyramidal system**, which initiates the contraction of the skeletal muscle that moves the body (Figure 14.1). The pyramidal system is so-called because it forms a pyramid shape as it passes down through the

DOI: 10.4324/9781003389118-14

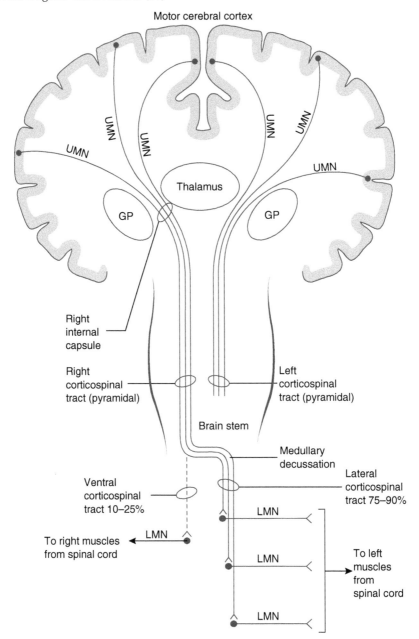

*Figure 14.1* The pyramidal tracts. The corticospinal (also known as pyramidal tracts) begin with widely distributed neuronal cell bodies within the motor cortex (which is the base of the up-side-down pyramid). Three of many thousands of motor neurons are shown on both sides. The axons collect together and pass between the globus pallidus (GP) and the thalamus at the internal capsule (the apex of the up-side-down pyramid). The fibres (70–90%) cross (decussate) to the opposite side (contralateral) in the medulla to form the lateral corticospinal tract. Ten to twenty- five per cent remain on the same side (ipsilateral) to form the ventral corticospinal tract. LMN: lower motor neuron; UMN: upper motor neuron.

brain. Consciousness suggests that each movement is purposefully thought about, but many movements are made *without* thinking. Most movements are pre-programmed and require little conscious thought. Pre-programming of movement is the essence of learning. The conscious aspect involves the ability to initiate the movement in response to sensory stimuli, to be aware of the movement as it happens and to modify the motor response according to sensory feedback. The muscle coordination, extent and smoothness of contraction, repetition of muscle action (as in running) and other features of movement are controlled at a subconscious level by the **extrapyramidal** system (extra = outside), i.e. a system outside the pyramidal system and functioning at an automatic level (see page 290).

### The pyramidal tract system

The cells of the primary motor cortex are positioned in a basic body plan (Figure 14.2). Larger surface areas with greater cell numbers occur on the cortex representing those parts where fine intricate muscle movement is required, notably the hands. The pathways descending from the motor cortex, the **pyramidal tracts**, pass through the brain down to the brainstem and onward into the cord (Figure 14.1). At the level of the medulla, about 75% of these fibres decussate – i.e. cross to the other side – and become **contralateral**, i.e. from the *opposite* side. The other 25% remain **ipsilateral**, i.e. from the same side. Since both cerebral hemispheres have a motor cortex, there are four pyramidal pathways descending the cord from the brain, two contralateral that have crossed, one from each side and two ipsilateral that have not crossed, one on each side. Neurons of the pyramidal tracts are called **upper motor neurons (UMNs)**, i.e. they extend from the brain to the cord within the **central nervous system, CNS**. The descending tracts

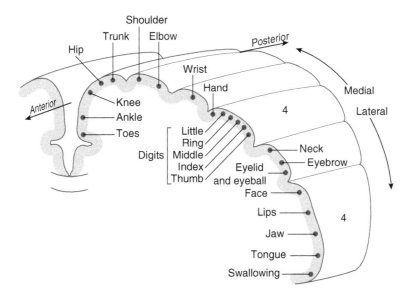

*Figure 14.2* The left main motor cortex (area 4) showing the layout of the cells according to function (i.e. the muscle they control). Notice the large area controlling finger and hand movements compared with the area for feet and toes, which indicates great manual dexterity.

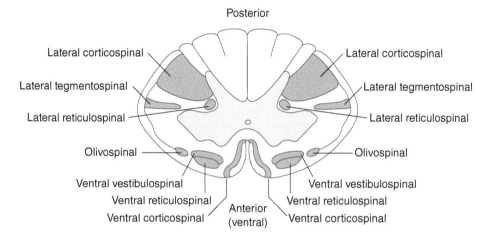

*Figure 14.3* Superior view of a cross section of the spinal cord showing the motor pathways within the white matter of the cord.

pass down the spinal cord in specific positions within the **white matter** (Figure 14.3). The fibres enter the anterior **grey matter** of the cord, where they synapse with other neurons at all the spinal levels, i.e. from high in the cervical (neck) region to low in the sacral (pelvic) region.

**Lower motor neurons** (**LMNs**) begin with cells in the anterior grey matter of the cord, and the fibres pass via the **anterior root** of the **spinal nerve** to the voluntary skeletal muscles of the body. The LMN is therefore part of the **peripheral nervous system** (**PNS**), being a component of the spinal nerves. So, the pyramidal system is two-neuronal, i.e. consisting of a UMN (brain to cord) and an LMN (cord to muscle; Figure 14.1).

The pyramidal system also operates through some of the **cranial nerves** that control muscles of the head, face and neck. The **corticobulbar tracts** (Figure 14.4) begin as neuronal cell bodies in the head and neck areas (lateral areas) of the motor cortex (hence *cortico*). These UMN fibres pass down to nuclei in the pons and medulla of the brainstem (*note*: the pons, part of the brainstem, is called *bulbar*, i.e. shaped like a bulb). From a nucleus in the *pons*, LMN fibres become components of the **trigeminal nerve** (cranial V) and pass to the muscles of the lower jaw, e.g. for eating. Also from the *pons*, LMN fibres form part of the **facial nerve** (cranial VII) and pass to muscles of the face e.g. for facial expression. Separate *medullary* nuclei give rise to LMN fibres within the **glossopharyngeal nerve** (cranial IX), to pharyngeal muscles, the **vagus nerve** (cranial X) to muscles of the pharynx, larynx, oesophagus and soft palate and the **spinal accessory nerve** (cranial XI) to the neck muscles.

### The extrapyramidal system

This system operates skeletal muscle at the subconscious level, i.e. it controls the automatic aspects of voluntary movement. The main areas of the brain involved are parts of the brainstem i.e. nuclei of the pons and medulla, which in turn are influenced by the basal ganglia, some sensory parts of the cerebral cortex, and parts of the thalamus and cerebellum, including all their pathways and feedback circuits (Figure 14.5).

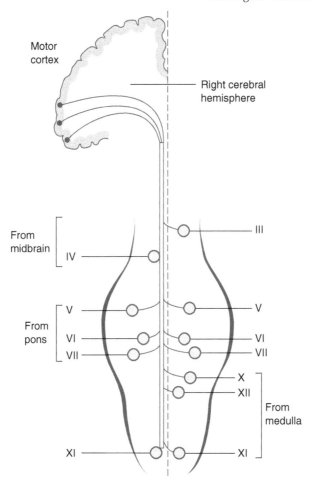

Motor
cortex

Right cerebral
hemisphere

From
midbrain

IV

III

From
pons

V

VI

VII

V

VI

VII

X

XII

From
medulla

XI

XI

*Figure 14.4* The corticobulbar tracts to the cranial nerves. This schematic diagram shows motor
pathways coming from the head and neck area of the right motor cortex (Figure 14.2)
and passing into the brainstem. The cranial nerve nuclei are indicated, showing their
brainstem locations, the corticobulbar input (unilateral or bilateral) and which ones
cross the midline. The left hemisphere (not shown) has a mirror image input.

Some pathways involved are:

1 *Primary* cells within the cerebral cortex that have fibres that end in the **red nucleus**
   within the midbrain, the **corticorubral tract**. In the red nucleus, *secondary* cells give
   rise to fibres that pass down the cord, forming the **rubrospinal tract**
2 Several nuclei towards the base of the brain are collectively called the **basal ganglia**
   (Figure 14.6). One of these nuclei, the **globus pallidus**, has *primary* cells providing
   fibres that terminate in some areas of the thalamus. From the thalamus, *secondary* cell
   fibres feed back to the motor cortex of the cerebrum, i.e. part of the basal ganglia motor
   loop (Figures 14.5 and 14.8 and see page 294)
3 Areas of the pons and medulla, known as the **reticular formation**, have *secondary* cells
   with fibres extending down the cord, creating the **reticulospinal tract**.

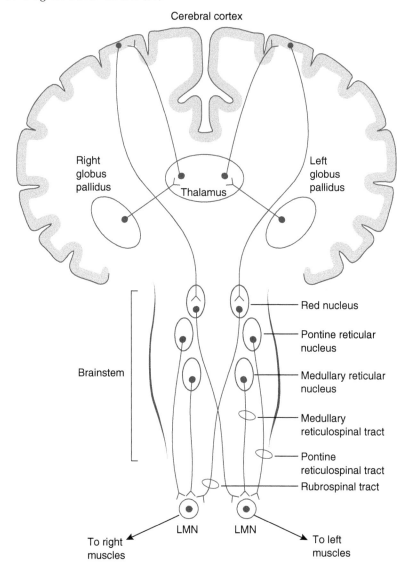

*Figure 14.5* Some extrapyramidal tracts. Pathways of the extrapyramidal system extend from the cerebral cortex to the red nucleus, and from the red nucleus to the contralateral lower motor neuron (LMN) in the cord, a pathway called the rubrospinal tract. Another pathway passes from the globus pallidus to the thalamus with feedback pathways to the cortex. Other pathways include those from the pontine nucleus to the ipsilateral LMN, called the pontine reticulospinal tract, and from the medullary reticulospinal nucleus to the LMN, called the medullary reticulospinal tract.

### The basal ganglia and thalamus

The five nuclei of the basal ganglia (Figure 14.6) have a major influence on movement, both **facilitatory** and **inhibitory** (Anderson and Kiehn 2004). Facilitatory promotes movement and inhibitory prevents movement. These nuclei have a role in slow, sustained movements and in maintaining **muscle tone** (Figure 14.7).

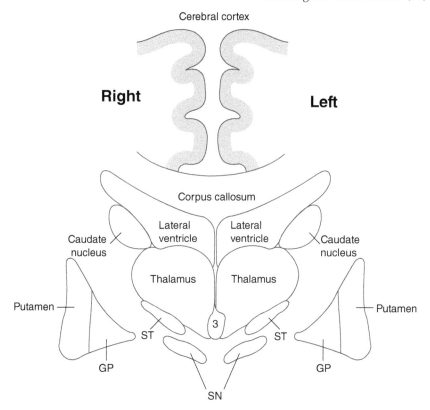

*Figure 14.6* Areas that make up the basal ganglia. GP: globus pallidus; SN: substantia nigra; ST: subthalamus; 3: third ventricle.

Muscle tone is a state of readiness for contraction, a tension within the muscle that is essential if the muscle is to function instantly when stimulated. Exercise increases muscle tone and a lack of exercise causes a loss of tone. Bed rest causes many complications, including muscle tone loss, i.e. loose, floppy muscles that do not function properly. The basal ganglia also provides *inhibition* (or *reduction*) of excessive muscle tone, and this is a major role of the **substantia nigra** (Figure 14.6 and see page 304). Excessive tone causes muscle stiffness and rigidity, as in Parkinson's disease (see page 303).

An important influence over movement is the **basal ganglia motor loop** (Figure 14.8), in which the globus pallidus *inhibits* part of the thalamus (the **ventral lateral nucleus**, or **VL**) during rest. Activation of the motor cortex of the cerebrum *switches on* another nucleus of the basal ganglia, the **putamen**, part of the **corpus striatum**. The putamen in turn *inhibits* the globus pallidus, thus removing the inhibition on the thalamus. Free now to act, the thalamus has considerable influence over an area close to the motor cortex, the **supplementary motor area** (**SMA**), which in turn focuses the activity of the main motor cortex. The loop is complete when the motor cortex activity switches on the mechanism that focuses that activity (Figure 14.8).

### The cerebellum

The **cerebellum** (Figure 14.9) contributes several aspects of movement, not least of which are **balance** and **posture**.

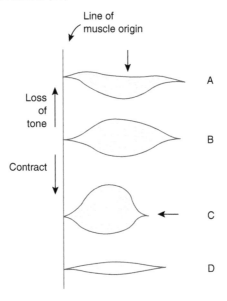

*Figure 14.7* Muscle tone. (A) Loss of muscle tone: the muscle is soft, loose and floppy, sinking in response to gravity (i.e. after long period of immobilisation). (B) Normal muscle tone: the muscle is firm and retains its shape, ready for contraction. (C) Contraction of the muscle, where the insertion (distal end of the muscle opposite to the origin) moves towards the origin (proximal end which does not move). (D) Muscle wasting, where muscle bulk is lost. Excessive muscle tone appears as the opposite of A, i.e. the muscle is tight and stiff and cannot contract normally.

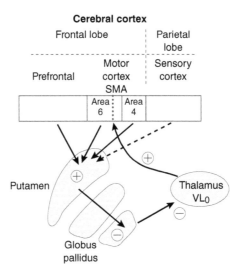

*Figure 14.8* Basal ganglia motor loop. Input to the putamen comes from the frontal cortex, with less input from the parietal sensory cortex. This activates (+) neurons running from the putamen to the globus pallidus, which, in turn, then deactivate (−) neurons linking the globus pallidus with the ventral lateral nucleus of the thalamus (known as $VL_0$). These globus pallidus neurons prevent (i.e. inhibit, shown as −) any feedback from the $VL_0$ to the cerebral cortex. However, deactivation from the putamen has removed this inhibition, and the $VL_0$ then has freedom to feedback to the cortex (+), more precisely the supplemental motor area (SMA) of area 6 of the motor cortex.

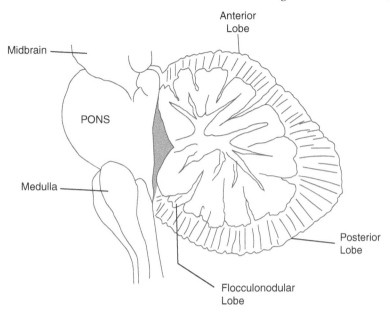

*Figure 14.9* Section through the cerebellum showing the lobes and brain stem (midbrain, pons and medulla).

The equilibrium of the body requires the **centre of gravity** (in the mid-lumbar spinal area) to remain within the base, i.e. the floor area occupied by the two feet. Should the centre of gravity drift outside the base, the individual will become unstable and will possibly fall to one side. To prevent this, many minute muscular adjustments are constantly being made to keep the body upright inside the base, correcting any defects in posture at the same time. These muscular adjustments are constantly changing as the body moves and the base constantly changes. Muscular contractions are coordinated by the cerebellum at an unconscious level, but they require *sensory* feedback to tell the cerebellum what the second-by-second state of the body's balance is. This sensory feedback on balance (known as **vestibular** stimuli) comes from the semicircular canals of the inner ear, via the **vestibulocochlear nerve** (cranial nerve VIII). Additional sensory information on balance comes from receptors in the joints and muscles called **proprioception**, and arrives in the brainstem via the spinal cord. Visual information is also used to assess balance (see *vestibulo-ocular reflex*, Chapter 15). The cerebellum, like the cerebrum, is divided into left and right **hemispheres**, both of which communicate with the rest of the brain entirely via the brainstem. Each cerebellar hemisphere is divided into three lobes: the **flocculonodular lobe**, the **anterior lobe** and the **posterior lobe** (Figure 14.9).

The vestibular stimuli from both ears arrive at the flocculonodular lobes in each hemisphere, the area ultimately responsible for balance. Proprioception stimuli arrive at the anterior lobe, where posture can be maintained. The posterior lobe receives impulses from the high centres of the cerebrum via the brainstem (Figure 14.10).

These cerebral connections allow the cerebellum to step in and control the fine coordination of voluntary movement at a subconscious level, i.e. the cerebellum makes muscle activity smooth, otherwise contractions would be jerky and erratic, especially for

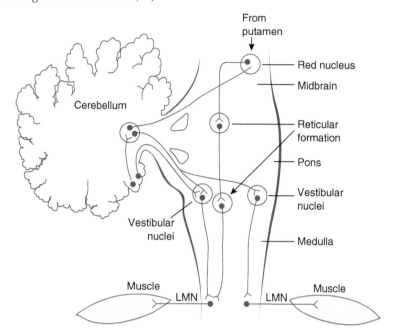

*Figure 14.10* The pathways from the cerebellum that control balance by adjusting the body's skeletal muscles (Figure 9.5, page 190). LMN: lower motor neuron.

fast movements. It also determines the extent and timing of muscle fibre contractions. It also *increases* muscle tone, providing a balance to the muscle tone function of the basal ganglia, which *decreases* muscle tone (see page 294, Figure 14.7). It also learns and perfects the skills of co-ordinating **synergy**.[2] Cerebellar synergistic skills involve the ability to coordinate muscle activity in relation to a moving object, using visual information from the visual cortex of the cerebrum to plot the direction and speed of the moving object. It works out the muscle response required to allow the chosen part, e.g. hand or foot, to intercept with that object. It means predicting ahead, since it takes time to move a limb to a new position, during which the object itself has moved. Children are born without these skills, and both synergistic skills and balance are learnt and practised from an early age. They are then pre-programmed, like many other motor skills, and function with very little or no conscious thought. Since visual information is crucial for this function, the cerebellum has some influence and control over eyeball movements, vital in tracking moving objects (see Chapter 13).

### Reflexes

Various reflexes exist to provide stability during movement and fast responses to adverse stimuli and are a safeguard against falling and injury (Pomfrett 2005). A reflex consists of a sensory input to the brain or cord, an integration or control centre and a motor response output to the relevant muscle group (i.e. the components of a **reflex arc**; Figure 14.11).

Painful sensory impulses pass into the posterior spinal cord and cross to the front on the same side via a **connector** (or **association**) neurone to the cell body of an LMN. The impulses from this LMN pass out of the cord to the muscle, which then contracts to pull

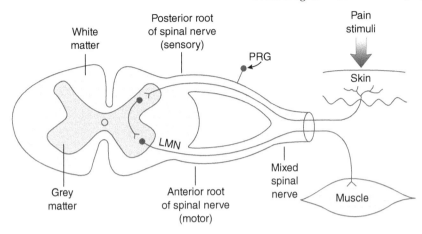

*Figure 14.11* The reflex arc. A special sensory neuron takes painful impulses from the periphery to the cord. Impulses pass to the brain, but at the same time interneurons cross the cord from the posterior sensory to the anterior motor areas of the grey matter, and the lower motor neuron conveys an impulse to the muscles to move the part from harm. LMR: lower motor neuron; PRG: posterior root ganglion (see Chapter 12).

the limb away from the source of the pain. **Deep tendon** (or **stretch extensor**) reflexes include the **patella reflex**, where the patella tendon is tapped below the patella bone with a clinical hammer. The **knee-jerk** that follows is caused first by stretching the sensory **muscle spindle** within the thigh muscle with the hammer tap, thus sending impulses into the cord. This then activates the LMN at the same level as the sensory input, and motor impulses are sent back to the same muscle, making it contract slightly to correct the original stretch. The **flexor** (or **withdrawal**) **response** is created by the application of painful stimuli to a limb, causing pain stimuli to pass into the cord. Again, an LMN fires in response to contract the flexor muscles of that same limb while relaxing the extensor muscles. At the same time, the impulse crosses the midline in the cord and causes the opposite response in the other limb, which then extends (called the **crossed extensor response**; Figure 14.12).

*The muscles*

The *end organ* of any motor system is the **muscle**, a specialist tissue with the function of contraction and in the process produces heat (see Chapter 1). Muscles are of three types: **skeletal muscle**, which is attached to the bones and serves to allow *voluntary* movement; **smooth muscle**, which forms the walls of internal *tubes*, such as blood vessels and the digestive tract and is *involuntary* and **cardiac muscle** in the heart wall, which contracts *involuntarily*. Muscle is the only tissue in the body that can itself move; anything else that moves, such as bones or blood, is moved by a muscle. Muscles *pull* but cannot *push*, but smooth muscle constructed into a distinct ring around a tube wall can constrict to close the tube lumen. This is called a **sphincter**.[3]

In the limbs, skeletal muscles are set in opposing positions around joints, called **antagonistic pairs** because these muscles have opposing functions: one muscle to *bend* the joint (the **flexor**) and one muscle to *straighten* the joint (the **extensor**; Figure 14.13).

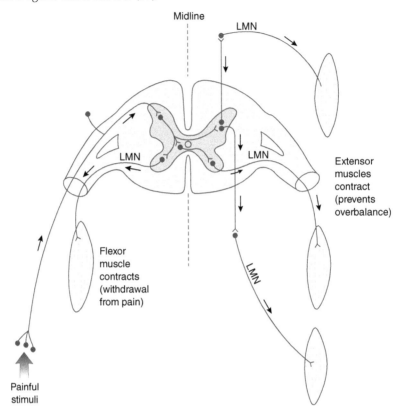

*Figure 14.12* The crossed extensor reflex. Painful stimuli affecting one side of the body cause flexion of the muscles on that side via the reflex arc (Figure 14.11) in order to withdraw from the pain. At the same time, impulses cross to the other side and stimulate extensor muscles at several levels above and below the level affected to prevent overbalancing.

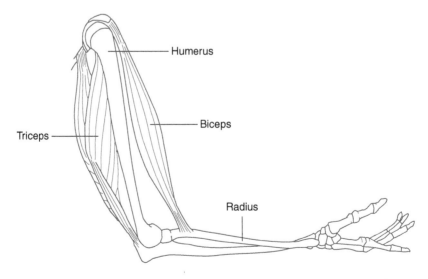

*Figure 14.13* Antagonistic muscle pairs. In this example, the flexor is the biceps and the extensor is the triceps muscles of the upper arm.

Once muscles have contracted they cannot return to a stretched state on their own. Therefore, contracting the flexor muscle stretches the extensor muscle, and vice versa. Muscle contraction involves moving the **insertion** (the *travelling* and mostly the lower end of the muscle) towards the **origin** (the *fixed* and mostly the upper end of the muscle). The nerve innervation of the various types of muscle are different: the skeletal muscle is *controlled* by the pyramidal and extrapyramidal tract systems, the smooth muscle is *controlled* by the **autonomic nervous system** (**ANS**) and the cardiac muscle is *regulated* by the ANS. Between the nerve and the *voluntary skeletal muscle* is the **neuromuscular junction**, a gap where a neurotransmitter called **acetylcholine** is active in passing the impulse from the neurone to the muscle cells.

## Movement observations

Disorders of movement can be classified according to the system that is causing the problem, i.e. *pyramidal* or *extrapyramidal* tract disorders, basal ganglia or cerebellar disorders, or diseases of the muscles themselves. Observations of movement are best achieved in conscious patients, either by watching as patients attempt movement or by requesting patients to undergo specific movements for the purpose of observation. Walking is a good opportunity to observe a patient's ability to move, whereby different forms of **gait** (i.e. the manner in which an individual walks) may be seen and balance can be assessed. Loss of consciousness removes all such *purposeful*[4] movements and would probably mean that any movements observed are likely to be spontaneous and probably reflex-type activities.

When assessing movement, the basic questions to establish are:

1 Can the patient walk properly, or are there noticeable difficulties with mobility (e.g. dragging one foot or being unable to balance)?
2 Can the patient talk properly, or are there noticeable problems with speech (e.g. slurring of words)? Remember, not all speech problems are due to abnormal muscle activity, but there is a major motor component to speech.
3 Does the patient show any abnormal (non-purposeful) movements (see footnote 4), such as shaking or inability to sit still?

Normal movements, i.e. the expected range and types of movement, are well understood. This expectation makes abnormal movements quite obvious as patients make efforts to get around and communicate.

Movement problems could be classified into *losses* and *excesses*. Losses (normal movements that have been lost) include:

- **hypokinesia,** a general reduction in the level of movement (kinetics = movement, hypo = lower than normal level)
- **akinesia,** the inability to *initiate* a movement, for example being unable to start to walk. The letter 'a' before a word means *without*, i.e. akinesia literally means *without movement* (due to being unable to start that movement)
- **paralysis**, a total loss of movement
- **paresis**, a weakness of muscle movement, a condition similar to – but less severe than – paralysis.

Excesses movements. i.e. unwanted movements that occur that the patient cannot control include:

- **dyskinesia**, an obvious abnormal movement
- **hyperkinesia**, an increase in *involuntary movements*, such as tremor, which is an uncontrolled shaking of limbs (hyper = greater than normal)
- **akathisia**, a motor restlessness that prevents the individual from sitting down.

### Movement losses

*Paralysis and weakness*

A total loss of the ability to move is paralysis, a major neurological deficit that may be local (e.g. in one limb) or involve wider aspects of the nervous system. **Hemiplegia**, a paralysis of either the left or right side of the body, may affect those suffering from a **cerebrovascular accident** (**CVA** – or **stroke**) to various degrees. CVAs are disruptions to the blood supply of the brain, resulting in brain damage. This very often involves the motor cortex and the major pathways from this area, the pyramidal tracts. Since these tracts mostly cross in the medulla (Figure 14.1), a *left* hemiplegia indicates a stroke on the *right* side of the brain, and vice versa. The degree of movement loss depends on the extent of the brain damage and its location within the brain. Small bleeds close to the brain surface may only result in *weakness* on one side, called a **hemiparesis**, with good prospects for some or total recovery. Larger or deeper bleeds may cause more profound paralysis with some permanent deficit. A CVA is an example of a UMN lesion leading to **spastic paralysis** in the longer term, where *spastic* means the stiffening and contracture of the muscles of the affected limbs if adequate preventative measures are not taken. The arm is usually held in a bent (= **flexed**) position and the spastic hemiparesis creates a characteristic gait where the leg *circles* stiffly outwards then inwards with a pointed toe while walking.

Unlike hemiplegia, **paraplegia** results in the loss of function of the lower limbs, and mobility often requires a wheelchair. Paraplegia is largely associated with spinal injuries where the cord is damaged, severing the pyramidal motor tracts at a point in the **thoracic** or **lumbar** regions. Such trauma cuts off any opportunity for the brain to control the muscles below the level of the injury. Of course, it could also affect the sensory neurons as well, causing sensation losses in the lower limbs. A similar injury higher up the spine in the **cervical** (neck) region may include a loss of movement below this level (i.e. a **tetraplegia**, involving all four limbs and the trunk). Another cause of lower limb paralysis is **poliomyelitis**, an infectious disease that damages the cell body of the LMNs or their axons passing from the cord. LMN lesions result in a **flaccid paralysis**, where muscles of the paralysed limbs become loose and floppy (loss of muscle tone) with complete loss of reflexes, and **foot drop**, a failure of the muscles that retain the foot at the normal right angle to the leg.

The loss of the ability to perform *purposeful* movements is **apraxia** (a = without, praxia = performing movements), i.e. the movements that occur are meaningless. The problem is *not* caused by simple paralysis or weakness, nor is it due to a lack of comprehension or motivation. It may be the result of a lesion in the parietal association cortex (see page 221) along with disturbance to sensory interpretation and integration. Different forms of apraxia may occur, and this depends on which side of the brain is affected. **Dyspraxia** (dys = difficulty, praxia = performing movements) is the difficulty in carrying out skilled movements with no evidence of disorder of the primary motor pathways. This is *not* the same as paralysis, which usually *does* involve the primary motor pathways. Apraxia and dyspraxia are functional developmental disorders of differing severity; apraxia is a total loss of purposeful movements and dyspraxia is a difficulty in carrying out skilled purposeful movements. Both disorders disturb the development of different systems, e.g. **verbal dyspraxia** (speech difficulty and delay), or **motor dyspraxia** (difficulty with body movement coordination, including balance and walking). A child with motor dyspraxia may be called a *clumsy child*.

Another motor problem is **multiple sclerosis (MS)**, an **autoimmune disease** of the neuronal myelin sheath, which breaks down and is replaced by scar tissue (i.e. it is a **demyelination** disease). Autoimmune diseases occur when the body's immune system identifies part of the body as foreign (or *alien*) tissue and begins to destroy it. The reason is not fully known but viral infections of the affected tissues are suspected. MS can affect any neuron, motor and sensory, and it causes a wide range of symptoms of varying degrees that can pass from *remissions* (periods of no or few symptoms) to *relapses* (periods of worse symptoms). Those signs affecting movement include spastic limb weakness with exaggerated reflexes (a UMN pyramidal sign) and an **ataxia** (i.e. loss of balance, a cerebellar sign; see page 296).

**Motor neuron disease** (**MND**) is another progressive degeneration of motor neurons, this time the pyramidal (corticospinal) tract fibres, some cranial nerve nuclei and some LMNs within the cord. It causes severe movement losses involving motor control of multiple muscles, including the swallow reflex, and death occurs within a few years. The usual age of onset is 40–60 years. There are now around 25 gene mutations identified in the causation of motor neuron disease. Some of these are inherited (i.e. run in families), which is estimated between 7 to 10% of cases. The following is some information on the main genes[5] involved (Corcia *et al*. 2008):

1 The gene **superoxide dismutase-1** (*SOD1*, found 1993) on chromosome 21q. It codes for the enzyme superoxide dismutase 1, which is a cellular defence against free radicals which damage cells. Over 150 gene mutations are known in this gene, one of the commonest being a codon change from alanine to valine.
2 The gene **angiogenin** (*ANG*, found 2006) is an autosomal dominant gene on chromosome 14q. It codes for a protein that is both an enzyme and a blood vessel growth factor (**angiogenesis** is the growth of new blood vessels). Patients with this gene mutation have predominant bulbar symptoms.
3 The gene **TAR DNA-binding protein** (*TARDBP*) on chromosome 1p. It codes for the protein **TAR DNA-binding protein 43** (**TDP-43**). Normally, this protein has important functions in gene transcription and translation.
4 The gene **chromosome 9 open reading frame 72** (*C9orf72*, found 2011) on chromosome 9p. This is a DNA sequence repeat. The gene normally has up to 20 repeats, while sufferers have hundreds of repeats. It affects about one-third of all familial MND sufferers.
5 The gene **fused in sarcoma** (*FUS*, found 2009) on chromosome 16p. It codes for a protein that has multiple functions within the nucleus of motor neurons, but mutations cause this protein to accumulate outside the nucleus.

Research on MND is also focused on **axonal transportation**. This is the transportation of substances, notably proteins, up and down the axon of neurons. This flow of proteins from neuronal cell body to the synapse and back is critical to synaptic and neuronal function. Disruption of this process leads to synaptic malfunction and ultimately to motor neuron losses.

Three different aspects characterise this disease:

1  **progressive muscular atrophy** (**PMA**)
2  **progressive bulbar palsy** (**PBP**)
3  **amyotrophic lateral sclerosis** (**ALS**, also known as **Lou Gehrig's disease**).

Most of the discovered genes are linked to the causation of ALS.
Patients with this disorder will first develop one of these three aspects first, either:

1  Muscular atrophy; i.e. loss of muscle bulk also called *muscle wasting*
2  Bulbar symptoms, i.e. paralysis of the mouth, throat or facial muscles, including difficulty in swallowing
3  Muscle weakness with twitching and some degree of paralysis.

These symptoms will remain dominant as other symptoms occur. Most patients will eventually show signs of all three to varying degrees. Those in whom PMA is dominant have the least severe form and can have a survival rate of up to 15 years or more. PBP causes deterioration of parts of the brainstem, and it has the worst symptoms and the shortest life expectancy. It causes deterioration of swallowing, with choking on food and muscle paralysis of the tongue and throat including speech loss. ALS is a progressive combination of **amyotrophy** (i.e. muscle wasting caused by a loss of LMNs) and **lateral sclerosis**, a loss of UMNs in the corticospinal tracts of the spinal cord. The main features are muscular weakness and **atrophy** (= wasting of muscles), with **fasciculation** (= twitching of muscles) in two or more limbs. The intellect and sensory systems are completely unaffected and remain intact throughout.

Unfortunately, there is currently no treatment available for MND, but extensive research is well underway and making progress towards a treatment.

*Muscular diseases*

Muscular diseases also cause weakness and paralysis. **Myasthenia gravis** is a disorder of the neuromuscular junction. Acetylcholine (see page 299) cannot bind to the receptors properly and muscle cells are unable to sustain repeated contraction during exercise so that they fatigue quickly. The receptors are blocked by antibodies, plus there is a reduced amount of acetylcholine available at the synapse. The **thymus gland**, part of the lymphatic and immune systems in the chest, may be the site of production of the antibodies concerned, and removal of this gland, plus drugs to improve acetylcholine function, are options for treatment.

The various **muscular dystrophies** form a group of disabling diseases involving the muscle itself. Several of these disorders are genetically inherited, such as **Duchenne muscular dystrophy** (**DMD**). This disease is the commonest in the group and affects mostly boys because the gene involved (the DMD gene) is on the X chromosome.[6] Normally, the gene codes for the protein **dystrophin** found in muscles. The role of dystrophin is to strengthen and protect muscle proteins as they contract and relax. In DMD, muscles become weakened and damaged due to the repeated muscle contraction, leading to deterioration in walking and other movement, with complete mobility loss by the time of adolescence. It can affect cardiac muscle, and life expectancy may be short, i.e. death by around 30 years.

**Myopathies** (myo = muscle, path = disease) is the term used to describe a failure of muscle development with weakness, muscle pain and cramps early in life, again often due to genetic inheritance. The weakness may be severe and cause major mobility difficulties that can be progressive throughout life.

*Increased muscle tone (rigidity)*

Disturbances to basal ganglia function, as in **Parkinson disease**, can cause an increase in muscle tone, known as **hypertonia**; i.e. muscles become stiff and rigid and fail to allow full body movement (Figure 14.14).

In Parkinson disease, the limbs are severely limited in function; the legs show a shuffling gait and sufferers cannot lift their feet properly. The body takes on a forward stance and often moves faster than their feet can. Patients may therefore lose their balance and fall forwards. Carers observing these patients should be aware of the potential for injury.

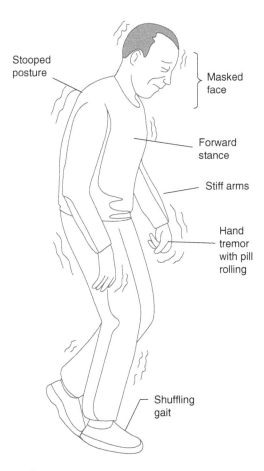

*Figure 14.14* The signs of Parkinson Disease.

The muscle tone increase is due to the failure of the basal ganglia's role of inhibiting excess muscle tone, causing stiffness in the muscles. James Parkinson, a Shoreditch apothecary surgeon, described the condition as *paralysis agitans*, i.e. agitated paralysis, which neatly describes the two main features: body rigidity and limb tremor, especially the hands along with 'pill rolling'.[7] They suffer gradual loss of speech and the ability to write. Parkinson's disease is progressive due to the relentless destruction of the **substantia nigra**,[8] with a corresponding gradual loss of the neurotransmitter dopamine in the pathway from the substantia nigra to the corpus striatum, the **nigrostriatal pathway**. The reason for the loss of cells in the substantia nigra is unknown and cannot be prevented and will eventually lead to the patient's death. It would appear that the symptoms do not occur until the dopamine loss reaches 80%, indicating the **asymptomatic** (= without symptoms) onset of this disease, which is very gradual over a number of years. On average, the age that symptoms become obvious is about 60 years or more, but the process leading to those symptoms must have started considerably earlier in life. Treatment is aimed at the replacement of the dopamine in this part of the brain, effectively reducing the symptoms – particularly the rigidity – and therefore improving the quality of life.

Other forms of rigidity are **decortication**, an *abnormal flexion response* and **decerebration**, an *abnormal extensor response* of the limbs (Figure 14.15). The symptoms of these disorders and their causes are shown in Table 14.1. Decerebrate symptoms can be severe enough to include stiff clenching of the jaw, neck extension and arching of the back.

Explanation of the terms in Table 14.1 are as follows:

* **Adduction**[9] is movement of a limb *towards* the midline of the body (i.e. held against the side of the body).
* **Internal rotation** is a twisting of the limb *inwards*.
* **Pronation** is a *palm downwards* position of the forearm and hand (see Figure 14.15).
* **Extension** is straightening of a limb.
* **Flexion** (or **hyperflexion**) is bending (or excessive bending) of joints.
* **Plantar flexion** is a downward movement of the foot; the toes point away from the body at an angle of as much as 45° from the normal right-angle position of the foot.

*Ataxia*

**Ataxia** is a difficult and abnormal gait, or walking, with specific forms of ataxia indicating certain neuromuscular disorders (Bastian 1997). The gait of spastic hemiparesis seen in CVA and the shuffling gait of Parkinson disease have both been described (see pages 300 and 303). **Cerebellar ataxia** is caused by a disorder of the cerebellum or its tracts. It produces an unsteady staggering gait with difficulty on turning, and balance loss when the feet come together, so the feet are usually held apart. This is often seen as a result of alcohol intoxication. **Sensory ataxia** is an unsteady gait where sensory feedback from the feet or legs to the cerebellum is lost. Again, the feet are held wide apart to help stabilise balance. During walking, each leg is lifted high followed by the foot being *slapped* on the floor. Since the patient is unable to feel the floor, it becomes necessary for the patient to watch the ground to ensure his/her foot is safely in contact before putting any weight on it. It is due to a destruction of the somatic sensory pathways of the spinal cord, as in **tabes dorsalis**, a spinal cord complication of the infectious disease **syphilis**. **Scissor gait** is caused by a bilateral spastic weakness of the leg muscles. The legs are moved slowly forwards over short steps; the thighs tend to cross over each other in turn.

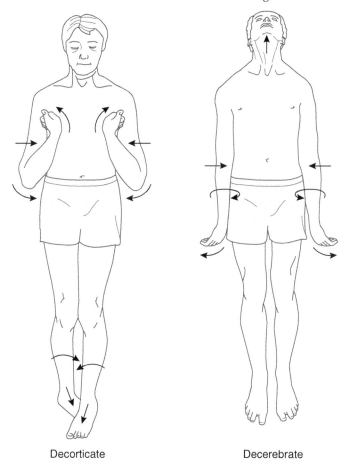

Decorticate                    Decerebrate

*Figure 14.15* Decorticate and decerebrate symptoms. In decorticate symptoms, the elbows, wrists and fingers are flexed with adduction of the arms, the legs are inwardly rotated, and the feet are plantar flexed. In decerebrate symptoms, the head is extended with the jaws clenched shut, the arms are adducted with stiffly extended elbows, the forearms are hyperpronated and the wrists and fingers are flexed, the legs are stiffly extended, and the feet are plantar flexed.

*Table 14.1* The symptoms and causes of decortication and decerebration

| Rigidity | Arms | Legs | Cause |
|---|---|---|---|
| Decortication | Hyperflexion of each of the joints with adduction of the limb | Extension of legs with internal rotation and plantar flexion of foot | A high cerebral lesion interrupting the corticospinal (pyramidal) tracts |
| Decerebration | Elbow extension, wrist flexion with limb adduction and pronated forearms | Stiff extension of legs with plantar flexion of foot | A hypothalamic or thalamic lesion involving the brainstem |

## Movement excesses

### Tremor

The uncontrollable and involuntary shaking seen in the limbs in Parkinson disease comes in two forms: a *coarse* tremor noticed in the whole limb and a *fine* tremor found in the hands and fingers (Figure 14.14). This fine tremor has been called *pill-rolling*, since this is the action taken during the manual production of pills before mechanisation and quality control. Parkinson's tremor disappears as the limbs are put into conscious motion but return at rest. Tremor is a very noticeable symptom and is very destructive of the patient's confidence, motor activities and natural behaviour patterns.

Tremor may also be the result of multiple sclerosis, strokes, brain injury, various neuro-degenerative disorders and even excess consumption of some drugs (e.g. amphetamines and caffeine), alcohol abuse and withdrawal, hypoglycaemia (low blood glucose levels), sleep deprivation, thyroid hormone excess, anxiety and stress. Some nutritional deficiencies (e.g. magnesium and niacin) also show tremor as a symptom.

### Athetosis, chorea and ballism

**Huntington disease** is a genetically inherited disorder caused by a gene mutation on the fourth chromosome (Bentley 1999). It results in a progressive degeneration of several areas of the brain, in particular the **corpus striatum** (composed of the **caudate nucleus** and **putamen**) of the basal ganglia, with cell losses in the frontal and parietal lobes of the cerebral cortex. Unwanted involuntary movements are a characteristic of this disease, and these are **athetosis** (slow writhing movements of the limbs, face and tongue) and **chorea** (fast twitching of whole limbs and body). If these two movements occur together, the words are combined (i.e. **choreoathetosis**). The major distinctions between them are the speed (*sudden* chorea movements compared with the *slow* athetosis movements) and the nature of the movement (in chorea, *jerky* and *twitching* movements; in athetosis, *writhing* movements). Observers will note that the patient appears to be unable to sit still. Chorea can sometimes occur in children (**Sydenham chorea**), often as a result of **rheumatic fever**, caused mostly by an immune response to the bacterium ***Streptococcus***. The child or adolescent shows sudden, irregular and uncontrolled movements of no real purpose, but unlike Huntington's disease this is not a permanent problem (Gasser and Kieburtz 2000).

Uncontrolled violent movements of a whole limb, involving flinging the arms suddenly in any direction, is called **ballism**. The appearance of this phenomenon may be sudden and frightening. **Monoballism** is the term used if a single limb only is involved, and **hemiballism** indicates that both limbs on one side are affected. The violent nature of this movement is due to the involvement of the **subthalamic nucleus** in the lesion.

## The immobile patient

Immobility reduces independence to varying degrees. Observations of the immobile patient are critical to understanding the patient's needs, for identifying the early stages of the complications of immobility and for maintaining the patient's progress towards mobility. In this observation checklist, the complications directly caused by immobility are shown in *italics*.

*Observations checklist*

1 Observation of the skin is vital for:

    a Assessing for any *dehydration* (i.e. when the skin is dry and can be pulled into folds that remain when released). Dehydration is a severe lack of fluids in the tissues, both the **intracellular** fluids (intra = inside, cellular = the cells) and the **extracellular** fluids (extra = outside; also known as **tissue fluid**; see Chapters 6 and 10)

    b Preventing **decubitus ulcers** (= *pressure sores*), caused both by constricted blood supply to the tissues when compressed by body weight and by friction eroding the surface of the skin when the patient is moved around the bed. Assessment of a patient's risk of skin breakdown is often made using the **Waterlow scale** (Baxter 2008) or the **Norton scale** (Lewko *et al.* 2005; see Chapter 10)

    c Assessing for *poor personal hygiene* and maintaining cleanliness.

2 Observing the mouth is vital for:

    a Preventing dehydration, which could result in a *dry mouth with poor saliva production* (see Chapter 6)

    b Preventing *infections*, which could cause red, swollen gums and halitosis (foul-smelling breath), pain and difficulty with eating, and the risk of complications, such as throat, chest, ear and brain infections.

3 Observing the urine is vital for:

    a Assessing the output to maintain fluid balance and reduce the risk of *renal disorders* (see Chapter 8)

    b Preventing *urinary tract infections* (see Chapter 8).

4 Observing the bowel function is vital for:

    a Assessing the output to prevent *constipation or diarrhoea* (see Chapter 9).

5 Observing the level of consciousness is vital for:

    a Prevention of *confusion or coma* (see Chapter 11).

6 Observing the respirations is vital for:

    a Maintaining adequate ventilation and oxygenation (see Chapter 5)

    b Preventing *chest infections* (see Chapter 5).

7 Observing body temperature is vital for:

    a Assessing the patient's ability to control body temperature (see Chapter 1)

    b Preventing or detecting any underlying *infections*.

8 Observing the ability to communicate is vital for:

    a Assessment of mental function, especially mood, which may be *depressed*

    b Assessment of problems such as *pain*, and maintaining a pain-free state (see Chapter 12).

9 Observing the ability to eat and drink is vital for:

    a Assessing the patient's nutritional status (see Chapter 7)

    b Preventing *hunger, dehydration* and *malnutrition*.

*Table 14.2* Red flag warnings of deteriorating mobility condition

**ꝗ Red Flag = serious situation which needs urgent medical attention.**

| *Flag warning* | *Details* |
|---|---|
| **ꝗ Red Flag** | **Rapid onset of weakness or paralysis of one side of the body (Chapter 11).** |

(After Hill-Smith and Johnson 2021, with permission)

10  Observing the sleep cycle pattern is vital for:

    a  Assessing that the patient has enough rest.

11  Observing the pattern of mobility possible in each limb and joint is vital for:

    a  Assessing what mobility the patient can achieve and maximising this to prevent *joint stiffness* and *muscle atrophy* (muscle atrophy = wasting of the muscles, or loss of muscle bulk; see page 302)

    b  Assessing what mobility assistance the patient will need in terms of professional help (such as physiotherapy) and mobility aids (such as a wheelchair) to prevent excessive periods of immobility.

Immobility disrupts all aspects of daily life, both physically and mentally. Given what is known about the complications of immobility, maximum possible mobility should be established and maintained. Immobility should not mean long periods confined to a bed or chair.

**Key points**

*The neurobiology of human movement*

- Pre-programming of movement is the essence of the learning process and allows movement to occur at a subconscious level.
- The motor cortex cells are arranged in a manner that reflects the basic body plan.
- The pyramidal tracts descend from the motor cortex.
- The pyramidal system is two-neuronal, consisting of an upper motor neurone (UMN) from brain to cord and a lower motor neurone (LMN) from cord to muscle.
- The extrapyramidal system controls voluntary movement at a subconscious level.
- The basal ganglia have a role in controlling slow, sustained movements and in maintaining muscle tone.
- Muscle tone is a state of tension of the muscle essential for contraction.
- The cerebellum is important for balance, posture, smoothing out muscle movements and synergistic skills.
- Reflexes provide stability during movement and fast responses to adverse stimuli. A reflex arc has a sensory input to the cord, a control centre and a motor output to the muscle.
- Muscles are of three types: skeletal muscle attached to bones, allowing voluntary movement, smooth muscle forming walls of internal tubes, allowing involuntary movement and cardiac muscle in the heart wall.
- The various types of muscle have different nerve innervation: skeletal muscle is controlled by the pyramidal and extrapyramidal systems, smooth muscle is controlled by the autonomic nervous system and cardiac muscle is regulated by the autonomic nervous system.

*Disorders involving movement*

- Paralysis is a loss of movement: hemiplegia is paralysis of either the left or right half of the body, paraplegia is paralysis of the lower half of the body and tetraplegia is paralysis of the body from the neck down.
- Cerebrovascular accident (CVA) or stroke is a bleed into the brain or an obstruction of the blood supply to the brain.
- Poliomyelitis is an infectious disease that damages the cell body of the lower motor neuron.
- Multiple sclerosis is an autoimmune disease of the myelin sheath, which breaks down and is replaced by scar tissue.
- Myasthenia gravis is the inability of acetylcholine to bind at the neuromuscular junction, which causes the muscles to be unable to sustain repeated contraction.
- Muscular dystrophies are often genetically inherited. Duchenne's muscular dystrophy affects mostly boys. Fat accumulates in the main muscles during childhood, leading to deterioration of walking with complete mobility loss by the time of adolescence.
- Parkinson disease is a degeneration of the basal ganglia, causing an increase in muscle tone resulting in rigidity and tremor.
- Decortication is an abnormal flexion response caused by a high cerebral lesion interrupting the corticospinal (pyramidal) tracts. Decerebration is an abnormal extensor response caused by a hypothalamic or thalamic lesion involving the brainstem.
- Ataxia is difficult or abnormal gait (method of walking).
- Motor neuron disease is a progressive degeneration of neurons of the pyramidal and bulbar tracts.
- Huntington disease is a genetically inherited disorder resulting in a progressive degeneration of the corpus striatum with cell losses in the frontal and parietal lobes.
- Unwanted involuntary movements are called chorea (sudden and jerky movements) and athetosis (slow writhing movements).

## Notes

1 Movements with regards to talking involves learning to speak a language as well as control of the lips, tongue, jaw and throat muscles.
2 Synergy is the combination of systems (e.g. multiple muscles) working together to achieve an outcome that is greater than what is possible with only one of those systems working alone (e.g. one muscle). On a broader scale, synergy is also the combination of *different* systems (e.g. muscular coordination with the visual system) to achieve a goal that one system alone cannot achieve (see *vestibulo-ocular reflex*, Chapter 15).
3 A sphincter is a distinct muscular ring strategically located at sites along a tube to act like a doorway (i.e. it opens or closes that tube). They are mainly smooth muscle but are differently arranged to the smooth muscle which is distributed throughout the tube wall and can act generally to squeeze the tube contents forwards. Some external sphincters are skeletal muscle (notable the external anal sphincter) and can be consciously controlled.
4 Purposeful movements are those that are deliberately and consciously carried out by the patient to achieve a purpose. Non-purposeful movements are those that occur automatically without conscious control and serve no purpose. Non-purposeful movements are often annoying to the patient and indicate a potential problem.
5 It is important to remember that these genes are present in everyone, and only cause disease when present as an abnormal mutation.
6 Females have two X chromosomes, so if one has the mutated gene then they most probably have an alternative normal gene on the second X. Males only have one X chromosome, so if that X has

the mutated gene then there is no alternative normal gene, and they will therefore show the signs of the disease.

7 Pill rolling dates from the time before mechanisation and quality control, when medication was rolled into balls by hand to form tablets.

8 Substantia nigra ('black substance') is part of the basal ganglia responsible for reducing muscle tone, among other functions.

9 Adduction should not be confused with abduction, where the limb is moved *away* from the midline.

## References

Anderson M.E. and Kiehn O. (2004) Motor systems. *Current Opinion in Neurobiology, 14*(6): 661–664. https://doi.org/10.1016/j.conb.2004.10.018

Bastian A.J. (1997) Mechanisms of ataxia. *Physical Therapy, 77*(6): 672–675.

Baxter S. (2008) Assessing pressure ulcer risk in long-term care using the Waterlow scale. *Nursing Older People, 20*(7): 34–38.

Bentley P. (1999) Dementia demystified. *Nursing Times, 95*(45): 47–49.

Corcia P., Praline J., Vourch P. and Andres C. (2008) Genetics of motor neuron disorders. *Revue Neurologique, 164*(2): 115–130.

Gasser T. and Kieburtz K. (2000) Huntington's disease and Sydenham's chorea. *Movement Disorders, 125*(19): 2214–2217.

Hill-Smith I. and Johnson G. (2021) *Little Book of Red Flags*. National Minor Illness Centre, Bedfordshire.

Lewko J., Demianiuk M., Krot E., Krajewska-Kułak E., Sierakowska M., Nyklewicz W. and Jankowiak B. (2005) Assessment of risk for pressure ulcers using the Norton scale in nursing practice. *Roczniki Akademii Medycznej w Bialymstoku Annales Academiae Medicae Bialostocensis, 50*(Suppl. 1): 148–151.

Pomfrett C.J.D. (2005) Neural reflexes. *Anaesthesia and Intensive Care Medicine, 6*(5): 145–150.

# 15 Pharmacology and drug side effects, interactions and allergies

- Introduction
- Pharmacology
- Drug side effects
- Drug interactions
- Drug allergies
- Key points
- Notes
- References

## Introduction

Drugs can cause unwanted side (or toxic) effects and allergic reactions and may also interact with each other when taken simultaneously. Such problems can cause health problems and sometimes even death (Gottlieb 2001). Serious side effects have caused patients to be reluctant to take their medication and sometimes being admitted to hospital (Gutierrez 2010). Some drugs were withdrawn from medical use because the side effects were unacceptable. Every effort is made to make medicines safe prior to their release.

## Pharmacology

**Pharmacology** is the study of drugs and includes several more specific sciences, the main ones being pharmacokinetics, pharmacodynamics and pharmacotherapeutics.

**Pharmacokinetics** ('drug movement') is the study of the way drugs move through the body, from the point of entry to the point of exit. There are four stages:

- Absorption is the point of entry to the body, usually through oral, intramuscular and intravenous administration.
- Distribution means transportation around the body, mostly in the blood.
- Metabolism can, for example, be chemical changes mostly in the liver.
- Elimination is the point of exit from the body, mostly through the kidneys.

DOI: 10.4324/9781003389118-15

Drug side effects, particularly drug interactions, can occur at any of these stages.

**Pharmacodynamics** is the study of how drugs work. Drugs work through multiple different ways depending on what they are prescribed for.

A useful way to distinguish pharmacokinetics from pharmacodynamics is to say the former is the way the *body handles the drug* and the latter is the way the *drug handles the body*.

**Pharmacotherapeutics** is the study of drugs used in clinical practice, including prescribing regimes and dosages, routes of administration, the storage of drugs and side effects.

The new science of **pharmacogenetics** puts the emphasis on prescribing 'tailor made' drug treatments to fit individuals rather than a blanket treatment approach to fit everyone. It is not available yet with all treatments.

Two things have made this approach possible:

1 *Advances in genetics*. Everyone is a unique combination of genes. Even identical twins have small variations in their genetic inheritance. Drugs and genes interact, if not directly, then through the protein products of genes. By understanding the genetic sequences of individuals, it has become possible to predict, to some extent, how a drug will work in that individual and the possible outcome
2 *Advances in drugs*. One of the problems noted about the blanket approach to treatment was that standard drug treatments are sometimes more affective in some people than in others. Factors such as age, gender, race and fitness all affect the way drugs interact with the body at cellular level, influencing how drugs do their job. Drug chemistry can be modified to fit individual requirements. The source for new drugs is almost unlimited, giving researchers many new compounds to explore and trial. The matching of chemical compounds with an individual genetic pattern is becoming a reality. Increases in computer power will make this a regular, everyday occurrence.

*Pharmacokinetics*

Most of our drugs can be administered by mouth. Oral drugs must be able to survive potential digestion by catabolic[1] enzymes and wide pH variations, from gastric acidity to bowel alkalinity. Some drugs must be given by injection, e.g. insulin, because these drugs would not survive catabolic enzyme destruction if ingested. Drugs injected into a muscle (i.e. intramuscular) will be absorbed slowly and that delays their activity over several hours or longer. Drugs injected directly into the blood (i.e. intravenously) bypass absorption entirely and this is the fastest route for instant drug delivery.

Oral drugs are transported to the liver via the hepatic portal vein[2] prior to release into general circulation (Figure 15.1). The liver carries out some metabolism on the drug prior to its release into the general circulation. This is called **first-pass metabolism**. This process may render a portion of the drug dosage useless. The surviving drug is called the **bioavailability**, i.e. it remains available for activity. If we consider the oral dosage of a drug as 100%, then first pass metabolism may reduce this by 15%,[3] with 85% leaving the liver unchanged (the bioavailability).

Most drugs are transported around the body in the blood stream. Whilst in the blood, most are carried bound to blood proteins, notably **albumin**, the commonest blood protein (see Chapter 4, Figure 4.1, page 67). Small quantities of drugs may be transported in the lymphatic system but ultimately return to the blood.

The product of drug metabolism is a **metabolite**. Most metabolites are no longer active as a drug and have been prepared for excretion (usually via the kidneys). They must then

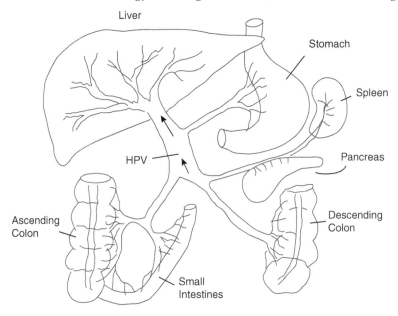

*Figure 15.1* Hepatic portal vein (HPV) from the gut to the liver.

be transported to the kidney for this purpose via the hepatic vein (see footnote 2) and the general circulation. In some cases, a drug metabolite is still active and continue to work as the original drug, i.e. it contributes to the bioavailability. In a few cases the original drug is not active until it has been metabolised. In this case the original (inactive) drug is called a **pro-drug**, and the actual (active) metabolite is the drug itself.

Injected drugs initially bypass the liver, and they are not subjected to first-pass metabolism. The original dose administered is also the bioavailability.

Eventually all drugs, after activity, are metabolised in the liver and prepared for excretion. How long drugs are active and remain in the blood depends on their **half-life**. The half-life of different drugs varies widely. For example, drug X has a half-life of 2 hours. The initial bioavailability is 100%. After 2 hours of metabolism (via the liver) and excretion (via the kidneys) the drug bioavailability in circulation is reduced to 50%. After the second 2-hour period of metabolism and excretion the bioavailability is further reduced to 25%. The third 2-hour period reduces this further to 12.5% and so on (Figure 15.2). Two things are shown by this:

1  The metabolism and excretion of the drug gradually slows down so only half of each of the preceding 2-hour period is removed from circulation
2  Because each 2-hour period removes only half of the preceding bioavailability, it becomes impossible to determine when zero is reached. Given enough time periods, the values reached are incredibly small, far below the levels required to be active, and it may therefore be necessary to take another dose.

Half-lives and first pass metabolism are known for different drugs, and these are taken into consideration when calculating drug dosage. Liver and kidney disease in some individuals will impinge on drug metabolism and/or excretion.

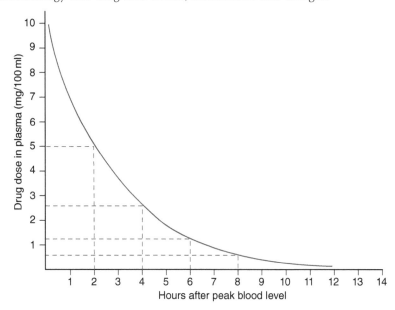

*Figure 15.2* The half-life of a drug. This graph shows the elimination pattern of a drug (e.g. drug X, with a half-life of two hours) from circulation. From peak plasma concentration (in this case 10 mg/100 ml) the first two hours sees an excretion of half the original concentration (down to 5 mg/100 ml). The second two-hour period sees an excretion of half this new value (i.e. half the 5 mg/100 ml, down to 2.5 mg/100 ml). This pattern is repeated every further two hours (i.e. removing half the concentration of the drug left at the start of that two-hour period) until the drug is virtually zero.

Drugs with short half-lives will require regular repeated dosages throughout the day, whilst those with long half-lives may only require a new dose daily or even longer. Drugs that are *slow release* provide the new dosages continuously themselves throughout the day with just one single administration daily, weekly or even monthly.

*Pharmacodynamics*

Pharmacodynamics describes how drugs work, i.e. their mode of action. It is beyond the scope of this book to examine how individual drugs carry out their function.
    Some important drugs are:

1  **Antibiotics**, which destroy bacterial infections by disrupting the structure or metabolism of the organism whilst avoiding any harm to human cells. They can affect the normal bacteria of the gut when taken orally, causing cause bowel function side effects. Some bacterial organisms can develop immunity to the antibiotics, the *'super bugs'*, making these infections much harder to treat. Antibiotics *do not* work against viral infections[4] (e.g. covid, the flu or the common cold) which will usually resolve on their own within five to ten days. Long-term or life-threatening viral infections, e.g. HIV (human immunodeficiency virus) will require treatment with *anti-viral* drugs.
2  **Analgesics**, or pain-killing drugs, discussed in Chapter 12, page 257
3  **Cardiac drugs**, which are discussed in Chapter 2 (page 36) and Chapter 3 (page 57)

4 **Respiratory drugs**, discussed in Chapter 5 (page 116)
5 **Elimination drugs**, discussed in Chapter 8 (page 177) and Chapter 9 (page 186).
6 **Ophthalmic drugs**, discussed in Chapter 13 (page 277).

A significant number of drugs work by binding to receptors on cell surfaces. Receptors are mostly proteins incorporated within the cell membrane with a binding site on the surface. There are many different receptors, some controlling channels in the membrane and therefore regulating substances entering through those channels. Others change the cellular metabolism through intermediary chemicals (called *messengers*). Receptors activate when a natural body substance (called the **ligand**) binds to the receptor. Different receptors have different ligands. Many drugs interrupt this binding process. **Antagonists** are drugs that bind to – and block – the receptor so the ligand cannot bind. This stops the action of the ligand. The opposite occurs when the drug is an **agonist**, which binds to the receptor and acts like the ligand to activate the receptor. Receptors tend to be specific to their own ligand, and for drugs to bind to a particular receptor it must have similar binding properties to those of the ligand, otherwise it would not bind. Side effects can occur when the same receptor is widely distributed across several organs or body systems. In this case, agonist or antagonist drugs given to affect the heart (for example) may also bind to the same (or similar) receptors on other organs as well, causing unwanted effects.

*Pharmacotherapeutics*

The way drugs are used in clinical practice is pharmacotherapeutics. It covers many aspects of clinical drug usage, including dosage, storage, prescribing, drug calculations, routes of administration, side effects, drug interactions, record keeping etc.

The prescribed dose of the drug is based on the **therapeutic window** (Figure 15.3). This is the window of dosage that will benefit the patient whilst creating the least amount of side effects. The lowest point of the window is the smallest dose that will have a beneficial

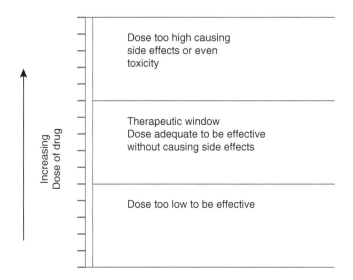

*Figure 15.3* The therapeutic window.

effect in the body, below which the effect is so small as to be of no value. The highest point of the window is the dosage that has the maximum effect, above which side effects (and possibly toxicity) will become a problem. It is the safe dosage window for prescribing (Figure 15.3). The ideal regime is to prescribe the drug at the lower end of the window so there is opportunity to raise the dose if required, but this depends on what drug is involved and the condition being treated.

### Drug side effects

Drug side effects (or 'toxic effects') are defined as those effects that the drug has which are unpleasant, unwanted and possibly harmful. They are mostly unrelated to the expected function of the drug. There are examples of drug side effects which can be beneficial or therapeutic. They usually occur through a different mechanism separate from that for which the drug was given i.e. a different pharmacodynamic activity.

Side effects involve almost every body system, but some systems are more affected than others. The most likely effect would be with the system responsible for the drug's entry into the body, i.e. the first point of contact. The digestive system is more affected because most drugs are administered by mouth, so it is the first system to contact the medication and the first system to process the drug. Topically administered drugs – i.e. drugs in creams rubbed in through the skin – and subcutaneous injections, i.e. injected just under the skin surface, can cause skin reactions.

#### *Gastrointestinal (GI) side effects*

**Gastrointestinal** (**GI**) side effects, such as nausea and vomiting, diarrhoea or constipation, are the most common side effects of drugs. Most GI side effects are mild and not life-threatening but can be unpleasant and debilitating. Intravenous injections can also cause GI side effects quite quickly by affecting the brain centres that control digestion (see Chapter 9).

#### *Nausea and vomiting*

**Nausea** (feeling of sickness) and **vomiting** are common side effects of drugs because oral drugs may irritate the mucosal lining of the stomach and because both oral and injected drugs may activate the **chemoreceptor trigger zone** (**CTZ**) in the brainstem (see Chapter 9, Figure 9.4, page 189). Digestive mucosal irritation sends sensory stimuli to the brainstem via the **vagus nerve** (**cranial nerve X**; see Chapter 9, Figure 9.6, page 190). Chapter 9 discusses vomiting and the main drugs that cause it.

#### *Diarrhoea and constipation*

Diarrhoea is the passing of loose, even liquid stool, often multiple times per day. Constipation is the retention of stools in the colon. The problems of constipation and diarrhoea are discussed in Chapter 9, including **morphine**, and other drugs known for their constipating side effects (see page 186). Drugs that cause diarrhoea include antibiotics since these not only kill the bacteria causing the infection; they also kill the normal bacteria that inhabit the gut (the **intestinal flora**; see *faeces*, Chapter 9).

*Indigestion (dyspepsia)*

**Dyspepsia** is a collection of stomach-related symptoms, including a feeling of bloating and being overfull from excess gas, '*heartburn*' (the burning pain caused by gastric acid refluxing into the lower oesophagus) and upper abdominal pain and distension. Acidic drugs, notably the **non-steroidal anti-inflammatory** (**NSAI**) drugs, may induce dyspepsia – and sometimes even gastric bleeding – by two different mechanisms. First, the acidic drug molecules can cause direct irritation of the stomach mucosa which is already subjected to a low pH (acidic) environment. Some aspirin products are **enteric-coated** which is a protective coating over the tablet to reduce this gastric irritation. The coating dissolves away once the tablet gets further down the digestive tract, where the environment is more alkali. Second, the drug inhibits the enzyme **cyclo-oxygenase** (**COX**; see page 258), which occurs in two forms, COX1 and COX2. By blocking these enzymes, there is a loss of production of certain **prostaglandins** (locally produced chemicals) that normally protect the gastric mucosa against stomach acidity. With this protection lost, the stomach lining is vulnerable, and becomes inflamed and irritated by its own hydrochloric acid (HCl) production. NSAIs that are COX2-specific are more gastric-protective with fewer GI side effects (see page 316 Makins and Ballinger 2003).

*Anorexia*

Anorexia is loss of appetite, and this would affect patients experiencing side effects of nausea and vomiting. The consequence of prolonged anorexia is weight loss and nutrient deficiencies, notably a loss of energy food (see Chapter 7).

The opioid drugs, such as morphine and diamorphine (heroin), are known to cause appetite loss. They bind to opioid receptors in the brain called **mu** (**μ**) **kappa** (**κ**) and **delta** (**δ**) (see Chapter 12, page 260, and *drowsiness*, page 324). Morphine activity on mu receptors in particular suppresses brain function because these receptors are inhibitory, i.e. they reduce brain function. Various parts of the brain are involved in appetite control (Blows 2022), and activation of mu receptors by opioid drugs will cause suppression of these appetite systems.

*Central nervous system (CNS) side effects*

Drug side effects involving the central nervous system occur in many different types and severity, dependent on which part of the brain is involved. Drugs must first cross the blood-brain barrier. This cellular barrier controls everything that crosses into the brain from the blood, including drugs. Some drugs can cross without needing help, but others do need help, via transport proteins, while some are unable to cross at all. Many drugs do cross into the brain unaided and contribute to both the beneficial and adverse effects on the brain.

*Antimuscarinic side effects*

**Acetylcholine** (**ACh**), a neurotransmitter, binds to two acetylcholine receptor types: the **nicotinic** and **muscarinic** receptors. They are named after two plant alkaloids, *nicotine* and *muscarine*, that bind to the receptors in laboratory conditions, although the natural binding agent, i.e. the **ligand**, in the brain is acetylcholine. Acetylcholine is the neurotransmitter found in the **autonomic nervous system** (**ANS**), i.e. the **sympathetic** and **parasympathetic** systems. Both these parts of the ANS are two-neuronal systems passing between the central nervous system and the target organ. The first synapse between the two neurons in both systems, are the **pre-ganglionic synapses** using acetylcholine. The terminal synapse at the target organ for the *parasympathetic* system also uses acetylcholine. The terminal synapse at the target organ for the *sympathetic* system uses noradrenaline (Figure 15.4).

Antimuscarinic drugs (i.e. **muscarinic antagonists**) block the muscarinic receptors and therefore block activity of the parasympathetic system. They are used to treat a range of conditions such as Parkinson disease and motion sickness and even in optical diagnostics (see *blurred vision*, page 320). Antimuscarinic side effects occur when other drugs, i.e. those *not* used for their acetylcholine effects, coincidentally bind to the

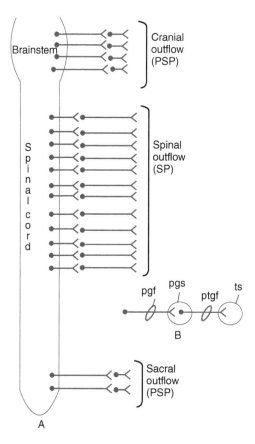

*Figure 15.4* The two parts of the autonomic nervous system (ANS). (A) The parasympathetic (PSP) cranial outflow comes from the brainstem (via cranial nerves III, VII, IX and X) and the sacral outflow comes from the lower end of the spinal cord. The sympathetic (SP) outflow comes from the thoracic section of the spinal cord. (B) Both systems involve two neurons from the source to the terminal organ. The preganglionic synapse (pgs) between the preganglionic fibre (pgf) and post ganglionic fibre (ptgf) uses acetylcholine (ACh). The terminal synapse (ts) at the target organ uses acetylcholine in the parasympathetic system and noradrenaline in the sympathetic system.

muscarinic receptor and prevent acetylcholine from binding. Antimuscarinic side effects include (Figure 15.5):

- **Dilated pupils** and **blurred vision**, due to reduced parasympathetic control of the intraocular eye muscles affecting the pupil size and the lens
- **Urine retention** happens when the parasympathetic bladder-emptying mechanism is lost and the bladder retains urine
- **Constipation** is due to loss of the parasympathetic bowel-emptying mechanism and the sympathetic takes over, retaining bowel content
- **Dry mouth** is due to changes in the salivary gland activity following loss of parasympathetic stimulation
- **Dry eyes** due to the lack of lachrymal gland activity which normally lubricates the eyes
- **Palpitations** may occur if the parasympathetic (vagus nerve, cranial nerve X) input is reduced to the heart and the sympathetic takes over, increasing the heart rate and force of contraction.

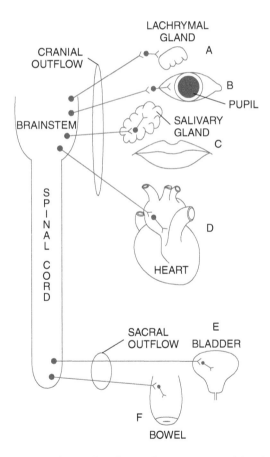

*Figure 15.5* The antimuscarinic drug side effects. These are caused by drugs blocking the muscarinic receptors in the parasympathetic system, and stopping acetylcholine (ACh) from binding. The effects of this parasympathetic blockade are: (A) Dry eyes, (B) Pupil dilation and blurred vision, (C) Dry mouth, (D) Palpitations (E) Urine retention and (F) Constipation.

*Dilated pupils*

Dilated pupils allow bright light to enter the eye causing adverse retinal effects. Pupil constriction is due to parasympathetic nervous system activity (see Chapter 13), and drugs blocking the muscarinic receptors prevent pupillary constriction. The sympathetic nervous system dominates, causing wide pupillary dilation.

*Blurred vision*

**Mydriatics** (*mydriasis* = pupil dilation) are antimuscarinics that dilate the pupil. **Cycloplegia** means paralysis of the ciliary muscles (see footnote 3, Chapter 13, page 285), which change the shape of the lens for accommodation, i.e. focusing. With paralysed muscles, the lens adopts a relaxed shape. The side effect of these intraocular changes of the lens shape is blurred vision. Since these drugs are given locally, i.e. into the eyes, they have little effect systemically.

*Urine retention and constipation*

In urine retention, the inability to pass urine, the accumulating urine in the bladder builds up to cause an acute emergency, requiring urgent treatment. Emptying the bladder (and the bowels) is a function of the parasympathetic nervous system (Figure 15.4), and muscarinic blockade by drugs reduces or even stops bladder and bowel emptying (i.e. constipation; Figure 15.5 and Figure 9.2, page 182).

*Dry mouth*

Dry mouth is due to the reduction of salivary gland stimulation by the parasympathetic nervous system. Parasympathetic normally produces a watery type of saliva, and the sympathetic produces a thicker form of saliva. Drugs that block the parasympathetic muscarinic receptors cause a reduction of watery saliva. This results in a dry mouth, and if not corrected, this ultimately leads to the complications of a dirty mouth (see Chapter 6, page 130).

*Dry eyes*

**Lachrymal glands** are producing lachrymal fluid that bathes the eyes. Antimuscarinic side effects cause **dry eyes** because the drug blocks the parasympathetic activity on these glands. Dry eyes can result in corneal ulceration and potential blindness if not lubricated often.

*Palpitations*

**Palpitations** are caused by antimuscarinic drugs reducing the parasympathetic vagus nerve to the heart. Normally the nerve slows the heart rate, but drugs reducing this activity allows the sympathetic to increase the heart rate and force of contraction. Increases in these cardiac parameters can cause the patient to experience beating or fluttering of the heart.

*Extrapyramidal effects*

The **extrapyramidal system** controls skeletal (voluntary) muscles subconsciously (see also *the extrapyramidal system*, Chapter 14, page 290). It involves the **basal ganglia**, i.e. five

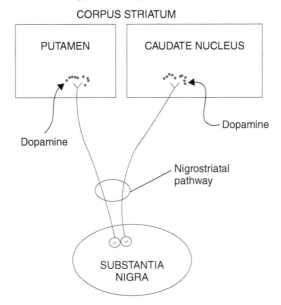

*Figure 15.6* The nigrostriatal pathway. This starts in the substantia nigra and passes to the corpus striatum (the putamen and caudate nucleus). It uses dopamine as the neurotransmitter at the synapses.

nuclei located deep in the brain. Two of these, the **putamen** and **caudate nucleus**, make up the **corpus striatum**. Between the corpus striatum and another area, the **substantia nigra**, is a neuronal pathway that uses **dopamine** as the neurotransmitter (i.e. its **dopaminergic**). This is the **nigrostriatal pathway** (*nigro* = starts in the substantia nigra; *striatal* = ends in the corpus striatum; Figure 15.6).

Being dopaminergic, it has dopamine receptors in the corpus striatum, and the pathway is susceptible to blockage by **dopamine antagonist** drugs, i.e. dopamine receptor blocking drugs, e.g. the antipsychotics.

*Tremor and rigidity*

**Tremor** is an involuntary, repeated muscle movement (shaking), mostly in the limbs, especially the upper limbs (see also *movement excesses*, Chapter 14, page 306). Fine tremor of the hands and fingers also occurs. **Rigidity** means stiff muscles with loss of movement and is due to excessive **muscle tone**. Drugs blocking the dopamine receptors in the corpus striatum reduce the activity of the nigrostriatal pathway, and this loss is the cause of these side effects. They are often referred to as **parkinsonism** because they resemble the symptoms of **Parkinson disease** (**PD**). Unlike the disease, parkinsonism can be reversed if the drug dosage is reduced or removed. The exception is **tardive dyskinesia**, a problem of uncontrollable, involuntary movements of the face, eyes, mouth, jaw, tongue and lips. It is seen in long-term use of dopamine antagonist (antipsychotic) drugs (i.e. *tardive* = very slow onset, 20 years or more). The long-term use of these drugs can cause permanent changes to the nigrostriatal pathway.

Other parkinsonism side effects include the following (*kinesia* = movement; *tonia* = muscle tone):

- **Akinesia**, inability to start movements, e.g. inability to rise from a chair or hesitating before walking. It could be due to low cell activity in dopamine pathways related to movement.
- **Akathisia**, motor restlessness, e.g. unable to sit still, seen mostly as a side effect of antipsychotic drugs but sometimes seen in Parkinson's disease. In akathisia, the brain shows raised levels of noradrenaline, and this may be due to a dysfunction of the N-methyl-D-aspartate (NMDA) glutamate receptors in the brain. Noradrenaline excites the brain into action, and motor restlessness appears to be the result of overactivity of either the motor cortex or the basal ganglia. Noradrenaline is regulated to some extent by glutamate acting on the NMDA receptor.
- **Dyskinesia** is a reduction of voluntary movements that are difficult to perform or distorted. This is often combined with some abnormal spontaneous involuntary movements such as chorea, i.e. regular involuntary movements of head, neck and trunk. It can be a side effect of antipsychotic drugs or levodopa, i.e. drugs affecting the basal ganglia.
- **Bradykinesia** is a full-range slowing of movements and is a key feature of Parkinson's disease but is rarely seen as a parkinsonism side effects.
- **Dystonia** is a wide range of muscle dysfunction and muscle coordination problems, causing postural abnormalities, muscle spasms due to involuntary movements and muscle pain. It can be due to antipsychotic drugs.
- **Ataxia** is abnormal gait (*gait* = the manner of walking) induced by a gross lack of muscle coordination. It involves brain areas that control involuntary muscle coordination, e.g. the cerebellum. As a drug side effect, it is seen mainly in as a result of drugs having a depressive effect on the brain. Alcohol intoxication is an important cause of ataxia, but it can occur with the anticonvulsant drugs, cannabis, lithium and some illicit drugs. Any drug that is an NMDA glutamate receptor antagonist can cause ataxia.

### Other CNS side effects

#### Fatigue

Fatigue (lethargy or exhaustion) is a profound feeling of tiredness and lacking energy. Different drugs are known to cause fatigue, in particular beta blockers and cancer chemotherapy, causing **cancer fatigue syndrome**, **CFS**. The mechanism by which drugs cause fatigue is elusive, involving many factors. Drug-induced **anaemia** is a major factor, i.e. a reduction in the oxygen-carrying capability of the blood by reducing the red blood cell numbers produced by the bone marrow. Other factors involve drug-related changes in hormones and cytokine production and the direct effect of drugs on some brain areas, e.g. parts of the cerebrum (the prefrontal and temporal cortex), the anterior cingulate and the cerebellum. It may be due to an abnormality with the use of fatty acids as an energy source leading to low neurotransmitter production (Kuratsune *et al.* 2002).

#### Tinnitus

**Tinnitus** is the presence of a constant noise in the ears, often a ringing sound or a buzzing or hissing noise. It may be quiet and ignored, or loud, causing distress. Some days can be worse than others. It occurs both as a symptom of disease or injury, or as a drug side effect, notably the NSAI dugs (e.g. aspirin). Many theories concerning the cause of tinnitus are proposed, some concerning the ear itself and others concerning the auditory pathways to the brain. The mechanism behind tinnitus, particularly drug-induced tinnitus, is poorly understood.

*Insomnia, drowsiness and nightmares*

**Insomnia** is unable to sleep. Sleep occurs as two phases: **rapid eye movement (REM)**, which is shallow sleep linked to dreaming, and **non-rapid eye movement (NREM)**, which is deeper sleep. These phases alternate throughout the night, starting and ending with REM (Figure 15.7).

Apart from insomnia, drugs can also affect this pattern of REM and NREM sleep. There are many drugs that list insomnia as a side effect, which is often referred to as *secondary insomnia*, i.e. secondary to taking the drugs. Some of the important drugs that cause insomnia are:

- **Psychoactive stimulants** (e.g. cocaine, caffeine, amphetamines and nicotine). Amphetamines and cocaine make it harder to get to sleep and cause shallow sleep rather than deep sleep. They increase dopamine accumulation in the brain, and high dopamine levels in turn cause brain excitement and overactivity, which is contrary to conditions needed for sleep. Caffeine blocks the brain receptors which bind the substance **adenosine**, i.e. caffeine is an adenosine receptor antagonist. Adenosine normally slows down neuronal activity and induces sleep. By blocking these receptors, caffeine prevents adenosine activity, and the individual remains awake.
- Some **anticonvulsants** (anti-epileptic drugs), notably the older medications, are reported to cause sleep pattern disturbances, including insomnia, with lengthening of the deepest levels of NREM sleep and reduced REM sleep.

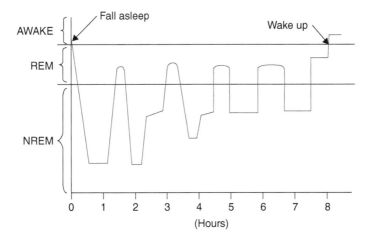

*Figure 15.7* The normal REM-NREM sleep pattern for a young adult. The normal sleep pattern alternates between rapid eye movement (REM) and non-rapid eye movement (NREM) sleep. REM occurs briefly first and then switches repeatedly with NREM. REM increases gradually as NREM reduces during the night, and the individual wakes from REM.

- **Beta-blockers** are drugs used for treating high blood pressure. They are **beta-adrenergic receptor antagonists** that block the action of noradrenaline on cardiac sympathetic receptors and thus reduce the force of ventricular contraction. As a side effect, these drugs, especially the **lipophilic** or fat-soluble drugs, reduce the amount of REM sleep and cause night-time waking.
- Some **statins**, i.e. drugs used to lower blood cholesterol, especially the lipid-soluble forms,[5] can cause insomnia. Lipid-soluble drugs cross the blood-brain barrier easier than the water-soluble drugs (Climent *et al.* 2021). They affect the neurons easier because cells have lipid membranes and myelin (lipid) sheaths. The exact mechanism by which fat-soluble statins cause insomnia is not fully known, but the problem is reduced with the water-soluble drugs. Statins have a wide range of side effects. These include depletion of **ubiquinone** (or **Coenzyme $Q_{10}$** or **$CoQ_{10}$**), which is a component of energy production in the cell. A depletion of $CoQ_{10}$ can lead to serious muscle and cardiovascular problems.

**Drowsiness** is often a side effect of pain-relieving drugs, notably the **opioid analgesics**. Opioid drugs bind to and activate the mu (μ) brain receptor (see also *loss of appetite*, page 317), which is inhibitory, i.e. it reduces neuronal function. Mu receptors are concentrated in the brainstem where activation can cause suppression of various brainstem activities. The brainstem contains the **reticular activation system** (**RAS**), which is involved in the sleep-wake cycle. The brainstem has the centres for consciousness (see *the biology of consciousness*, Chapter 11). Opioid drugs active on the brainstem mu receptors may suppress consciousness and cause drowsiness.

Other drugs causing drowsiness include the **anxiolytic** drugs, i.e. anti-anxiety drugs, mostly the **benzodiazipines**, alcohol, barbiturates and the antihistamines. The benzodiazepines, barbiturates and alcohol work by binding to a particular **gamma-aminobutyric acid** (**GABA**) receptor called **$GABA_A$**. When activated by binding GABA, the receptor opens a chloride ionic channel ($Cl^-$), which causes suppression (inhibition) of brain impulses (or **action potentials**) across that synapse. This sedates brain activity. Benzodiazepines, barbiturates and alcohol promote the GABA inhibitory activity of this receptor, sedating the brain and causing drowsiness.

**Antihistamines** are drugs given to reduce the effects of an allergic reaction where histamine has been released from mast cells (see page 331). They are **H1 receptor antagonists**, i.e. they block the H1 histamine receptor, and this reduces inflammation. However, this desired effect is mediated mainly through the *peripheral* H1 receptor, i.e. those in body tissues. But there are also *central* H1 receptors in the brain, and these drugs, particularly the older generation of antihistamines, cross the blood-brain barrier and block brain H1 receptors. This causes disruption to neurotransmission in the cerebral cortex involving blockage of sodium channels, leading to drowsiness.

**Nightmares** are unpleasant and often frightening dreams that can be caused by some medicines, mostly the dopamine agonists, hypnotics, beta blockers and amphetamines. The mechanism is unknown because the physiology of nightmares is unknown. With amphetamines and the dopamine agonists it may be due to excess dopaminergic activity on dopamine receptors caused by these drugs.

*Dizziness, vertigo, hypotension and fainting*

**Dizziness** is a difficulty with body stability – i.e. disturbed balance or equilibrium – and a feeling of being giddy. **Vertigo** is a feeling of motion when nothing is moving. Either the patient is feeling they are moving in a non-moving environment or they feel that their environment is moving when it is not. Vertigo can often be accompanied by feelings of nausea and vomiting (see also *vertigo* later).

**Hypotension** is low blood pressure, and drugs that cause reduced blood pressure (e.g. **vasodilators**) can cause dizziness and **fainting** (**syncope**). Three symptoms are linked, i.e. a *drop in blood pressure* causes reduced blood flow to the brain, and this then causes *dizziness*, and *fainting*. A drug-induced fall in blood pressure is the result of **vasodilation**, i.e. dilating the **peripheral arterioles**, which then lowers the **peripheral resistance** and reduces the blood pressure (see Chapter 3, page 47):

Cardiac output (CO) × peripheral resistance (PR) = blood pressure (BP)

Therefore:

CO × reduced PR ($\downarrow$) = reduced BP ($\downarrow$)

A similar situation can occur with drugs affecting the heart by reducing its output from the ventricles (i.e. the *cardiac output*, CO):

($\downarrow$) CO × PR = reduced BP ($\downarrow$)

Examples are drugs such as **beta blockers** which slow the heart rate and reduce the force of contraction.

Drugs can cause dizziness by interference with the **vestibular** (i.e. balance) mechanism (Chapter 9, Figure 9.5, page 190). This involves the **vestibular apparatus** of both ears (i.e. the **semicircular canals**), which detect changes in movement and body position. The eyes give information of position and movement in relation to the environment. The sensory nerves from the joints and tendons (called **proprioception**) inform the brain about the position and movement of limbs. Finally, skin pressure detectors (nerve endings; Table 10.1, page 201) inform the brain about limb and body position in relation to gravity.

Vertigo is the result of conflicting information about movement sent to the brain at the same time from any of these sensory systems. For example, information about movement comes from the eyes and the vestibular apparatus arrives at the brain simultaneously, but the two bits of information do not match up, i.e. conflicting information; vertigo is the result. The term 'vertigo' is often used incorrectly by being muddled with a fear of heights (which is **acrophobia**). Certainly, looking down from a height can trigger a sensation of movement, causing vertigo, but vertigo can also be triggered at any height, even at ground level, as in drug side effects (see also Chapter 9, page 189). The **vestibulo-ocular reflex** (**VOR**) is a good example of how vestibular (balance) and ocular (visual) information work together and how disturbance of this system can cause vertigo (Figure 15.8).

The VOR allows for fixation of the gaze on an object during head movement (see Chapter 13, page 281). The semi-circular canals detect rotational movement of the head and convert the movement into nerve impulses, which are then sent via the eighth cranial (**vestibulocochlear**) nerve to the **vestibular nuclei** of the brainstem (*neuron 1*). From here, the pathways cross before passing out to the nuclei of the eye muscles (*neuron 2*) via the third (oculomotor) and sixth (abducens) cranial nerves (*neuron 3*). The VOR works in response to vertical head movements as well as horizontal. The eyes move in the same manner as the head, but in the opposite direction, in order to maintain the gaze on the

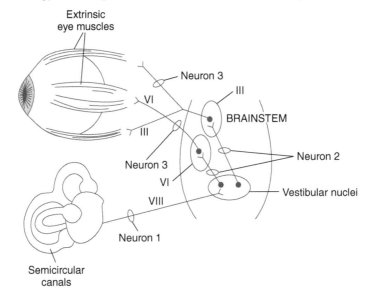

*Figure 15.8* The vestibulo-ocular reflex (VOR). Neuron 1 runs from the semicircular canals of the vestibular apparatus, taking head movement information to the vestibular nuclei of the brainstem. Neuron 2 takes the information to the brainstem nuclei that control the external eye muscles (i.e. the nuclei of cranial nerves III and VI). Neuron 3 runs from the brainstem nuclei to the eye muscles. The purpose is to allow the eyes to sustain a fixed gaze on an object while the head turns. Some drugs can affect this system and cause vertigo.

object despite the head movements. Vertigo can be caused by disturbance of the neuro-transmitters that occur in the synapses between the three-neuronal system of the VOR, which could be caused by drugs. These neurotransmitters include glutamate, acetylcholine, gamma-aminobutyric acid (GABA), dopamine, noradrenaline and histamine.

### Psychosis

Any drugs that stimulate dopamine receptors in the brain are potential causes of acute psychoses. Cocaine ('cocaine psychosis'), amphetamines and cannabis ('cannabis psychosis') are drugs that regularly cause psychotic episodes (Blows 2022). More than 80% of hospital admissions for acute psychosis each year in the UK are drug-induced. The dopamine receptors (especially D2 and D3) in the mesocortical pathways of the brain become overstimulated and cause hallucinations, delusions, thought disorder and mania. Cannabis is known for causing a high degree of paranoia.

### Headache

Drug-related headaches can occur as a drug side effect, as a feature of chronic drug overuse or as a result of drug withdrawal (e.g. alcohol).

Those medications that increase blood flow to the brain (**vasodilators**) and the amphetamines are especially known to cause headaches. Why a raised blood flow to the brain causes throbbing headaches is not fully understood. It follows drug-induced vasodilation of the cerebral vascular system. It may be due to a rise in intracranial pressure since normal cerebral blood flow contributes about 10% of the intracranial pressure, and vasodilation is likely to increase this percentage. It may be due to stretching of the arterial wall inside the skull. The throbbing (pulsatile) nature of the headache indicates the involvement of arterial blood flow. **Glyceryl trinitrate** (**GTN**) is a vasodilator drug used in treating the cardiac disorder called **angina** and has headaches as a main side effect. The initial (primary) headache can be immediate or soon after administration, and it tends to be relatively mild with no other symptoms. A secondary headache is delayed and more severe, with symptoms of nausea, vomiting and **photophobia** (a dislike of light). **Nitric oxide** (**NO**) is the active metabolite derived from glyceryl trinitrate and is the cause of the vasodilation that leads to the headache. The delayed secondary headaches are caused by the release of other chemical mediators, including the neurotransmitter glutamate (Bagdy *et al.* 2010).

Chronic daily use of normal-dose analgesia can cause rebound headaches (known as **medication overuse headaches**, **MOH**). The problem occurs with other drugs as well, notably the **opioids** and the **triptans** (i.e. drugs used to treat migraine). The headache causes the patient to take the analgesic, but when the drug wears off the headache returns and the patient then repeats the drug. If this continues over a period of days or weeks, a state occurs where the headache will automatically return at any time the drug is withdrawn. The reason for this is not fully understood but does appear to involve a genetic predisposition and changes in receptor and enzyme physiology in the brain.

Substance withdrawal headaches are known to occur if a substance (e.g. a medication or alcohol) is taken for longer than three months then stopped. Soon after stopping, the headaches begin, but if the patient can remain off the substance long enough (usually no longer than three months) the headaches will subside. The problem is due to tolerance, where the brain has got used to the presence of the substance and suddenly finds it is missing. These substances include opioid drugs, caffeine, alcohol and oestrogen medications.

### Skin side effects

Skin side effects are usually the first to be identified as they are the quickest to occur and the most visible. They are the result of rapid immune reactions (e.g. rashes).

### Rash

Redness (**erythema**) and rashes begin usually within the first few days of starting a drug, and often within hours, depending on the level of sensitivity to the drug (see also Table 10.2, page 204). The penicillins and sulphonamide antibiotics are a common cause of rashes. The mechanism involves one of four types of immune reaction (see page 330) causing vasodilation (redness), skin eruptions (rashes) and local skin oedema (swelling; Lee and Thomson 2006; see *drug allergies*, page 330).

There are non-immune causes of skin rashes, including drugs such as the NSAI (see page 257) that directly release histamine from mast cells i.e. not through the immune system (see page 331).

### Hair loss

**Alopecia** (hair loss) is a known side effect of some drugs, especially anti-cancer drugs (i.e. **chemotherapy**). Hair grows from rapidly reproducing cells in the skin follicles.

Anti-cancer drugs kill rapidly reproducing cells, therefore, hair follicle cells are vulnerable to these drugs.

Hair growth follows two phases; the **anagen phase** (3 to 4 years long) is the period of hair growth, followed by the **telogen phase** (about 3 months long), when hair growth stops and the hair 'rests'. At the end of the telogen phase, the hair falls out and the cycle starts again. Drugs can cause one of two types of alopecia. **Telogen effluvium**, the most common form of drug-induced hair loss, occurs when the hair passes quickly into the telogen phase and falls out early (about 100 to 150 hairs lost per day). **Anagen effluvium**, the main cause of alopecia in chemotherapy, is hair lost during the hair growth phase. Here, the drugs destroy or disrupt the fast reproduction of hair follicle cells. It occurs quicker than telogen effluvium, and it can be very severe, causing total hair loss across the body.

## Drug interactions

Adverse drug interactions *may* occur when two or more drugs are taken together. The interaction involves one drug impeding or enhancing the action of another (Rodrigues 2008). Many oral medications can be taken safely together, but if any interactions do occur, they can sometimes be harmful or even fatal. The elderly have a greater risk of this problem because they are more likely to be prescribed multiple medication (called **polypharmacy**) and because their metabolic and excretory pathways are less efficient due to the ageing process (Blows 2022; Seymour and Routledge 1998). About 20% of the UK population aged 60 years or older consume 56% of all the dispensed medication, and the elderly population is growing. There are recommendations that the over-60 population should not be prescribed more than 3 medications at any one time because of the risk to health from drug interactions, but this is not always possible. Each additional drug added to the mix increases the risk of an interaction. It is not just prescribed medications that are involved. A mix of 'over-the-counter' self-medication – or several illicit drugs used together during addiction – can cause an interaction.

Smoking can also cause drug interactions when medication is taken at the same time, since nicotine is a drug. Smoking induces metabolic enzymes (see page 329), and this interferes with the metabolic process of other drugs (see *pharmacokinetic interactions* later). Nicotine also has pharmacodynamic interactions (see page 329) with a wide range of drugs, and this causes changes with the activity and efficacy of those drugs.

### Pharmacokinetic interactions

During **absorption**, some oral drugs may compete for uptake into the blood from the digestive tract. If one drug is absorbed first, this may block the absorption of another drug, causing it to be delayed in the gut. When this happens, the therapeutic effect of the delayed drug is reduced and it may be eliminated from the bowel before being fully absorbed. Alternatively, some drugs bind with specific foods, and this delays or prevents the drug's absorption. Those foods must be avoided when taking the drug. An example is the antibiotic tetracycline that binds to calcium, and so the drug must not be taken with calcium-rich foods such as milk.

During **distribution**, drugs in circulation bind to blood proteins. Some drug combinations result in drugs competing for the same binding sites on the proteins. This competition causes some drugs to displace others for protein binding sites, and this changes the activity level (the **bioavailability**) of the displaced drugs.

During **metabolism**, multiple drugs may compete for the various enzyme systems, i.e. multiple enzymes working together. This can alter the enzyme activity (Scully 2008; Zhang *et al.* 2008). Most drug metabolism takes place in the liver, and enzyme systems in the liver vary the metabolic process depending on what drugs are present. For example, some drugs *increase* enzyme activity (called **enzyme induction**) or *decrease* enzyme activity (called **enzyme inhibition**), and this may affect the metabolism of other drugs using those same enzymes systems. These other drugs may be delayed or accelerated in their metabolism. Delayed metabolism of a drug increases that drug's concentration in the blood, and this then risks reaching toxic levels, especially if subsequent doses are taken. Metabolic interactions are particularly important, mainly because one liver enzyme system, called the **cytochrome P450 oxidases** (**CYP**), is involved in the metabolism of the majority of drugs and therefore is prone to enzyme induction or inhibition. Alcohol is metabolised by this enzyme system and also causes induction of some P450 enzymes, therefore disturbing the metabolism of any other drugs administered at the same time. Usually, the alcohol competes with the drug and displaces the drug, which is therefore delayed in its metabolism. This delay causes the drug to lengthen its period of activity, indicated by an increased drug **half-life** (Figure 15.2), and this prolongs and increases the drug's activity. Chronic alcoholism and smoking cause specific P450 enzymes induction to remain high. This will speed up the metabolism of other drugs faster than normally expected.

Smoking causes a very large range of undesirable chemicals to enter the circulation, among which the **polycyclic aromatic hydrocarbons** provide powerful induction of some P450 enzymes. This has a profound effect on drug metabolism, a case of smoking speeding up the metabolism and therefore the clearance of drugs quickly, shortening the drug's therapeutic life.

During **elimination**, some drugs may cause other drugs to be eliminated quicker or slower than they should be. Those eliminated too slowly will accumulate in circulation and may reach toxic levels. An example is the drug digoxin, which is delayed in its excretion by the presence of a range of other drugs, which must then be avoided to prevent digoxin toxicity.

*Pharmacodynamic interactions*

Pharmacodynamic interactions occur when two or more drugs administered together interfere with each other's mode of action, i.e. they alter in some way the mechanism by which one or both drugs carry out their function. Receptors are usually the main site for interactions to occur. Several drugs administered together may become competitive at the same receptor site (Figure 15.9).

This means that one drug can easily affect the activity of another by preventing its binding. If two **agonists**, i.e. drugs that stimulate or activate a receptor type, are given at the same time, this may increase the normal expected activity, i.e. it will cause an *additive* effect, and that can lead to toxicity. Similarly, two **antagonists**, i.e. drugs that block receptors, given at the same time could reduce the receptor function to dangerously low levels. If an agonist and antagonist for the same receptor were given together, they would basically cancel each other out with little therapeutic value.

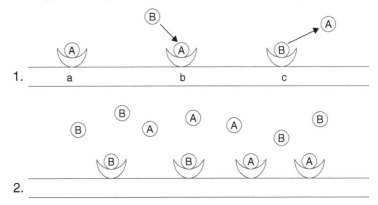

*Figure 15.9* Pharmacodynamic drug interaction between two drugs. Drugs A and B are shown binding to the same cell surface receptors. 1. (a) Drug A has bound to the receptor. (b) Drug B is competing with drug A for the receptor. (c) Drug B has displaced drug A and now occupies the receptor. This means that drug B affects the function of drug A. 2. Both drugs A and B bind to the same receptors. When both occur together, some of each will bind, affecting the total function of both drugs. If both drugs had opposing effects on the receptors, they may cancel out each other's effect.

## Drug allergies

Allergies occur when a foreign substance (an **antigen**) enters the body and sets up an immune response. Drugs may react with proteins of the immune system (called **antibodies**, or **immunoglobulins**, **Ig**). This is a type I response, but equally there are 3 other drug allergic responses possible, i.e. type II, type III and type IV (see below). Drugs become the **antigen**[6] in all these immune reactions. The allergic response occurs each time the drug enters the body and the reaction triggers several chemical chain reactions, including histamine release, causing inflammation.

The four types of allergic responses with medication are:

- **Type I** reaction is an acute response (i.e. rapid onset) causing skin rash, **urticaria** (inflamed patches of skin with red, raised, itchy bumps; also called **hives**), tissue swelling (due to local oedema; see Chapter 6, page 129), respiratory difficulties (due to bronchoconstriction; see Chapter 5) and even **anaphylaxis**, i.e. a severe shock caused by extensive peripheral vasodilation leading to a loss of peripheral resistance and therefore collapse of blood pressure (see Chapter 3 and page 55). Anaphylaxis is potentially fatal if not treated urgently. Type I is IgE-mediated, i.e. the drug (the antigen) has caused an increase in the production of the antibody IgE that is specific to the drug's chemical properties. IgE binds to cells in the tissues called mast cells. **Mast cells** are specialised cells that can release **histamine** which causes local inflammation. When the drug is introduced into the body, it binds to the IgE on mast cells in a cross-linked manner (Figure 15.10). Mast cells then release their histamine and inflammation occurs. Type I reactions are the fastest type of drug allergy, and include reactions to any medication containing a protein (acting as the antigen), such as insulin.
- **Type II** reaction is a delayed response where drugs bind to and modify the body's cellular proteins, which then appear as cell surface antigens in the body and cause an

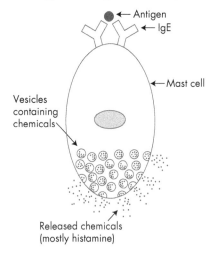

*Figure 15.10* The release of histamine from mast cells by an immune response. The antibody IgE
binds to the mast cell surface and cross-links an antigen, a foreign substance from
outside the body, which can be a drug. This cross-linkage causes release of vesicles
containing chemicals, mostly histamine, a cause of inflammation (i.e. an inflammatory mediators).

immune reaction. The immune system responds to these modified cells through activation of B-cell lymphocytes, which then release antibodies (IgG) to attack the antigenic
(drug-modified) proteins. This leads to activation of K cells (K = killer) that have a cytotoxic effect, i.e. they kill the cells that are bearing the antigens. It also triggers a chemical reaction in the **complement system**. This series of blood proteins, when activated,
produces substances that result in the destruction of the cell by **lysis** (i.e. breaking up
the cells; Figure 15.11). Drugs that can do this include some antibiotics such as the
penicillins, cephalosporins and the sulfonamides.

- **Type III** reaction is where drugs in circulation (the antigens) form complexes of different sizes with the antibodies **IgM** or **IgG**. The drug antigen is usually present in much
larger quantities than the antibodies. The large immune complexes formed can be
cleared by **macrophages** (phagocytic cells), but small complexes cannot be cleared, a
condition called **serum sickness**. The complexes create problems with:

1  The renal **nephrons** causing **glomerulonephritis**
2  The tiny blood vessels causing **vasculitis**
3  The joints, causing joint pain (**arthralgia**).

The salicylates (e.g. aspirin) and chlorpromazine can cause this type of reaction.

- **Type IV** reaction is a delayed hypersensitivity caused by drugs applied to the skin
surface, as in **contact dermatitis** or injected subcutaneously into the skin, as in
some skin tests, which then react with **T-cells**. This is the most common type of
drug reaction in skin reactions (e.g. rashes), including many topically applied skin
medications.

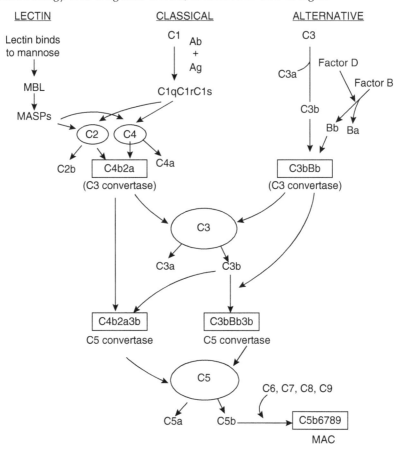

*Figure 15.11* The complement system, a chain reaction occurring between various plasma proteins (C proteins) leading to a membrane attack complex (MAC). The common pathway can be activated by any of three initial pathways, the classical, lectin and alternative pathways. The classical pathway begins with antibodies binding to the antigen creating the C1qC1rC1s complex. The lectin pathway begins with lectin binding to the sugar mannose on the antigen surface to form mannose binding lectin (MBL). This forms a complex with mannose-binding lectin-associated serine proteases (MASPs). C1qC1rC1s complex and MASPs act on C2 and C4 to form C4b2a, C4a and C2b being discarded. The alternative pathway starts with C3 which is split into C3a and C3b. C3a is discarded. Factor B and factor D join to split factor B into Ba and Bb. Bb joins C3b to form C3bBb. C4b2a and C3bBb are enzymes that act on C3 (i.e. C3 convertase). This splits C3 into C3a and C3b. The C3b forms a complex with C4b2a to form C4b2a3b, and C3 also forms a complex with C3bBb to form C3bBb3b. Both C4b2a3b and C3bBb3b are enzymes acting on C5 (i.e. C5 convertase), splitting C5 into C5a and C5b. C5a is discarded. C6, C7, C8 and C9 are added to C5b to form the membrane attack complex (MAC) (i.e. C5b6789) which breaks down antigen cells.

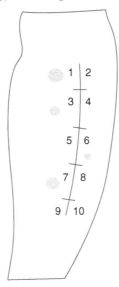

*Figure 15.12* Type IV skin test reactions. A tiny dose of a drug is dropped on the labelled skin, in this case samples of 10 different drugs labelled 1 to 10. The skin reaction is observed after a few minutes. Here there is a strong reaction to drugs 1 and 7, with minor reactions to drugs 3 and 6, and no reaction to the others. This type of skin test is most often done with food samples to test for food allergies.

*Table 15.1* Red flag and warnings of deteriorating condition

**Ᵽ Red Flag = serious situation which needs urgent medical attention**.

| Flag warning | Details |
| --- | --- |
| **Ᵽ Red Flag** | **Missed dosage of drugs, the problems that result depends on the drug missed. Accidental or deliberate overdose of drugs may be life threatening, again depending on which drugs and how much was taken. Treat all overdoses as requiring urgent medical attention.** <br> **Any drug, including illicit drugs, causing mental health issues, e.g. psychosis.** <br> **Some severe allergic reactions to drugs may be life threatening, e.g. anaphylactic shock.** |

(After Hill-Smith and Johnson 2021, with permission)

## Key points

*Pharmacology*

- Pharmacology is the study of drugs and involves pharmacokinetics (drug movement), pharmacodynamics (drug action) and pharmacotherapeutics (clinical use of drugs).
- Half-life is the time period required to reduce the blood level of a drug by half, then reduce the level by half again within the same time period. This is repeated until only a tiny trace of the drug remains.
- Agonists increase receptor activity, antagonists block receptor activity.

- Therapeutic window means the dosage of a drug which is physiologically active but not causing dangerous side effects or toxicity.

*Drug side effects*

- Drug side effects are unwanted adverse effects that usually occur from a mechanism unrelated to the desired effect of the drug.
- Many side effects are mild and transient, but others are very unpleasant and can be harmful.
- Gastrointestinal side effects, especially nausea and vomiting, are common for many drugs, especially oral medication.
- Central nervous system side effects are also common and occur in many different types, depending on the brain area involved.

*Drug interactions*

- Drug interactions occur when two or more drugs are given together, and one drug then causes unwanted changes in the action of the other drug.
- Pharmacokinetic interactions can occur during absorption, distribution, metabolism or excretion of the drugs.
- These interactions allow one drug to change the activity of the other drug.
- Metabolic interactions often involve one drug affecting the activation of liver enzyme systems, which then affects the metabolism of a second drug.
- Pharmacodynamic interactions mean that two or more drugs given simultaneously may block or enhance each other's function.
- Most pharmacodynamic interactions occur at cell surface receptors.

*Drug allergies*

- Drug allergies can be mild or serious and even fatal.
- Drugs are sometimes treated by the immune system as antigens, i.e. they can cause an allergic response as a foreign substance entering the body.
- There are four allergic responses possible when drugs cause allergic reactions: type I, type II, type III and type IV.

## Notes

1 Catabolic enzymes are those that breakdown substances, and in the case of the digestive system they breakdown food (catabolism = the metabolic process for reducing large complex substances to smaller simpler substances).
2 The hepatic portal vein should not be confused with the hepatic vein. The former takes blood (and the products of food digestion plus oral drugs) to the liver from the gut. The latter takes blood (and the products of liver metabolism, including drug metabolites) from the liver into general circulation. Two portal veins exist in the body: (1) The large hepatic portal vein, from the gut to the liver and (2) The tiny hypothalamo-hypophyseal portal vein from the hypothalamus to the pituitary gland.
3 This is an arbitrary value in this example since the actual amount differs between different drugs.
4 Viruses have the type of structure that antibiotics cannot affect. Sometimes a viral infection may be followed by a bacterial *secondary* infection, and antibiotics may then be of value in stopping the secondary infection.

5  Lipophilic (fat-soluble) statins are simvastatin, fluvastatin, and atorvastatin. Hydrophilic (water-soluble) statins are rosuvastatin and pravastatin.
6  Antigen is any foreign substance that enters the body and causes an immune response, usually via antibody production.

## References

Bagdy G., Riba P., Kecskemeti V., Chase D. and Juhasz G. (2010) Headache-type adverse effects of NO donors: Vasodilation and beyond. *British Journal of Pharmacology*, *160*(1): 20–35.

Blows W.T. (2022) *The Biological Basis of Mental Health* (4th edition). Routledge, Abingdon.

Climent E., Benaiges D. and Pedro-Botet J. (2021) Hydrophilic or lipophilic statins? *Frontiers in Cardiovascular Medicine*, *8*(Article 687585): 1–11. https://doi.org/10.3389/fcvm.2021.687585

Gottlieb S. (2001) Drug effects blamed for fifth of hospital deaths among elderly. *British Medical Journal*, *323*(7320): 1025.

Gutierrez D. (2010) Drug side effects blamed for 20 percent of hospital readmissions. *Natural News*, 4 January. www.naturalnews.com/027866_drugs_side_effects.html

Hill-Smith I. and Johnson G. (2021) *Little Book of Red Flags*. National Minor Illness Centre, Bedfordshire.

Kuratsune H., Yamaguti K., Lindh G., Evengård B., Hagberg G., Matsumura K., Iwase M., Onoe H., Takahashi M., Machii T., Kanakura Y., Kitani T., Långström B. and Watanabe Y. (2002) Brain regions involved in fatigue sensation: Reduced acetylcarnitine uptake into the brain. *NeuroImage*, *17*(3): 1256–1265.

Lee A. and Thomson J. (2006) Drug-induced skin reactions, in Lee A. (ed.) *Adverse Drug Reactions* (2nd edition). Pharmaceutical Press, New York.

Makins R. and Ballinger A. (2003) Gastrointestinal side effects of drugs. *Expert Opinion on Drug Safety*, *2*(4): 421–429.

Rodrigues A.D. (2008) *Drug – Drug Interactions*. Informa Healthcare, London.

Scully C. (2008) Drug interactions. *Drug Metabolism Reviews*, *41*(3): 486–527.

Seymour R.M. and Routledge P.A. (1998) Important drug – drug interactions in the elderly. *Drugs & Aging*, *12*(6): 485–494.

Zhang H., Sinz M.W. and Rodrigues D. (2008) Metabolism-mediated drug – drug interactions, in Zhang D., Zhu M. and Humphreys W.G. (eds.) *Drug Metabolism in Drug Design and Development: Basic Concepts and Practice*. Wiley, New York.

# 16 Physiological changes occurring in pregnancy

- Introduction
- Cardiovascular changes
- Respiratory changes
- Hormonal changes
- Biochemical changes
- Renal and fluid balance changes
- Pre-eclampsia and eclampsia
- Key points
- Notes
- References

## Introduction

The maternal changes that occur in pregnancy are all adaptive to accommodate and sustain a developing child. While most of these changes take place gradually as the child grows, nearly all of them will return to the pre-pregnant conditions relatively quickly after the birth. They should leave behind few, if any, permanent effects. This indicates that these changes are normal, and they should be easily distinguished from anything that is pathological. All organs and body systems are affected to a greater or lesser degree; the most important of these changes are discussed in this chapter (Soma-Pillay *et al.* 2016).

Pregnancy is divided into three stages i.e. the first, second and third **trimesters**. The first trimester covers weeks 1 to 12, starting from the date of the last menstruation. The second trimester covers weeks 13 to 27 and the third trimester covers weeks 28 to birth, which is sometime around week 40.

## Cardiovascular changes

Blood is a key factor that changes during pregnancy to provide the foetus with nutrition and fluid and to remove waste. Plasma volume increases gradually throughout normal

DOI: 10.4324/9781003389118-16

pregnancy, having expanded about 50% by the thirty-fourth week of gestation. This dilution of the blood by additional plasma, known as **haemodilution**, exceeds the red cell mass, and therefore it lowers the haemoglobin (Hb) concentration, the haematocrit and red blood cell (RBC) count (see Chapter 4, page 91). The mean corpuscular Hb (MCV) and the mean corpuscular Hb concentration (MCHC) both remain unchanged (see Chapter 4, page 92).

The platelet count drops as pregnancy progresses but usually stays above the normal minimum. However, up to 10% of pregnant women will develop a platelet count of $100-150 \times 10^9$ cells/litre at full term, but this is not considered to be pathological. To be thrombocytopenic, the platelet count in pregnant women would have to fall below $100 \times 10^9$ cells/litre.

Blood clotting factors increase to prepare for haemostasis immediately after birth. Factors VIII, IX and X are all raised, and fibrinogen is increased by 80% (Chapter 4, Figure 4.7, Table 4.8). Factors preventing blood clotting, such as protein S and antithrombin, are reduced. This increases the risk of venous thrombosis from the first trimester through to 12 weeks after birth. Thrombosis risk increases further due to venous blood flow slowing down, particularly in the lower limbs, and there may be some degree of actual venous blood stasis.

Changes occur in the heart as well. It becomes slightly enlarged during pregnancy and provides a greater force of contraction. Coupled with peripheral vasodilation, this increased force of ventricular contraction raises the cardiac output (CO) by about 20% at 8 weeks gestation and increases it by a total of 40% overall. This CO increase is due to an increase in both the stroke volume (SV) and the heart rate (HR) (see Chapter 3, Figure 3.7, page 48). CO reaches a maximum at 20–28 weeks and falls again by full term. The stroke volume also decreases by full term but an increase in heart rate stabilises the raised CO.

Blood pressure normally falls a little during the first half of the pregnancy (up to week 20) despite the blood volume increase noted earlier. This is because of progesterone, which relaxes the smooth muscle of the blood vessels causing vasodilation, therefore lowering the peripheral resistance. This may occasionally result in feeling faint, especially when rising from a bed. The blood pressure returns to normal by 6 weeks after pregnancy (Figure 16.1).

Labour also changes the cardiac parameters. The cardiac output increases by 15% during the first stage of labour and by 50% during the second stage. Pain and anxiety raise the heart rate and blood pressure via a sympathetic response. Between 300 and 500 ml of blood return to the maternal circulation during uterine contraction, boosting the mother's blood volume. After delivery, this return of blood to the mother's circulation, plus the loss of the uterine weight that had been compressing the inferior vena cava, restores the maternal circulation to normal quite quickly, and the cardiac output is raised by 60–80%. Cardiac output is fully back to pre-pregnant values by 14 days post-delivery in all women who have had no cardiovascular complications.

Cardiac auscultation (listening via a stethoscope) and electrocardiogram (ECG) examination may show variations in pregnancy that could be misinterpreted as pathological. These include additional or loud heart murmurs. The ECG may show ectopic beats, small Q waves and inverted T waves in lead III, or depression of the ST segment (see Chapter 2).

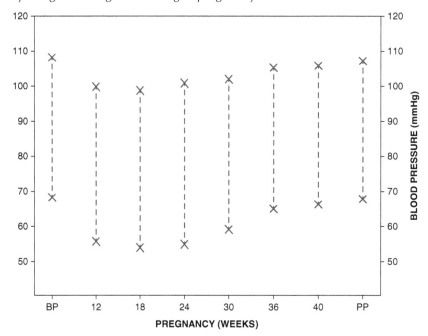

*Figure 16.1* The normal maternal blood pressure through pregnancy. The blood pressure before pregnancy (BP) is shown on the left. Further blood pressure readings taken at 12 and 18 weeks gestation shows a dip, but this gradually recovers from weeks 24 to 40 and is fully restored to pre-pregnant levels by 6 weeks post-partum (PP).

### Respiratory changes

Due to a 15% increase in metabolic rate during pregnancy, there is a 20% increase in oxygen consumption. This is provided by an increase in tidal volume and results in a raised maternal arterial $pO_2$ with a corresponding fall in arterial $pCO_2$ (see Chapter 5). Serum bicarbonate also falls, and this leads to a mild respiratory alkalosis (slightly raised blood pH) in normal pregnancy. Pregnant women may feel slightly breathless, usually during the third trimester, and this is considered normal.

### Hormonal changes

**Progesterone** is the 'pro-gestation' hormone, hence the name, meaning 'in favour of gestation'. It is initially produced by the corpus luteum of the ovary, i.e. the remaining follicle after the ovum has been released during ovulation. This hormone maintains the uterus for pregnancy by preventing the inner lining (the **endometrium**) from being lost, i.e. an absence of the next menstruation. Without the endometrium, the fertilised ovum could not implant or develop. Progesterone remains high throughout pregnancy in order to maintain the endometrium, but it cannot continue to come from the corpus luteum for long. Once the placenta is established, it takes over production of the hormone and the role of the corpus luteum is then complete.

Not only does progesterone maintain the endometrium; it also promotes blood vessel growth to the uterus, thus increasing uterine blood flow, and stimulates endometrial glands that produce essential nutrients for the foetus.

Progesterone is ultimately produced from cholesterol, and the placental cells can start this role at some point between six and nine weeks into the pregnancy. Progesterone also stabilises the uterus by preventing premature contractions and stops early lactation.

**Oestrogen** is the hormone required to promote progesterone production, and levels of oestrogen rise steadily throughout the pregnancy. There are three types of oestrogen i.e. **oestriol**, **oestrone** and **oestradiol**, all of which are derived from cholesterol. Oestradiol is the primary active hormone, with functions including the normal development of the foetal organs and bone density, promoting growth and function of the placenta and increasing growth of maternal breast tissue in preparation for lactation. Oestrogen and progesterone both inhibit actual lactation during pregnancy, but once blood levels of both these hormones have fallen after delivery of the placenta, breastfeeding is able to commence.

The adrenal cortex increases production of **cortisol** due to a raised level of **adrenocorticotropic hormone** (**ACTH**) from the pituitary gland. ACTH is raised because of a rise in the level of **corticotropin-releasing hormone** (**CRH**), and this stimulates extra production and release of ACTH. The whole system (i.e. CRH → ACTH → cortisol) is the product of the **hypothalamus-pituitary-adrenal** (**HPA**) **axis**, which increases activity under stress conditions, cortisol being raised in stress. CRH normally comes from the hypothalamus, but the rise in pregnancy is because it also comes from the placenta. CRH may be important in ensuring the foetus survives by suppressing the maternal immune system that otherwise may cause rejection of the foetus (Table 6.1). It is also involved in regulating blood flow to the foetus, essential for foetal organ maturity, and it may influence the timing of the birth. Cortisol levels rise from the second trimester and are three times higher than the non-pregnant values by the time of delivery. Over the last few weeks of pregnancy, cortisol may play a role in brain development and maturity of the lungs to enable them to cope with the change to breathing air.

Throughout pregnancy, although the cortisol levels are higher than non-pregnant levels, the normal 24-hour rise-and-fall cycle of cortisol is maintained. Cortisol may help the mother cope with the stress of delivery, and CRH may be involved in preparing the maternal brain for motherhood.

The pituitary gland enlarges in pregnancy due to increased numbers of cells in the anterior lobe that produce **prolactin**. This is the '*pro-lactation*' hormone, i.e. in favour of lactation, that promotes breast milk production. By the end of pregnancy, prolactin levels are 10 times higher than in the non-pregnant state. **Follicle-stimulating hormone** (**FSH**) and **luteinising hormone** (**LH**) remain at very low levels throughout pregnancy since their role in controlling ovum production and release from the ovary is suspended throughout pregnancy. **Growth hormone** (**GH**) production switches largely to the placenta, resulting in lower pituitary production but an overall rise in serum levels.

**Oxytocin**, a hormone from the hypothalamus via the posterior lobe of the pituitary gland, increases gradually in circulation throughout pregnancy, but it reaches a peak at the onset of labour. Oxytocin is a key hormone in both triggering and sustaining labour. It also increases the feelings of motherhood and bonding with the child. Oxytocin causes regular uterine contractions and is important in softening and dilating the cervix for the foetus to pass. Other hormones that increase during labour aid in this process. These include some prostaglandins and **relaxin**, a hormone that expands the lower pelvic muscles and prolongs the cervical changes. Oxytocin continues to contract the uterus after the birth in order to expel the placenta and to help prevent bleeding. The contracting uterine muscles tend to close the ends of blood vessels to stop further haemorrhage. Figure 16.2 is a summary of the major hormonal changes that occur during pregnancy.

*Table 16.1* The foetus contains 50% genes from the father. These could render the foetus as foreign material which could be rejected by the mother's immune system. Here are some reasons why the maternal immune system does not attack and reject the foetus, i.e. the foetus becomes an *immunological privileged site*

| Subject | Mechanism |
| --- | --- |
| Placenta | Forms a barrier to the immune system between the mother and the foetus. |
| Neurokinin B | This comes from the placenta and contains phosphocholine which binds with proteins to form compounds that suppress the maternal immunity. |
| Trophoblasts | Produced by the placenta, these cells lack certain HLA[1] molecules. These HLA molecules would trigger an immune response from the mother. Their absence allows the foetal cells to prevent an attack from maternal immunity cells. |
| Lymphocytic suppressor cells | These cells block maternal immunity T-cells[2] from destroying the foetus. |
| Syncytium[3] | The placental cells have very little extracellular space between them. This results in a barrier that prevents potential antigenic cells from moving out of the placenta and reaching the maternal immune system. |

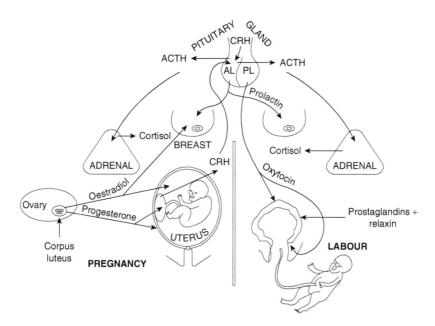

*Figure 16.2* The main hormones in pregnancy and labour. Left: During pregnancy, the ovarian corpus luteum produces oestrogen (oestradiol) and progesterone until it is replaced by the placenta, which takes over the production of these hormones, and the corpus luteum then disappears. The placenta also produces corticotropin-releasing hormone (CRH), which stimulates adrenocorticotropic hormone (ACTH) from the pituitary gland (anterior lobe, AL), and this then stimulates cortisol from the adrenal cortex. Prolactin, also from the pituitary gland (anterior lobe, AL), prepares the breasts for lactation. Right: During labour, oxytocin, from the pituitary gland (posterior lobe, PL), contracts uterine muscles to expel the baby, along with some prostaglandins and the hormone relaxin and also allows the cervix to dilate.

**Thyroid-stimulating hormone** (**TSH**) from the pituitary is raised slightly at the end of the first trimester but is otherwise remains stable in pregnancy. The free **thyroid hormones** ($T_3$ and $T_4$; see Chapter 4) are normally a little lower in the second and third trimesters.

## Biochemical changes

Iron, folate and iodine requirements during pregnancy are increased. **Iron** intake should increase by as much as 2 to 3 times when pregnant. Iron is required for both maternal and foetal haemoglobin.

**Folate** (vitamin $B_9$) intake should increase by 10 to 20 times. Folate is essential to prevent foetal **neural tube defects** (**NTDs**) such as **spina bifida** (a defect of the spinal cord) and **anencephaly** (a serious defect of the head and brain). Additional supplements of folic acid in the maternal diet, starting just before becoming pregnant, and for up to 12 weeks of pregnancy, are usually recommended.

**Iodine** intake during pregnancy should rise from the average 100 mg/day before pregnancy to 150–200 mg/day during pregnancy. Iodine in pregnancy is required for the foetus, and a shortage in the diet may induce a maternal goitre (i.e. enlargement of the thyroid gland).

Twice as much **vitamin B**$^{12}$ (see Table 7.3, page 142) than normally consumed is also required during pregnancy to prevent maternal anaemia and for the foetal blood.

**Glucose** and **lipid metabolism** undergo significant changes during pregnancy in order to supply both mother and foetus with glucose for energy. These changes involve an increase in **pancreatic beta cells** producing higher levels of **insulin**. However, insulin resistance starts to occur in the second trimester and peaks during the third trimester. This resistance is due to a cocktail of hormones, including progesterone and cortisol, that disturb peripheral insulin receptor efficiency. Foetal glucose uptake and additional glucose storage as glycogen in the maternal tissues may contribute to a relative hypoglycaemia. Lipolysis provides an additional source of energy as serum cholesterol, notably **low-density lipoproteins**, **LDL** (see Figure 4.5, page 75) and triglycerides rise during pregnancy. The higher LDL level becomes important as a substrate in the production of steroidal hormones in the placenta. The rise in triglycerides may provide more of the energy needs for the mother, thus allowing the foetus to use the glucose.

**Protein** metabolism mainly involves providing the additional required amino acids for foetal growth and development. Much of these extra amino acids will come from the maternal diet by increasing protein intake. The normal turnover and breakdown of the mother's protein is reduced to allow fat reserves to be preferentially used for maternal energy.

**Calcium** is required for foetal growth, particularly during the third trimester when development of the skeleton is increasing. The main source of calcium is the maternal diet, and calcium absorption from the digestive tract is significantly increased after 12 weeks gestation. Maternal bone absorption and replacement also increases in the third trimester, providing additional calcium for the foetus.

## Renal and fluid balance changes

The hormone **relaxin** is produced by the corpus luteum and placenta, and the level rises to a peak in the first trimester. Relaxin stimulates the production of other hormones called **endothelins** (ETs), the most important being ET-1. These bind to two types of endothelin receptors, $ET_A$ and $ET_B$. The binding of ET-1 to these receptors in smooth muscle causes arterial vasoconstriction, and therefore a rise in blood pressure. In cardiac muscle it increases the force of contraction. $ET_B$ receptors are also found on the endothelial lining cells of arteries. When endothelin binds to the endothelial $ET_B$ receptors, nitric oxide (NO) is produced, and this reduces ET-1 production causing vasodilation and reducing the blood pressure. This is particularly important regarding the renal arteries, which dilate, creating an increase in the renal blood flow during pregnancy (Figure 16.3).

The result of increased renal blood flow is a rise in the **glomerular filtration rate (GFR)** (see Chapter 8). The kidneys enlarge slightly to accommodate the increased vascular glomeruli and raised urinary volumes. Dilation of the urinary collecting system within the kidneys can lead to a mild **hydronephrosis**, an accumulation of urine in the kidney, in as many as 80% of pregnant women, with some degree of urinary stasis. Glucose is normally excreted by the glomerulus and then fully reabsorbed (see Chapter 8), but in pregnancy the reabsorption is not as effective, and therefore about 90% of pregnant women have some glucose in their urine. This should return to normal after delivery. High levels of glucose in the urine may be the sign of **gestational diabetes**.

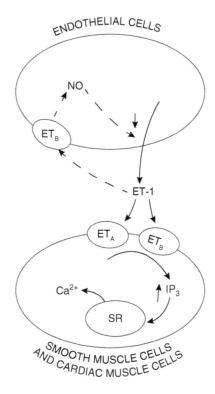

*Figure 16.3* Endothelin (ET-1) is released from endothelial cells lining blood vessels and binds to two ET receptor types, $ET_A$ and $ET_B$ on vascular smooth and cardiac muscle cells. ET-1 binding to both receptor types raises ($\uparrow$) $IP_3$, an intracellular messenger molecule. Raised $IP_3$ causes release of calcium ($Ca^{2+}$) from the cell's sarcoplasmic reticulum (SR) and this causes smooth muscle contraction (i.e. vasoconstriction) and increased cardiac muscle contraction (i.e. increased cardiac output) both leading to raised blood pressure. ET-1 binding to $ET_B$ receptors on the endothelial cells causes production of nitric oxide (NO) which reduces ($\downarrow$) ET-1 production.

This may return to normal or it may require investigation and treatment (NHS 2022). Similarly, protein and uric acid may appear in the urine when the kidney's ability to prevent this loss is compromised.

Antidiuretic hormone (ADH), a hormone from the hypothalamus via the posterior pituitary gland, increases in pregnancy, causing water retention and hypervolaemia. The maternal blood volume increases by 45%, with plasma volume increasing by 30–40%, rising to 50–60% by the end of pregnancy. Extracellular fluid also increases by 30–50%. The volume increase in circulation is important for the maintenance of the blood flow to the uterus and placenta.

**Sodium** retention in pregnancy is the result of activation of the **renin-angiotensin-aldosterone cycle** (see Figure 3.6, page 47). Aldosterone conserves sodium from the second convoluted tubules and collecting ducts of the nephron (see page 162), and the level of aldosterone in circulation rises steadily throughout pregnancy. Sodium retention is partly the reason for the hypervolaemia since higher levels of sodium in the blood attracts water back into circulation (see Chapters 3 and 8). However, sufficient sodium is still lost in the urine to prevent sodium overload, and this is the result of the increased GFR, which is excreting more sodium, combined with the anti-aldosterone effect of progesterone.

### Pre-eclampsia and eclampsia

As identified above, normal blood pressure falls by mid-pregnancy and then returns to normal by full term (Figure 16.1). **Pre-eclampsia** is a condition that occurs in 5–7% of pregnant women, mostly in late pregnancy (after 20 weeks gestation). It is characterised mainly by high blood pressure (Tables 16.2 and 16.3) and protein in the urine. It may progress, and it sometimes leads to the onset of seizures (called **eclampsia**).

The symptoms of pre-eclampsia include any combination of the following:

- high blood pressure (see Chapter 3 and Tables 16.2 and 16.3)
- protein in the urine (called **proteinuria**; see Chapter 8) and reduced urine output (**oliguria**; see Chapter 8)

*Table 16.2* The systolic and diastolic pressure values for normal blood pressure, mild, moderate and severe hypertension

| Blood pressure | Systolic (mmHg) | Diastolic (mmHg) |
| --- | --- | --- |
| Normal | 110–120 | 70–80 |
| Mild hypertension | 140–149 | 90–99 |
| Moderate hypertension | 150–159 | 100–109 |
| Severe hypertension | > 160 | > 110 |

*Table 16.3* Terms used for hypertension at different stages of pregnancy. Chronic hypertension is probably pre-existing before pregnancy and is therefore unrelated to the pregnancy. Gestational hypertension is due to the pregnancy

| Gestation (week when first discovered) | Type of hypertension |
| --- | --- |
| 0–20 | Chronic (pre-existing) |
| 20–40 | Gestational |

*Table 16.4* Red and amber flag warnings of deteriorating condition

🏴 **Red Flag = serious situation which needs urgent medical attention.**

🏴 **Amber Flag = important to get a medical assessment as soon as possible.**

| Flag warning | Details |
|---|---|
| 🏴 Red Flag | **Abdominal pain or asthma attack during pregnancy.** <br> **Vaginal bleeding or discharge.** <br> **Seizures during pregnancy (eclampsia).** |
| 🏴 Amber Flag | **Contact with chicken pox, measles, scarlet fever, rash, influenza or shingles during pregnancy.** <br> **Fever during pregnancy.** <br> **Diarrhoea, vomiting with weight loss or headache during pregnancy.** <br> **Urinary infection.** <br> **Symptoms of high blood pressure (pre-eclampsia).** |

(After Hill-Smith and Johnson 2021, with permission)

- severe headaches
- excessive vomiting and nausea (see Chapter 9)
- dizziness (**vertigo**; see Chapter 9)
- rapid weight gain and swelling of the legs, feet and hands, caused by fluid retention (see Chapter 6)
- abdominal pain.

Pre-eclampsia must be recognised as early as possible and intervention is required quickly. Complications include liver and kidney malfunction, **hypercoagulability** of the blood (due to raised levels of clotting factors) leading to increased risk of circulatory **thrombosis**, pulmonary oedema and the risk of seizures (eclampsia). The mother and baby may both be at risk of harm.

The pathology of pre-eclampsia is complex and not fully understood, but it does appear that the placental is central to the problem (Hladunewich *et al.* 2016). Abnormal arterial disease within the placenta prevents adequate blood flow through the placenta, reducing oxygen and nutrient exchange with the foetal circulation. The very early stages of the disease may be asymptomatic, and this may be the reason diagnosis is delayed until later in the pregnancy. Termination of the pregnancy (and therefore removal of the placenta) at the earliest possible time preterm, provided the child is survivable outside the uterus, may be the only way available to safeguard the mother and child against further harm.

**Eclampsia** is the presence of **tonic-clonic** seizures (see Chapter 11, page 235) during pregnancy as a result of raised blood pressure. It is a severe complication of pre-eclampsia and affects about 1 in 200 pregnant women who had previously developed pre-eclampsia.

Key points

- The maternal changes in pregnancy are normal, and they accommodate and sustain a developing child.
- There are three stages of pregnancy, the first (weeks 1 to 12), second (weeks 13 to 27) and third (weeks 28 to 40) trimesters.

- Blood changes during pregnancy provide the foetus with nutrition and fluid.
- Blood pressure drops slightly over the first half of pregnancy but restores to normal by full term.
- The heart becomes enlarged during pregnancy, with a greater force of contraction and in labour cardiac output increases by 15% (first stage) and by 50% (second stage).
- Blood clotting factors increase in pregnancy to prevent bleeding during birth, but this leads to an increased risk of thrombosis.
- There is 20% increase in oxygen consumption during pregnancy.
- Progesterone remains high in pregnancy to maintain the endometrium, and oestrogen rises.
- Oxytocin reaches a peak at the onset of labour and causes uterine contractions and dilation of the cervix.
- Folate (vitamin $B_9$) intake should increase in pregnancy in order to prevent foetal neural tube defects. Iron and iodine intake should increase also.
- Glucose and lipid metabolism changes occur in pregnancy to supply energy to mother and foetus.
- Renal changes in pregnancy include an increase in the glomerular filtration rate (GFR), sodium and water retention due to increased aldosterone, and the loss of some glucose in the filtrate.
- High blood pressure and protein in the urine are symptoms of pre-eclampsia.
- Eclampsia means seizures occur as a result of the high blood pressure.

## Notes

1 HLA is a group of human leukocyte antigens which nucleated cells produce on their surfaces. They are part of the cells ability to regulate the immune system.
2 T-cells are part of the body's immunity which can destroy cells that are foreign (antigenic cells).
3 Syncytium is a collection of cells closely united and acting together as a single unit.

## References

Hill-Smith I. and Johnson G. (2021) *Little Book of Red Flags*. National Minor Illness Centre, Bedfordshire.

Hladunewich M., Karumanchi S.A. and Lafayette R. (2016) Pathophysiology of the clinical manifestations of preeclampsia. *Clinical Journal of the American Society of Nephrology*, 2(3): 543–549. http://doi.org/10.2215/CJN.03761106

National Health Service (NHS) (2022) www.nhs.uk/conditions/gestational-diabetes/ (Accessed 3rd March 2023). Due for update 8th December 2025.

Soma-Pillay P., Nelson-Piercy C., Tolppanen H., Mebazaa A., Tolppanen H. and Mebazaa A. (2016) Physiological changes in pregnancy. *Cardiovascular Journal of Africa*, March–April, 27(2): 89–94. http://doi.org/10.5830/CVJA-2016-021

# Index

9 781032 484402